FREE Study Skills DVD Offer

Dear Customer,

Thank you for your purchase from Mometrix! We consider it an honor and privilege that you have purchased our product and want to ensure your satisfaction.

As a way of showing our appreciation and to help us better serve you, we have developed a Study Skills DVD that we would like to give you for <u>FREE</u>. **This DVD covers our "best practices" for studying for your exam, from using our study materials to preparing for the day of the test.**

All that we ask is that you email us your feedback that would describe your experience so far with our product. Good, bad or indifferent, we want to know what you think!

To get your **FREE Study Skills DVD**, email <u>freedvd@mometrix.com</u> with "FREE STUDY SKILLS DVD" in the subject line and the following information in the body of the email:

    a.   The name of the product you purchased.

    b.   Your product rating on a scale of 1-5, with 5 being the highest rating.

    c.   Your feedback. It can be long, short, or anything in-between, just your impressions and experience so far with our product. Good feedback might include how our study material met your needs and will highlight features of the product that you found helpful.

    d.   Your full name and shipping address where you would like us to send your free DVD.

If you have any questions or concerns, please don't hesitate to contact me directly.

Thanks again!

Sincerely,

Jay Willis
Vice President
<u>jay.willis@mometrix.com</u>
1-800-673-8175

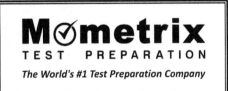

PANCE
SECRETS

Study Guide
Your Key to Exam Success

PANCE Exam Review for the
Physician Assistant National Certifying
Examination

Published by
Mometrix Test Preparation
PANCE Exam Secrets Test Prep Team

Written and edited by the PANCE Exam Secrets Test Prep Staff

Printed in the United States of America

Mometrix offers volume discount pricing to institutions. For more information or a price quote, please contact our sales department at sales@mometrix.com or 888-248-1219.

Mometrix Media LLC is not affiliated with or endorsed by any official testing organization. All organizational and test names are trademarks of their respective owners.

ISBN 13: 978-1-5167-0819-2
ISBN 10: 1-5167-0819-9

Dear Future Exam Success Story:

Congratulations on your purchase of our study guide. Our goal in writing our study guide was to cover the content on the test, as well as provide insight into typical test taking mistakes and how to overcome them.

Standardized tests are a key component of being successful, which only increases the importance of doing well in the high-pressure high-stakes environment of test day. How well you do on this test will have a significant impact on your future, and we have the research and practical advice to help you execute on test day.

The product you're reading now is designed to exploit weaknesses in the test itself, and help you avoid the most common errors test takers frequently make.

How to use this study guide

We don't want to waste your time. Our study guide is fast-paced and fluff-free. We suggest going through it a number of times, as repetition is an important part of learning new information and concepts.

First, read through the study guide completely to get a feel for the content and organization. Read the general success strategies first, and then proceed to the content sections. Each tip has been carefully selected for its effectiveness.

Second, read through the study guide again, and take notes in the margins and highlight those sections where you may have a particular weakness.

Finally, bring the manual with you on test day and study it before the exam begins.

Your success is our success

We would be delighted to hear about your success. Send us an email and tell us your story. Thanks for your business and we wish you continued success.

Sincerely,

Mometrix Test Preparation Team

Need more help? Check out our flashcards at: http://MometrixFlashcards.com/PANCE

TABLE OF CONTENTS

Top 20 Test Taking Tips

1. Carefully follow all the test registration procedures
2. Know the test directions, duration, topics, question types, how many questions
3. Setup a flexible study schedule at least 3-4 weeks before test day
4. Study during the time of day you are most alert, relaxed, and stress free
5. Maximize your learning style; visual learner use visual study aids, auditory learner use auditory study aids
6. Focus on your weakest knowledge base
7. Find a study partner to review with and help clarify questions
8. Practice, practice, practice
9. Get a good night's sleep; don't try to cram the night before the test
10. Eat a well balanced meal
11. Know the exact physical location of the testing site; drive the route to the site prior to test day
12. Bring a set of ear plugs; the testing center could be noisy
13. Wear comfortable, loose fitting, layered clothing to the testing center; prepare for it to be either cold or hot during the test
14. Bring at least 2 current forms of ID to the testing center
15. Arrive to the test early; be prepared to wait and be patient
16. Eliminate the obviously wrong answer choices, then guess the first remaining choice
17. Pace yourself; don't rush, but keep working and move on if you get stuck
18. Maintain a positive attitude even if the test is going poorly
19. Keep your first answer unless you are positive it is wrong
20. Check your work, don't make a careless mistake

Task Areas

History Taking and Performing Physical Exams

Cholesteatoma

The patient with a history of ear infections who presents with foul ear drainage, pain in or behind the ear, dizziness, hearing loss, or partial loss of muscle control on the affected side should be evaluated for cholesteatoma. This abnormal growth in the middle ear can cause severe pain and hearing loss that, if treated, can often be corrected. Evaluation might include a hearing and balance test, and a computed tomography (*CT*) scan of the mastoid. Treatment initially focuses on resolving drainage and treating infection. Surgical removal may also be required. If left untreated, cholesteatoma can lead to permanent hearing loss through bone deterioration, abscess, meningitis, and even death.

Ganglion cyst

Also referred to as a bible cyst, a ganglion cyst is more common in women than men and most often located on the back of the wrist. It can also be found on the underside of the wrist, in the finger, knee, ankle, and toe joints. Manifestation can be gradual or rapid and is most often accompanied by pain that gets worse with joint use. The normal size is 1 to 3 cm, and it can appear as one large, immovable lump or a cluster. The lump may grow more prominent when the joint is engaged. Thick, clear fluid can be aspirated from the cyst. Ultrasound can also be useful in determining the makeup of the cyst. If not painful or interfering with function, usually treatment is just to follow course. If problematic, crystalline glucocorticoid injection and fine needle aspiration are usually performed. Surgical removal may eventually be needed for some.

Paronychia

Paronychia is the most common form of finger/toe nail infection. Infection often occurs after trauma to the area by moisture or physical or chemical damage. The nail bed becomes red, swollen, and painful to the touch. If left untreated, yellow-green pus will begin to collect and form an abscess. This infection can spread to the entire finger. This type of infection may or may not cause systemic fever or chills. If the infection reoccurs after treatment, suspect a fungal causative agent.

Celiac disease

Mild symptoms can include a sense of abdominal discomfort and an increase in flatulence. Increasing severity manifests with abdominal distention, bloating, diarrhea, steatorrhea, weight loss, fluid retention, anemia, osteoporosis, abnormal bleeding, nerve damage, infertility, muscle weakness and cramping, and bone fractures related to malabsorption. Stools are often liquid, greasy, light-colored, very foul-smelling, and tend to float on top of the toilet water. Confirmation of celiac disease can be obtained through biopsy of the small intestine or testing for anti-tissue transglutaminase antibody (anti-tTG) or endomysial antibody (EMA). Supporting data are obtained through complete blood count (CBC), chemistry panel, cholesterol and triglyceride, and thyroid and bone density tests.

Lyme disease

The patient often presents with a history of tick bite; note a history of outdoor activities even if a bite doesn't seem evident. The ELISA test for Lyme disease confirms antibody presence. During the first stage of onset, the lesion will show a clear center and reddened edges at the point of the bite within the first week. The patient may complain of itching, chills, fever, malaise, headache, faintness, muscle pain, and stiff neck. In stage two (weeks to months after the bite), the bacteria has begun to spread throughout the body, causing increased muscle weakness in the face, pain and swelling in large muscles or joints, and an irregular heart rate. Widespread infection indicates stage three (months to years after infection). The first line of treatment is doxycycline possibly in combination with rifampin for two to four weeks. Stages 2 and 3 Lyme disease are treated with intravenous (IV) ceftriaxone. Erythromycin is used in the presence of a penicillin allergy.

Diverticulitis

More than half of Americans older than age 60 will have some degree of diverticulitis. The patient with diverticulitis generally presents with loss of appetite, bloating, cramping, and lower-left-quadrant abdominal pain. The pain is not exacerbated by meals, but nausea and vomiting can be present. Confirm the presence of fresh blood in the stool, rebound tenderness, and fever. Lab work will show an elevated white blood cell count. A computed tomography (CT) scan with contrast can help with confirmation and the extent of disease by showing inflammation, perforation, diverticulosis, and fatty deposits within the colon.

Trigeminal neuralgia

Trigeminal neuralgia creates extreme pain, often described as stabbing or electric-shock-like, along one side of the maxillary and mandibular (near the nose and mouth) first brachial branch. This pain is typically sporadic at first but may become constant. Triggers of the pain may include sound, touch, or stimulation of the area through brushing teeth, chewing, drinking, eating, or shaving. Often, no cause is found. Underlying causes are more likely to be determined in patients younger than 40, generally multiple sclerosis or a swollen blood vessel or tumor providing pressure on the trigeminal nerve. Testing often includes magnetic resonance imaging (MRI) and trigeminal reflex testing. Treatment might include antiseizure medications, muscle relaxants, or tricyclic antidepressants. More aggressive treatment entails cutting or destroying part of the trigeminal nerve, electrostimulation, microcompression, tumor removal, or microvascular decompression.

Fibrocystic disease

Fibrocystic disease can occur in women as young as 18, but it is most common in women 30 to 50 years of age, and it can effect up to 70% of women. Bilateral breast changes are described as lumpy, bumpy, ropelike, or an uneven texture of the breast tissue. This texture is often classified as nodular or glandular. Nipple discharge may also be present. Nodules are most noticeable in the upper outside area of the breast and can radiate to the underarm area. These changes are considered a normal deviation and not indicative of any actual disease. However, it is important to emphasize self-exams and mammograms because these textures can mask the development of abnormal lumps. Swelling, increased definition of the lumps, and tenderness can occur premenstrually. Symptoms and palpable changes tend to disappear after menopause.

Mitral stenosis murmur

The best way to detect a mitral stenosis murmur is to have the patient roll slightly onto their left side (left lateral decubitus position) and use the bell of the stethoscope over the apex. This allows you to easily detect a loud S1 followed by low-pitched rumbling sounds distinctive to mitral stenosis. These sounds can also be brought on during a stress test or exercise. Exertional dyspnea will also be present. Patches of pink-purple discoloration (mitral facies) in the cheek area may occasionally be present; a bounding jugular pulse may also be visualized. The exam should also assess for heart failure, atrial fibrillations, infection, and embolism.

Best locations to auscultate the four cardiac valves

The S1 or "lub" sound is created by the mitral and tricuspid valves. The S2 or "dub" sound is created by the aortic and pulmonary valves. Heart sounds are created by the blood flow through the valves, not the valves themselves. So the best auscultation will occur where those reverberated sound waves produce the greatest effect, not at the anatomical point of the heart valve itself.
- Aortic valve: Right second intercostal space, right-upper sternal border
- Pulmonary valve: Left second intercostal space, left-upper sternal border
- Mitral valve: Left fifth intercostal space, medial to left midclavicular line
- Tricuspid valve: Xiphisternal junction, lower-left sternal border

Mesenteric ischemia

There are three major arteries feeding the small and large intestines; when one or more develops restricted blood flow, mesenteric ischemia results. The stomach and liver may also be affected. This disease is more common in patients older than the age of 60; in smokers; and in those who have coronary artery disease, peripheral vascular disease, high blood pressure, and elevated cholesterol. Other conditions that may contribute to the development of mesenteric ischemia include chronic low blood pressure, congestive heart failure, aortic dissection, coagulation, and blood vessel disorders. Chronic symptoms often begin as vague complaints; acute problems occur suddenly. Symptoms include severe postprandial pain, bloody diarrhea, and in acute cases caused by a clot, vomiting may also be present.

Uterine fundal height during normal pregnancy

Fundal height is measured from the top of the pubic bone to the top of the uterus. It's a simple and noninvasive way to help judge the health and growth of the fetus. Variances can indicate a breech or transverse presentation; oligohydramnios, hydramnios, or polyhydramnios; multiple births; or engagement into the pelvis in preparation of birth. Measured in centimeters, fundal height should closely correspond to the number of weeks in the pregnancy. The top of the fundus should be palpable above the pubic symphysis at 12 to 15 weeks, at the level of the umbilicus by 20 to 22 weeks, and finally at the level of the xiphisternum by 36 to 38 weeks.

Communication regarding sexual history

Be comfortable with your own sexuality, and maintain an objective, nonjudgmental attitude. Clearly specify the privacy of information that the patient can expect during and after the interview. Do not assume marital status or orientation. Ask open-ended questions, provide examples that illustrate an acceptance, and signify a "no-wrong-answer" attitude that gives the patient permission to speak freely. Use terms that the patient understands, and be clear in your use of terms. Clarify any terms the patient uses that might be ambiguous.

Anorexia nervosa

Weight loss that continues even as the patient continues to express intense fear of gaining weight or being overweight, even if he or she is already underweight. The patient may have a history of an anxiety disorder as a child, an extreme need for perfection, or an absorption in exercise. Note poor memory or judgment, emaciation, dysmenorrhea, orthostatic hypotension, bradycardia, hypothermia, dry skin, and thinning or brittle hair and nails. Lab results can show decreased white blood count, hypochloremia, hypokalemia, increased blood urea nitrogen (BUN), and metabolic acidosis.

Heavy alcohol use

Health effects of alcoholism include:
- Anemia and malnutrition.
- Cancer. Scientists believe that the increased cancer risk is related to the conversion of alcohol into acetaldehyde, a potent carcinogen, in the body. This risk is also increased by smoking. The most common types include, mouth, throat, larynx, esophagus, liver, breast, and colorectal.
- Cardiovascular disease, high blood pressure, and abnormal clotting that increase the risk of myocardial infarction or stroke. Atrial flutter can occur with excessive use or withdrawal symptoms.
- Cirrhosis and pancreatitis.
- Dementia and other forms of impaired thinking.
- Depression.
- Seizures, even in the absence of epilepsy. Alcohol can also alter the effectiveness of seizure medications.
- Aggravated gout.
- Suppressed immune system and nerve damage.

Comprehensive cardiac/vascular patient assessment

The following are the four basic components of a comprehensive cardiac/vascular patient assessment:
1. Patient history: The best source of information about the history of his condition is the patient himself. Other resources might include past medical records and involved family members.
2. Physical exam: Execute a full, head-to-toe and symmetrical exam including inspection, palpation, percussion, and auscultation methods as appropriate.
3. Laboratory results: Typical laboratory tests include cardiac enzymes, clotting function, cholesterol levels, and therapeutic medication levels.
4. Diagnostic tests: Diagnostic tests can include x ray, computed tomography (CT) scan, magnetic resonance imaging (MRI), electrocardiogram (ECG), echocardiography (ECHO), myocardial perfusion imaging, and cardiac catheterization.

Assessment of qualities of pain

The following are qualities of pain that should be assessed in a thorough patient history:
1. Quality: Have the patient describe the quality of the pain using words such as dull, stabbing, sharp, aching, throbbing, and burning.
2. Severity: Pain can be rated on a scale of 1 to 10 or by another assessment tool.
3. Location: Where on the body is the pain located, and does it radiate or shift?
4. Timing: When did the pain begin; is it constant, or does it come and go with a predictable or random frequency?
5. Causative factors: Is the patient able to pinpoint a precipitating event prior to the onset of pain?
6. Aggravating factors: Does the quality or severity of pain change with activity, position, stress level, or other varying conditions?
7. Alleviating factors: What effects do medications, position, or other noninvasive treatment interventions have on the amount of pain?
8. Related S/S: Is the pain accompanied with nausea, dizziness, shortness of breath, or other closely related symptoms?

Methods of questioning to encourage accurate, in-depth personal history

The following lists methods of questioning that encourage the patient to give an accurate, in-depth personal history:
- Open discussion: Promotes patient comfort by encouraging questions and feedback during the interview.
- Ask leading questions: Ask questions that require more than a "yes" or "no" answer, and give clear permission for the patient to speak freely about their health.
- Restate and summarize provided information in another way: Allows you to verify that your understanding of the given information is correct.
- Focus: Assisting the patient to concentrate on identifying his highest healthcare needs or make connections between healthcare behavior and larger priorities.
- Order and sequence: Verify cause and effect and timing of the events given in a patient history.
- Encourage self-evaluation: Allow patients to draw their own conclusions regarding information, and do not judge or try to educate at this point.
- Make observations: Providing commentary on the patient's physical, mental, and emotional demeanor to help them focus and give permission to discuss further aspects of their health or immediate needs.

Breast cancer

When assessing for signs indicating breast cancer, the practitioner should feel for a painless mass in the breast or surrounding tissue. The most common locations are directly beneath the nipple and the outer-axillary portion of the breast. Other indications can include changes in the appearance or texture of the breast and nipple. There may be an obvious lack of symmetry between breasts. Nipple areas can change color, texture, and orientation as well as produce discharge. Breast cancer most commonly metastasizes to the bone, liver, brain, and lung. Breast cancer patients face issues associated with body changes – loss of femininity and loss of sexual appeal and function.

Prostate cancer

The most common symptoms noted by the patient with prostate cancer are difficulty urinating and sexual dysfunction. Urination difficulties can include difficulty starting or stopping the flow of urine, decreased force of urine stream, or dribbling. With a loss of sexual function, many men also experience a perceived loss of masculinity. Blood may be detected in both urine and semen, and the patient may experience weight loss and painful bowel movements. Bone pain in the lower back or pelvis indicates metastasis. Rectal exam reveals a palpable prostate that is enlarged, hardened, with a lumpy or uneven surface. Prostate-specific antigen (PSA) blood levels will also be elevated.

Tuberculosis

Tuberculosis is common among immune-suppressed patients. Physical symptoms include night sweats, unexplained weight loss, and fatigue. Pulmonary tuberculosis also shows a chronic cough with active sputum production. If left untreated, tuberculosis may also spread to other organs and cause neurological diseases such as meningitis, bone infections, and urinary bleeding. A positive tuberculin skin test signifies a previous exposure to tuberculin organisms. However, it cannot pinpoint a recent change from a negative status unless the positive test is a follow-up to previous negative test results. The skin test alone cannot accurately pinpoint the time of exposure. An initial tuberculosis diagnosis to identify the presence of an active disease state can be obtained by finding acid-fast bacilli in stained smear samples from sputum or other body fluids. The initial diagnosis is confirmed by isolating *Mycobacterium tuberculosis* on culture or rapid nucleic acid test probes.

Core principles of pain assessment and management

All patients have the right to appropriate assessment and management of pain. Caregivers should encourage all patients to report their pain and follow through with pain-relieving treatments. Assessments for pain must be appropriate for the individual patient and address all aspects of their pain. Both the patient and family should be included in the assessment process. The most accurate indicator of pain is the patient's own description. It is always subjective: The clinician should accept and respect the patient's report of pain. Each person's pain experience is unique and dependent on many contributing factors such as heredity, energy level, coping skills, and prior experiences. Physiological and behavioral observations should not replace information obtained directly from the patient when it can be communicated. Pain can be present without physiological evidence or cause; pain in such cases should not be immediately assigned to psychological causes. Chronic pain can create an overall lower threshold of tolerance for pain and other stimuli. Unrelieved pain has adverse effects on all aspects of the patient's life.

Order of procedure for physical examination

The order of procedure for a physical examination is as follows:
- Inspection: Visual inspection with the naked eye and specialized equipment such as an ophthalmoscope to view physical features such as height, body mass, skin condition and color, breath frequency and quality, hair distribution, balance, gait, and presence of tremors or physical injuries.
- Palpation: Examination by touch for pulses, organ size and location, pain response, temperature, and distinguishable masses.
- Percussion: Further touch intervention using the fingers to create sound.

- Auscultation: Auditory assessment with and without the assistance of a stethoscope generally focusing on cardiac, respiratory, and digestive systems. Other useful tools might include the use of Doppler to locate pulses that were difficult to palpate.

This general procedure varies slightly during assessment of the abdomen, placing auscultation before palpation and percussion. Other systems may not require the use of all four examination elements.

Obsessive-compulsive disorder

Obsessive-compulsive disorder (OCD), also known as obsessive-compulsive anxiety disorder, is defined as a series of unreasonable thoughts that lead the patient to execute repetitive behaviors. Whether or not the patient believes these actions will alter the imagined fears, they are unable to ignore or stop the action. Completing the compulsion allows them to lower their anxiety and stress levels. OCD may occur when there is a family history of the disorder or as a result of stressful life changes. Test results may show decreased serotonin levels, increased activity in the frontal lobe (thought to trigger the obsessions), and increased caudate nucleus activity (responsible for the resulting compulsions).

Disorders associated with history of smoking

The diseases most commonly associated with smoking are lung cancer and chronic obstructive pulmonary disorder (COPD). Tobacco use is also responsible for an increased risk of mouth, throat, bladder, kidney, liver, stomach, and pancreatic cancers. It decreases blood flow by damaging both peripheral and cerebrovascular vessels, increasing the risk of heart disease, myocardial infarction, and stroke. Respiratory conditions include chronic bronchitis, emphysema, pneumonia, exacerbation of asthma, as well as respiratory infections and colds. It can also cause infertility, miscarriage, stillbirth, premature and low-birth-weight infants, as well as impotence in men.

Macular degeneration

Macular degeneration, also referred to as age-related macular degeneration (AMD), is the leading cause of vision loss in the patient older than 55 years of age. Risk factors that increase the likelihood of a patient developing AMD include smoking, Caucasian descent, high blood pressure, increased cholesterol levels, and genetics. The macula, the most sensitive part of the retina, which provides sharp, central vision, is destroyed. Progression is often very slow and therefore goes undetected for an extended period. If the progression is faster, it is more likely to affect the vision in both eyes. Central vision and the ability to focus on fine detail are lost. This makes it difficult for the patient to drive, recognize facial features, read, or do other close-up work.

Disorders associated with obesity

A patient who is more than 20% over the highest weight allowance for his or her height is considered obese. In other terms, an adult is considered overweight when their body mass index (BMI) is between 25 and 29.9. Obesity is defined as a body mass index (BMI) of more than 30. These patients are more at risk for heart disease; high blood pressure; stroke; diabetes; colon, breast, uterine, kidney and esophageal cancer; gallstones; osteoarthritis; gout; polycystic ovary syndrome (PCOS); sleep apnea; and asthma than the patient within normal weight parameters. These conditions often coexist. Metabolic syndrome describes the patient with a grouping of obesity, hypertension, and elevated lipids and blood sugar.

Endometriosis

Endometriosis occurs when the endometrial cells that make up the lining of the uterus begin to invade and grow in areas outside of the uterus. The tissue often implants itself on the ovaries, bowel, rectum, bladder, and the lining of the pelvis. Normal endometrial cells respond to the hormone changes by being sloughed off during the woman's period. Cells that have migrated may bleed, but they are not released from the body. They continue to grow with each new menstrual cycle. Pain is the presenting factor for this disease and can be present during the patient's period and for up to two weeks prior to the period. Pain may also be present during sexual intercourse or bowel movements. It may also present as back pain that appears unrelated to hormonal changes. The patient with endometriosis is likely to have begun menstruation at a young age, is nulliparous, and has frequent, prolonged periods.

Using Laboratory and Diagnostic Studies

Coarctation of the aorta

Magnetic resonance angiography is preferable in the older patient. Echocardiography is not conclusive, but it can be used to help measure peak pressure gradients. Computed tomography (CT) angiography is an option in postoperative patients with stents and surgical clips. It can also be ordered to identify associated lower extremity damage. X-ray identifies related cardiomegaly, pulmonary edema, and congestive heart failure (CHF). Laboratory workups might include cultures, urinalysis, electrolytes, blood urea nitrogen (BUN), creatinine, glucose, arterial blood gases, and serum lactate.

KOH preparation

Any patient presenting with a scaly rash should undergo a KOH test. A KOH (potassium hydroxide) preparation is an inexpensive and noninvasive test used to detect the presence of fungal infections on skin, hair, nails, and vaginal discharge. A minute scraping from the infected area is placed on a microscope slide with KOH and the solvent dimethyl sulfoxide (DMSO). Skin cells will be quickly dissolved, leaving behind only fungal cells that appear as thin branching structures (septate hyphae).

Hydrogen breath test

Excess hydrogen is produced when there is an overabundance of undigested sugars and carbohydrates present in the small intestine. This hydrogen passes through the small intestines into the main blood supply and then to the lungs to be excreted during exhalation. This excess amount can be measured as a convenient and reliable method to diagnose lactase deficiency, lactose intolerance, bacterial overgrowth in the small intestine, or abnormal rate of digestion. The patient is asked to fast for 12 hours prior to the testing. An initial breath sample is taken by having the patient blow into a balloon. A small amount of sugar is then administered, and the hydrogen levels on the breath are then measured at intervals of 15 minutes for up to 5 hours. Any increase in hydrogen production means that there is a problem with the sugar digestion. An extremely rapid increase may indicate food is traveling through the small intestines too quickly; two separate spikes in hydrogen production may indicate a bacterial infection of the small intestines.

Pertussis

Testing procedures differ between private clinical and public health settings. For the private clinic, the goal is to rapidly diagnose and treat any patient who may be at risk (PCR). At a public health level, more discrimination against false negatives is required (culture). The polymerase chain reaction (PCR) is a rapid method of diagnosis that detects the presence of the DNA sequences particular to *Bordetella pertussis* bacteria without requiring the presence of live bacteria. Inaccurate results are still possible however. Best results are obtained within the first three weeks of signs and symptoms (cough) appearing and must be performed before antibiotic treatment begins. Swabs or aspiration of mucus is obtained from the nasal passage. Cultures should be started immediately after collection, and all mucus should be disposed of properly within 24 hours of collection.

Hypothyroidism

The older woman presenting with fatigue, dry skin, constipation, and/or a hoarse voice should be screened for hypothyroidism. Thyroid stimulating hormone (TSH) is the most sensitive test. A high TSH result (4.0 and above) is indicative of a thyroid with reduced function. Other laboratory workups might include triiodothyronine, thyroxine, triiodothyronine uptake, thyroxine-binding globulin, and anti-thyroid peroxidase (anti-TPO). Ultrasound of the thyroid may also be considered. Infertility, pregnancy, and mental and cardiac health also require a higher level of monitoring.

Cystic fibrosis diagnosis

Cystic fibrosis is an autosomal recessive disease with mutation of chromosome 7. This particular chromosome is responsible for the transport of chloride across membranes. Failure to move chloride appropriately results in increased lung secretions and eventual fibroid and cyst formation. The immunoreactive trypsinogen (IRT) blood test is a standard screening procedure for newborns. High IRT test results warrant further testing through the sweat chloride test, the industry standard diagnostic test. X-ray and CT scan show tubular, air-filled pockets, normally in the upper lobes of the lungs. Lung, pancreas, and intestinal function tests, and a fecal fat test may also be ordered and monitored.

Spirometry

Spirometry is an inexpensive and rapid way of assessing the extent and severity of airway obstruction causing a patient with asthma, chronic obstructive pulmonary disease (COPD), bronchitis, emphysema, or pulmonary fibrosis to be unable to expire as forcefully or as quickly as a normal person. These measurements are taken at the time of initial diagnosis and are then monitored periodically to track disease progression. Decreased forced expiratory volume (FEV-1), a measure of the amount of air expelled in a single second, decreased forced vital capacity (FVC), a measure of the largest amount of air you are able to expel, and a decreased FEV1:FVC ratio all indicate the severity of the breathing restriction. Measurements may be also reevaluated 15 minutes after administration of an inhaled bronchodilator to assess its specific effectiveness.

Holter monitor

A Holter monitor is worn continuously for 24 to 48 hours. This is helpful when a regular, brief electrocardiogram (ECG) has not shown any abnormalities, but the patient is presenting with symptoms such as pain, dizziness, palpitations, or a change of consciousness that could still be cardiac health related. While it does allow for an extended view and perspective on heart health, it is also partially dependent on accurate reporting/journaling on the part of the patient while wearing the monitor. It may also be a little bothersome to the patient, and he or she will not be able to shower or bath until the monitor is removed at the end of testing.

Clostridium difficile infection

Clostridium difficile (*C. diff*) is a gram-positive, anaerobic, spore-forming bacillus that causes diarrhea and colitis. The proliferation of *C. diff* is usually the result of antibiotic therapy and is seen most often in the elderly patient. There can be an extended period of time (weeks to even months) before the patient even shows signs and symptoms of the infection. The bacteria release toxins that increase mucosal inflammation and damage to the colon. The patient presents with frequent diarrhea, and abdominal discomfort. In advanced cases, fever, nausea, dehydration, weight loss, and blood or pus in the stool will also be present. If symptoms are severe or persistent, they may need to be treated with metronidazole (first choice) or vancomycin.

Imaging findings in rheumatic heart disease

Rheumatic heart disease, caused by a streptococcal infection (generally in children), most frequently affects the mitral valve causing stenosis and regurgitation. Stenosis is created by inflammation of the valve leaflets, fibrin deposits on the cusps, fusion of leaflet adhesions (commissures) and formation of the classic "fish-mouth deformity" to the valve. X ray, computed tomography (CT), and magnetic resonance imaging (MRI) will show edema or inflammation in the acute phase, calcifications, cardiomegaly, specific chamber enlargements in established disease, and in severe cases pericardial effusion and alveolar hemorrhage.

CT scan

A computed tomography (CT) scan is a more detailed and intricate series of x-rays that allow for examination of bones and soft tissues. While there are often more cost-effective screening methods, CT scan is the first choice in the presence of a head injury. Other uses might include diagnosing muscle and bone disorders, internal injuries, and bleeding. It can also detect and monitor tumors, infection, blood clots, and heart and lung disease. A CT scan is not recommended in the pregnant patient. CT creates radiation exposure and creates a risk of an allergic reaction to any contrast used.

Electrocardiogram

Electrocardiography, or the electrocardiogram (ECG), is the study of electrical impulses through the heart. Correct placement of the 12 monitor leads must be executed in order to receive accurate results. Leads are divided into three divisions:
- Limb leads—leads I, II, and III.
- Augmented leads—aVR, aVL, and aVF.
- Precordial leads—V1 to V6.
  - V1 is placed at the fourth intercostal space, to the right of the sternum.
  - V2 is also in the fourth intercostal space, to the left of the sternum.
  - V3 is located directly between V2 and V4.
  - V4 is placed in the fifth intercostal space at the midclavicular line.
  - V5 is also in the fifth intercostal space at the anterior axillary line directly between V4 and V6.
  - V6 is also in the fifth intercostal space at the midaxillary line.

Additional leads are placed on each limb.

CBC

Normal diagnostic ranges of a complete blood count (CBC) are as follows:
- White blood cells - 4500 to 11,000/mm³
- Red blood cells -
  - male, 4.3 to 5.9 million/ mm3
  - female, 3.5 to 5.5 million/ mm3
- Hemoglobin - Carries oxygen and is decreased in anemia and increased in polycythemia. Normal values:
  - Males >18 years: 14.0-17.46 g/dl.
  - Females >18 years: 12.0-16.0 g/dl.
- Hematocrit - Indicates the proportion of RBCs in a liter of blood (usually about 3 times the hemoglobin number). Normal values:
  - Males >18 years: 45-52%.
  - Females >18 years: 36-48%
- MCV - Indicates the size of RBCs.
  - Males > 18 years: 84-96 μm3.
  - Females >18 years: 76-96 μm3.
- MCH - 25.4 to 34.6 pg/cell
- MCHC - 31% to 36% Hb/cell
- Platelets - 150,000 to 400,000/mm3

Risks associated with endoscopy

A patient consenting to endoscopy needs to be aware of the risks of an adverse reaction to the sedation used, arrhythmia, infection, pain, bleeding, or perforation. Upper endoscopy [esophagogastroduodenoscopy (EGD)] can also lead to aspiration or respiratory depression. Lower endoscopy (colonoscopy, sigmoidoscopy, and enteroscopy) can cause dehydration and an uncomfortable blotting from the gases used during exploration and polyp removal. These risks are greater in those with preexisting conditions such as lung, liver, or cardiac disease. A thorough history and screening for potential problems should be completed and prophylactic intravenous fluids and antibiotics considered.

Clean-catch urine specimen

The following are the instructions that should be given to a patient on how to gather a clean-catch urine specimen:
- Begin with clean hands.
- For females, instruct them to sit on the toilet and spread apart the labia with two fingers. They should then gently cleanse the inner labia, from front to back, twice. Continue to hold open the labia, then begin urinating. Stop the urine flow, and hold the collection container a few inches away from the urethra before beginning the stream of urine again. Only a few inches of urine need to be collected in the specimen cup. Cover and label the specimen clearly.

- For males, clean the head of the penis. Retract the foreskin as needed and begin cleaning at the urethral opening and continue down and away from the head of the penis. Begin urinating. Stop the urine flow, and hold the collection container a few inches away from the penis before beginning the stream of urine again. Only a few inches of urine need to be collected in the specimen cup. Cover and label the specimen clearly.

Pathophysiological mechanisms of dyspnea

The vascular bed begins to decrease from thromboemboli, tumor emboli, vascular obstruction, radiation, chemotherapy toxicity, or concomitant emphysema. As the vascular bed decreases, the physiological dead space causes increased ventilation demands. This results in hypoxemia and severe deconditioning with metabolic acidosis, alterations in carbon dioxide output (VCO_2), and arterial partial pressure of carbon dioxide (PCO_2). This also increases neural reflex activity, anxiety, and depression. Inspiratory muscle weakness from cachexia, electrolyte imbalances, neuromuscular abnormalities and steroid use, pleural or parenchymal disease, reduced chest wall compliance, and airway obstruction (such as asthma, tumor growth, and COPD) can produce impaired mechanical responses and ventilatory pump impairment.

CK results following MI

The expected pattern of creatine kinase (CK) results in the hours and days following a myocardial infarction (MI) are as follows:
- CK and CK-MB levels are evaluated every 6 to 8 hours in a suspected myocardial injury. Total CK and CK-MB (specific to cardiac cells) initially rise within the first 4 to 6 hours of an MI. A normal range would be 30 IU/L to 180 IU/L for CK and CK-MB totaling 0% to 5% of the CK level.
- Assuming no further damage is sustained, peak levels (in excess of six times the normal range) are reached between 12 to 24 hours after the injury.
- CK levels will return to normal within 3 to 4 days of the event.
- Small spikes in CK level might also occur following invasive cardiac procedures.

Hyperkalemia

A normal potassium level is between 3.5 to 5 mEq/L. Elevated potassium, or hyperkalemia, is normally classified as a level greater than 6mEq/L. It is possible to see a false-high potassium level if the blood cells rupture during or after the lab draw. Hyperkalemia is caused by renal disease, adrenal insufficiency, metabolic acidosis, severe dehydration, burns, hemolysis, and trauma. It rarely occurs in the absence of renal disease but may be induced by drugs such as NSAIDs and potassium-sparing diuretics. Untreated renal failure results in reduced excretion of K. Patients with Addison's disease and deficient adrenal hormone levels experience a sodium loss that results in potassium retention. Along with elevated blood potassium levels, the electrocardiogram will show peaked T waves, flattened P waves, prolonged PR interval, and wide QRS complexes. The patient may also complain of muscle fatigue, weakness, partial paralysis, or nausea.

Sleep studies

Sleep study options include the polysomnogram (PSG), multiple sleep latency test (MSLT), maintenance of wakefulness test (MWT), actigraphy, and home-based portable monitoring devices. The PSG test requires an overnight sleep center visit. It monitors bodily functions (electroencephalogram, heart rate, respirations, oxygen level) during sleep in order to identify and properly diagnose sleep-related disorders such as sleep apnea, restless leg syndrome (RLS), and related conditions such as sleep-triggered seizures. Home-based monitoring may be an abbreviated option for extensive PSG studies. The MSLT and MWT are daytime measurements of wakefulness. Actigraphy is a portable, continuous monitoring system of activity levels and sleep patterns. Sleep studies may be considered if a patient mentions having trouble falling asleep or staying asleep, snores, or complains of extreme tiredness and fatigue during most waking hours.

Initial testing for shock

Shock can be classified into several causative categories: hypovolemic, hemorrhagic, cardiogenic, neurogenic, glycemic (hypo- or hyper-), and anaphylactic. Shock is treated as an emergency situation, with the highest priority going toward assessing and maintaining the ABCs (airway, breathing, circulation). While some needed additional information may vary depending on whether or not the type of shock is known, other information is universally gathered. This testing includes vital signs, electrolytes, glucose, ABGs, urinalysis, serum creatinine, CBC, blood type and match, coagulation studies, pulse oximetry, and blood gases. Blood lactate, BUN and creatinine, ionized calcium, C-reactive protein, cultures (when indicated), total bilirubin and alainin aminotranferase may also be useful to assess septic shock. Chest xray may be useful in patients with hypovolemic shock who do not show improvement after being given fluids. In hypovolemic shock with possible hemorrhage, PT/INR and focused assessment with sonography for trauma are useful as well. In patients with cardiogenic shock, EKG and possible echo are useful in diagnosis.

WBC count and differential

White blood cell (leukocyte) count is used as an indicator of bacterial and viral infection. WBC is reported as the total number of all white blood cells:
- Normal WBC for adults: 4,800-10,000.
- Acute infection: 10,000+, 30,000 indicate a severe infection.
- Viral infection: 4,000 and below.

The differential provides the percentage of each different type of leukocyte. An increase in the white blood cell count is usually related to an increase in one type and often an increase in immature neutrophils, known as bands, referred to as a "shift to the left", an indication of an infectious process:
- Immature neutrophils (bands):
  - Normal - 1-3%.
  - Changes - Increase with infection.
- Segmented neutrophils (segs):
  - Normal - 50-62%
  - Changes - Increase with acute, localized, or systemic bacterial infections.
- Eosinophils:
  - Normal - 0-3%
  - Changes - Decrease with stress and acute infection.
- Basophils:
  - Normal - 0-1%
  - Changes - Decrease during acute stage of infection.
- Lymphocytes:
  - Normal - 25-40%
  - Changes - Increase in some viral and bacterial infections.

- Monocytes:
  - Normal - 3-7%
  - Changes - Increase during recovery stage of acute infection.

Formulating Most Likely Diagnosis

Hyphema

Hyphema refers to the presence of blood in the front area of the eye. This blood is normally the result of mild trauma to the eye. Other causes might include blood vessel abnormalities, infection or inflammation, or ocular cancer. Patients may complain of eye pain, vision changes, and sensitivity to light. In most cases, the blood will be reabsorbed within a few days without treatment of any kind. If natural healing does not occur, the patient may need to undergo intraocular pressure measurement, ultrasound, vision, and glaucoma screenings. Also note a history of sickle cell disease.

Cystocele and rectocele

When the vaginal wall becomes weakened, a cystocele and/or rectocele results. When the weakness occurs on the side against the bladder, it is called a cystocele or prolapsed bladder. Muscle weakness can result from straining during childbirth, chronic constipation, coughing, or heavy lifting. Patients might present with complaints of pressure within the vagina; a feeling of discomfort when sitting; pain when bearing down, having intercourse, coughing, or lifting; multiple urinary tract infections; or urine leakage. A rectocele is a weakness on the posterior wall against the rectum that occurs from the same types of injury. There is a complaint of vaginal fullness, discomfort when sitting, and difficulty passing stool.

Major depressive disorder and depressive disorder with a seasonal pattern

Depressive disorder with a seasonal pattern patient's complaints include lethargy, depression, and loss of interest in normal activities that normally manifests in the fall and increase into the winter months then lessen in the spring and summer. Symptoms may be lessened during daylight hours and worsen on dark days and at night. Patients complain of hopelessness, irritability, increased appetite, and weight gain. Major depressive disorder can manifest from substance abuse, medical conditions, medications, prolonged sleep deprivation, and recent stressful life events. It creates a distortion of thought, hopelessness, agitation, irritability, change in thought processes, lethargy, and an extreme change in appetite and sleep patterns. Both types of depression are more common in women than men.

Tourette syndrome

Tourette syndrome (TS) is a neurological disorder that manifests repetitive, involuntary movements, and vocalizations. These are referred to as tics. Simple tics might include eye movements, grimacing, shrugging, jerking, grunting, throat-clearing, or sniffling. Complex tics are created with combined, coordinated activities, full words, or phrases. These symptoms first appear in the preschool or early elementary school child and are more common in males than females. There is often a worsening of the condition during puberty with a gradual resolution into adulthood. Treatment is not required unless the tics interfere with normal daily functioning. Medication with neuroleptics may then be considered as a means of providing some control.

Galactorrhea

Galactorrhea refers to an abnormal milky discharge from the nipple of one or both breasts that is not related to lactation. It can occur spontaneously or be produced by manual manipulation. Discharge can be continuous or intermittent. This condition is more common in women, but it may occur in men or infants. This condition can be brought on by excessive breast stimulation, side effects of certain medications (hormone supplements, tranquilizers, antidepressants, blood pressure medications, and some herbal supplements), or pituitary gland disorders. Patients presenting with this complaint may also be experiencing dysmenorrhea, headache, or vision changes. If the discharge is other than a milky substance, it may indicate a more significant underlying disease state such as cancer.

Right- and left-sided heart failure

Right-sided heart failure (cor pulmonale) generally results from long-term high blood pressure or chronic lung disease, such as chronic obstructive pulmonary disease (COPD). It is a failure of the right side of the heart to efficiently retrieve blood from the body, and it causes fluid retention. Symptoms can include an activity-dependent altered level of consciousness, complaints of chest pain or discomfort, dependent edema, and altered breathing state (wheezing or cough). Patients may also present with ascites, gastrointestinal complaints, cyanosis, swollen liver, abnormal heart sounds, and neck vein distension. Right-sided heart failure can also result from preexisting left-sided heart failure.
Left-sided heart failure is a result of a dysfunction in the heart's ability to pump blood to the rest of the body correctly (the responsibility of the left ventricle). This causes fluid retention in the lungs (pulmonary edema). The patient may present with cardiomegaly and marked dyspnea.

Paronychia with herpetic whitlow

Herpetic whitlow can form tiny pustules resembling blisters (clear fluid), and their location is further away from the nail bed than paronychia lesions (deeper yellow-green abscess). Herpetic whitlow often affects more than one finger at a time, paronychia is generally focused on one nail bed. Paronychia is caused by fungus or bacteria with complete resolution with treatment. Herpetic whitlow is a herpes simplex viral infection, which will remain dormant in the body. Herpetic whitlow is not treated by draining the infected area as paronychia often is; herpetic whitlow will often resolve itself.

Aphthous ulcers and oral herpes

Aphthous ulcers (also known as canker sores) are small, shallow, round or oval lesions occurring inside the mouth. Canker sores are not contagious and are more likely to be the result of injury to the area, malnutrition, or stress. Cold sores (oral herpes) most often occur on the lips, have a more blister like appearance, and are highly contagious. Only oral herpes is caused by the herpes virus, which lies dormant within the body and manifests during times of illness or high stress levels. Both conditions can be painful and create difficulties eating, drinking, and talking. Both types of lesions will heal on their own within two weeks.

Esophageal achalasia

Esophageal achalasia is a disorder of the esophagus that affects motility. It may be primary or secondary to other conditions. Achalasia is most common in middle-aged and older adults. It can also be a genetic trait. Achalasia can be present in esophageal tumors, Zenker diverticulum, Chagas disease, nutcracker esophagus, and diffuse esophageal spasms.

S/S: Patients present with dysphagia with both solids and liquids. Other symptoms might include pain, heartburn, cough, or a slight regurgitation of food. Diagnosis includes barium swallow to rule out a mass or tumor. Laboratory results may also show anemia or malnutrition. Diagnosis is confirmed when there is incomplete lower esophagus sphincter relaxation and aperistalsis in the lower portion of the esophagus per manometry. The most effective treatments are pneumatic dilation and surgical myotomy. Other options are Botox injections, and medications aimed at esophageal sphincter relaxation.

Types of transplant rejection

Hyperacute rejection occurs within minutes to hours of the transplant. This type of reaction occurs when the donated tissue (or blood cells) has not been properly matched to the new host. Acute rejection happens within days and up to three months after transplant. Acute rejection is the most common form. Most patients will experience at least some degree of acute rejection, and the primary focus of immunosuppressive medication regimes. Chronic rejection occurs after four months and up to years after the transplant after a slow and constant fight by the body against the tissue that is foreign to the system.

Viral meningitis

There are approximately 10,000 cases of viral meningitis in the United States each year. Viral meningitis is most common in those younger than five years old or those with compromised immune systems. The most common forms result from infection with enteroviruses, arboviruses, and type 2 herpes simplex virus. Viral meningitis is transmitted through contact with the mentioned viruses, or through contamination with saliva, sputum, mucus, or fecal matter of an already-infected person. The patient presents with fever, nausea, vomiting, light sensitivity, head and neck pain, and a change in mental status. Viral meningitis will often run its course without medical intervention other than monitoring fluids and using universal precautions. Complications include seizures, hearing loss, brain damage, kidney failure, and death.

Psoriasis

Psoriasis is a very common, chronic disease affecting 1% to 2% of the United States population. The cause is unknown, but current theories support an autoimmune origin and/or genetics. Psoriasis results from an accelerated skin reproduction cycle. It occurs most frequently on elbows, knees, scalp, intergluteal cleft, penis, and lumbosacral areas. Advanced lesions show abscesses, parakeratotic scales with thinned or absent stratum granulosum. Bacterial and fungal diseases may aggravate psoriasis but are not the primary cause. Other triggers can include stress, skin irritation, sunlight, alcohol consumption, AIDS, chemotherapy, or other autoimmune conditions. There are a variety of forms of psoriasis including nail, inverse, guttate, pustular and Erythrodermic psoriasis. The most common form of psoriasis is called chronic plaque psoriasis, which accounts for about 75% of cases.

With chronic plaque psoriasis, there are erythremic, raised, sharply defined plaques that are symmetrically distributed. Many times a thick scale with a silver color may be present. The plaques are asymptomatic or pruritic in most cases. Diagnosis is made by history and clinical assessment. Treatment includes creams and ointments, phototherapy, or meds such as adalimumab, alefacept, etanercept, infliximab, and Stelara. Complications include increased risk of psoriatic arthritis, MI, metabolic syndrome, autoimmune disorders, and kidney disease.

Bacterial meningitis

Approximately 4,000 cases of bacterial meningitis occur yearly within the United States, resulting in 500 deaths each year. Even in the presence of recovery, there are often lasting consequences of the disease, including brain damage, hearing damage, and learning disabilities. Leading causes include *Haemophilus influenza*, *Streptococcus* strains, *Listeria monocytogenes*, and *Neisseria meningitides*. Contamination results from contact with bacterial-infected saliva, sputum, and mucus. The patient presents with fever, nausea, vomiting, light sensitivity, head and neck pain, and a change in mental status. Immediate treatment with antibiotics is needed. Prevention can also be initiated with vaccination.

Hodgkin disease

Hodgkin disease (Hodgkin lymphoma) is a painless lymphoma in the cervical or supraclavicular region. Palpable nodules in the lymphatic system may be found in the neck, armpits, and groin. The patient may also present with fever, night sweats, weight loss, dry cough, and pruritus. Diagnosis includes biopsy and identifying the presence of the Reed–Sternberg cell. If caught in the early stages, most cases of Hodgkin disease are curable. It spreads first to other nearby lymph nodes and eventually spreads to the lungs, liver, or bone marrow. Treatment includes chemotherapy and/or radiation. Complications include impaired immune system and infection and other types of cancers.

Angina pectoris and myocardial infarction

Angina pectoris often serves as a warning sign for myocardial infarction. Angina is chest pain occurring from reduced blood flow to the myocardium. Stable angina is described as squeezing, pressure, or burning and is focused on the chest cavity. It is intermittent, often correlating with increased activity and dissipating with rest and/or the use of nitroglycerin. Unstable angina will present with the above symptoms, but the symptoms do not abate with rest or medication. Myocardial infarction occurs when the lack of oxygen perfusion to the heart causes myocardial tissue death. This pain is more extreme, often referred to as crushing, and it extends beyond the chest to radiate out toward the back, shoulder, neck, and jaw. Rest and nitroglycerin will have no effect on this type of pain. Initial treatments will include oxygen, repurfusion, and medications (nitrates, beta blockers, antiplatelets, anticoagulants). Morphine can be given for extreme pain control. In an ST-elevated myocardial infarction (STEMI), an electrocardiogram will show ST changes and laboratory results will show elevated troponin and creatinine levels. Unstable angina and a non-ST elevated MI (NSTEMI) may present very similiarly in pain and other factors, but will primarily be able to be told apart by the elevation of cardiac biomarkers that will be present in an MI.

Irritable bowel syndrome and inflammatory bowel disease

Irritable bowel syndrome (IBS) is the most common intestinal disorder in America. It does not actually affect the actual tissue of the bowel, although there may occasionally be an infection present. The actual cause is unknown, and it occurs in women more than men. The patient may present with complaints of abdominal pain, cramping, bloating, and changes in bowel habits. Inflammatory bowel disease (IBD) is an actual inflammation or abnormality of the bowel caused by an immune response, such as Crohn's disease or ulcerative colitis. The initial cause is also unknown. Symptoms may include fever, stomach cramps, and bloody diarrhea. Joints, eyes, skin, and liver may also show signs of the disease, and it increases the patient's risk for colon cancer.

Myasthenia gravis

Myasthenia gravis is an autoimmune disorder affecting the neuromuscular system. Myasthenia gravis causes skeletal muscle weakness by blocking neurotransmitters and interrupting messages from nerve cells to the muscle. Signs and symptoms may worsen with activity and recover with rest. The main symptom is skeletal muscle weakness and fatigue. This may be fluctuating. This can include difficulty breathing, chewing, swallowing, talking, performing exertive motions, or controlling eye movements. Ptosis and diplopia are found in half of patients. Indications of these symptoms should prompt further clinical assessment to include the bedside ice test on patients with ptosis. Confirmation of diagnosis is usually through a positive MuSK-Ab or AChR-Ab assay. For symptomatic issues, treatment is anticholinesterase. Both chronic and rapid immunomodulating treatments are used including glucocorticoids and plasmapheresis. Surgically, a thymectomy may be performed, and in some patients, this will improve the disease. Complications include respiratory and other muscle failures, thymomas.

Cholecystitis

Most cases of acute cholecystitis are caused by gallstones. Cholecystitis pain is most often found in the right upper quadrant. The pain can be described as sharp, cramping, dull, or constant and may radiate to the back or just below the right shoulder blade. The patient may have complaints of pain after eating, but often the pain is delayed by two to four hours. Other symptoms include pale, gray, or clay-colored stools; jaundice; fever; nausea; and vomiting. Patients with right upper quadrant abdominal pain with a positive Murphy's sign are suspected. Diagnosis is confirmed usually by ultrasound showing thickening of the gallbladder wall, a sonographic ultrasound, or inefficient filling of the gallbladder by cholescintigraphy. Treatment consists of control of pain, and fluid and electrolyte balance and stabilization of the patient if needed. If sepsis is suspected or if gallbladder ischemia is seen on radiology, empiric antibiotics should be started, usually a beta-lactam/beta-lactamase inhibitor is used. Definitive intervention, such as cholecystectomy, cholecystostomy, or endoscopic sphincterotomy is recommended due to the likelihood of recurrence and complications, but may be post phoned depending on the patient. Emergent cholecystostomy is usually done for patients that are hemodynamically unstable or who have evidence of perforation or necrosis of the gallbladder. Complications include gangrene in the gallbladder, pancreatitis, or peritonitis.

Gonorrhea and chlamydia

Gonorrhea is a bacterial infection caused by *Neisseria gonorrhoeae* and is spread through oral, vaginal, penile, or anal contact. Symptoms may appear within two days of infection, or be delayed up to a month in men. Female symptoms include vaginal discharge and pain in the lower abdomen/pelvis, with urination and during intercourse. Male symptoms can also include discharge and pain during urination and swollen and tender testicles. Gonorrhea and chlamydia coexist in 50% of cases. Diagnosis is made by cervical or urethral culture or NAAT. Treatment consists of ceftriaxone 250 mg IM in 1 dose AND azithromycin 1 g orally in 1 dose **OR** Ceftriaxone 250 mg IM in 1 dose AND doxycycline 100 mg twice daily for seven days.

Chlamydia is an STD caused by *Chlamydia trachomatis*. It is the most common STD in the United States. Signs and symptoms in males are urethritis, epididymitis, proctitis, or Reiter syndrome (urethritis, rash, conjunctivitis). In females signs and symptoms include mild cervicitis with vaginal discharge and dysuria, but complications can lead to infertility and pelvic inflammatory disease. Many are asymptomatic. Diagnosis is confirmed by nucleic acid amplification test (NAAT). Treatment includes Azithromycin 1 g orally in 1 dose **OR** Doxycycline 100 mg orally twice daily for 1 week. Avoid sexual contact for 1 week. Treatment of the infected person's sexual partner is very important to avoid reinfection after treatment.

Migraine and cluster headaches

A migraine is classified as a throbbing headache accompanied by nausea, vomiting, photophobia, and sensitivity to sound that can last for hours or days. The headache may be preceded by a sensory warning, an aura, a smell, a change in vision, or a sensation on the skin. Each patient's sensory warning is unique. There may also be other subtle changes in bowel habits, mental outlook, appetite, and mood in the day or two prior to each episode. Migraines are more common in women. Cluster headaches are so named because of their tendency to occur in "clusters." Attacks will happen frequently over a few weeks or months and then go into a remission period. There is no defining aura or warning sign of pending attacks. The patient is often awakened in the night to the pain on one side of their head. Cluster headaches are more common in men.

Syphilis

Direct visualization of *Treponema pallidum* is possible by preparing a slide from a specimen taken from the suspect lesion. It is then viewed with direct darkfield microscopy, immunofluorescence, immunoperoxidase, or silver staining. Serologic tests include nontreponemal and treponemal tests. The nontreponemal [Venereal Disease Research Laboratory, (VDRL)] test is best for testing for secondary syphilis. Specific treponemal testing [fluorescent treponemal antibody absorption (FTA-ABS)] can be used for diagnosing secondary and tertiary syphilis. Pregnant women, men in same-sex relationships, those infected with HIV, or those with partners testing positive for the disease should be screened for syphilis. Cases of syphilis are reported in every state and tracked by the Centers for Disease Control (CDC).

Infections and malignancies associated with AIDS

The AIDS patient is highly susceptible to many bacterial, viral, fungal, and parasitic infections as well as certain types of cancers, such as Kaposi's sarcoma, central nervous system lymphoma, and non-Hodgkin's lymphoma. Bacterial infections include streptococcus pneumonia, *Mycobacterium avium* intracellulare (MAI) and *Mycobacterium avium* complex (MAC), tuberculosis (TB), salmonellosis, syphilis, and bacillary angiomatosis. Viral infections include cytomegalovirus (CMV), viral hepatitis, herpes simplex virus (HSV), human papillomavirus (HPV), and progressive multifocal leukoencephalopathy (PML). Fungal infections include *Candida albicans, Histoplasma capsulatum,* and cryptococcal meningitis. Parasitic infections include *Pneumocystis carinii* pneumonia (PCP), toxoplasmosis, and cryptosporidium. The rates of contamination with these types of infections in AIDS patients far exceed the rates found within the general population.

Leukemia

Leukemia is a condition in which the proliferating cells compete with normal cells for nutrition. Leukemia affects all cells because the abnormal cells in the bone marrow depress the formation of all elements, resulting in several consequences, regardless of the type:

- Decrease in production of erythrocytes (RBCs), resulting in anemia.
- Decrease in neutrophils, resulting in increased risk of infection.
- Decrease in platelets, with subsequent decrease in clotting factors and increased bleeding.
- Increased risk of physiological fractures because of invasion of bone marrow that weakens the periosteum.
- Infiltration of liver, spleen, and lymph glands, resulting in enlargement and fibrosis
- Infiltration of the CNS, resulting in increased intracranial pressure, ventricular dilation, and meningeal irritation with headaches, vomiting, papilledema, nuchal rigidity, and coma progressing to death.
- Hypermetabolism that deprives cells of nutrients, resulting in anorexia, weight loss, muscle atrophy, and fatigue.

Leukemia occurs when one type of WBC proliferates with immature cells, with the defect occurring in the hematopoietic stem cell, either lymphoid (lympho-) or myeloid (myelo-). With acute leukemia, WBC count remains low because the cells are halted at the blast stage and the disease progresses rapidly. Chronic leukemia progresses more slowly and most cells are mature.

Sickle cell disease

Sickle cell disease is a recessive genetic disorder of chromosome 11, causing hemoglobin to be defective so that red blood cells (RBCs) are sickle-shaped and inflexible, resulting in their accumulating in small vessels and causing painful blockage. While normal RBCs survive 120 days, sickled cells may survive only 10 to 20 days, stressing the bone marrow that cannot produce fast enough and resulting in severe anemia. There are 5 variations of sickle cell disease, with sickle cell anemia the most severe. Different types of crises occur (aplastic, hemolytic, vaso-occlusive, and sequestrating), which cause infarctions in organs, severe pain, damage to organs, and rapid enlargement of liver and spleen. Sickle cell disease occurs almost exclusively in African Americans in the United States, with 8% to 10% carriers. This sickle shape shortens the lifespan of the hemoglobin causing a chronic anemic state. Pallor, jaundice, weakness, and fatigue are common symptoms. A crisis occurs when the cells clump together causing thrombi and vascular occlusions, leading to hypoxia and even myocardial infarction. It is also associated with multiple acute pain events. Pain episodes are individualized and can vary in both frequency and severity. A sickle cell crisis is identified by pale lips, tongue, palms, or nail beds; lethargy and difficulty awakening; listlessness; irritability; severe pain; or high fever for at least two days. In the patient older than 20 years of age, more than three hospitalizations in a year may be an indication of impending death.

ALS

Amyotrophic lateral sclerosis (ALS) is a progressive degenerative disease of the upper and lower motor neurons, resulting in progressively severe *symptoms*, such as spasticity; hyperreflexia, muscle weakness, and paralysis that can cause dysphagia; cramping; muscular atrophy; and respiratory dysfunction. ALS may be sporadic or familial (rare). Speech may become monotone; however, cognitive functioning usually remains intact. Eventually, patients become immobile and cannot breathe independently. Diagnosis is based on history, electromyography, nerve conduction studies, and MRI. Treatment includes riluzole to delay progression of the disease. Treatment includes nebulizer treatments with bronchodilators and steroids, antibiotics for infection, and mechanical ventilation. Assisting the patient to set up a living will or medical power of attorney is crucial for this patient, as respiratory failure will eventually happen. Complications include acute respiratory failure and aspiration pneumonia.

Parkinson's disease

Parkinson's disease is an extrapyramidal movement motor system disorder caused by loss of brain cells that produce dopamine. Symptoms result from an imbalance between dopamine-activated and acetylcholine-activated neural pathways in the basal ganglia and are generally found in people older than 65. Signs and symptoms include tremor of face and extremities, rigidity, bradykinesia, akinesia, poor posture, and lack of balance and coordination, causing increasing problems with mobility, talking, and swallowing. Some may suffer depression and mood changes. Tremors usually present unilaterally in an upper extremity. Diagnosis is made with the Cogwheel rigidity test: extremity put through passive range of motion, which causes increased muscle tone and ratchet-like movements, physical and neurological exam, and complete history to rule out drug-induced Parkinson akinesia. Treatment includes symptomatic support, dopaminergic therapy: levodopa, amantadine, and carbidopa, anticholinergics: trihexyphenidyl, benztropine. If it is drug-induced Parkinson disease, terminate drugs. Drug therapy tends to decrease in efficiency over time, and patients may present with marked increase in symptoms. Discontinuing the drugs for 1 week may exacerbate symptoms initially, but functioning may improve when drugs are reintroduced.

Stroke

Within the United States, stroke is the third leading cause of death. A stroke or cerebrovascular accident (CVA) occurs from damage and death of brain cells from clots or plaque within a blood vessel, or the rupture of a vessel. The extent of the damage, including patient death, and the symptoms presented are dependent upon the location and size of the vascular compromise. Common symptoms can include weakness, loss of voluntary movement, paralysis, or a loss of sensation on one side of the body. These conditions can result in other problems such as speech and swallowing problems with increased drooling, as well as impairing the balance and vision and their breathing. If damage is extensive enough, unconsciousness or death can occur.

ADLs assessment tools

All of these assessment tools are used to help determine a patient's overall ability to function in general activities of daily living (ADLs) and review the patient's ease in meeting his or her own needs:

- The Karnofsky Performance Scale (KPS) is based on a 0 to 100 scale rating the patient's success in completing his or her own ADLs. Higher scores indicate higher levels of competence with 100 representing full ability without patient complaint. As the numbers decrease, so does the patient's need for outside help with ADLs.
- Eastern Cooperative Oncology Group (ECOG) Performance Status uses a 0 to 5 scale as a correlation between the patient's disease process and its effects on his or her own ADL competencies. Lower numbers indicate a lower level of restriction related to the disease process.

- The Palliative Performance Scale (PPSv2) rates the patient's abilities in only the following five areas: ambulation, activity, current disease manifestations, self-care, nutritional intake, and level of consciousness. These are rated as a percentage that correlates to their success in these functions.

Dementia

Dementia is defined as a progressive, irreversible state of decline in mental function. The state of dementia is chronic and irreversible. Its onset is quiet and slow. Symptoms do not change over the course of the day. Mental clarity remains intact until the later stages but may be complicated by delirium. Short-term memory may be affected early on, but attention span generally remains intact until later stages. Orientation to person, place, and time remain unaltered until later stages when the person may have difficulty recognizing familiar and common objects (anomia) or recognizing familiar people (agnosia). The patient experiences aphasia, a difficulty finding appropriate words and expressing thoughts clearly. Delusions and hallucinations are most often absent. Psychomotor activity is generally unaffected, but the patient may exhibit signs of apraxia, a difficulty initiating purposeful movement. Sleep and wake cycles become fragmented.

Cirrhosis of the liver

When toxins, inflammation, or metabolic changes within the liver create nodules and fibrosis, cirrhosis is the resulting condition. Cirrhosis of the liver is incurable, although in some cases a liver transplant might be considered as an option. The nodules and fibroids interfere with blood flow through the liver that can cause blood to back up in the spleen. When blood pools within the spleen, it becomes enlarged and blood platelet counts fall. Cirrhosis can also cause gastric and esophageal varices. If not treated, these varices can rupture and bleed, which can result in death. Abdominal ascites and peripheral edema often result from the blood flow restrictions as well. The patient begins to exhibit jaundice coloring in the eyes and then in the skin. Rectal hemorrhoids are also common. Hormonal, metabolic, and kidney disturbances can also result from cirrhosis. *Treatment* varies according to the symptoms and is supportive rather than curative as the fibrotic changes in the liver cannot be reversed: Options include abstaining from alcohol use or hepatotoxic drugs. Medications such as prednisone, ursodiol (Actigall), lactulose, and azathioprine (Imuran) can be administered, diet alterations include low-sodium and low-protein diets with increased vitamin K intake, dietary supplements and vitamins, diuretics (potassium sparing), such as Aldactone® and Dyrenium®, to decrease ascites, colchicine to reduce fibrotic changes, liver transplant (the definitive treatment).

Depression

The depressed patient may present with any number of the following: depressed mood; insomnia or hypersomnia; an absence of pleasure in previously enjoyed activities; psychomotor retardation; fatigue; feelings of worthlessness and guilt; and an inability to concentrate, make decisions, or remember important information. The patient may experience significant and unexplained weight loss or weight gain. In severe cases, he or she may also disclose recurrent thoughts of death or suicide. Severity is assigned by the presence of an expressed intent with a plan and means to carry out a suicide attempt, as well as previous attempts. The hallmark symptoms of depression are appetite and sleep changes and decreased energy and concentration. However, in the presence of physical illness, these symptoms can be masked or created by the disease process or corresponding treatments. With preexisting illness, symptoms such as fearfulness, depressed or changed appearance, social withdrawal, brooding, self-pity and pessimism, and a depressed mood or affect that cannot be changed or lifted may be more reliable indicators of depression.

Anxiety

Anxiety is marked by feelings of excessive worry, irritability, restlessness, intense feelings of danger, and agitation. The source of the disquiet is unknown or very vague. The patient may have trouble falling or staying asleep and experience interference with other normal activities in their daily lives. Physically, the patient may be identified as having frequent crying spells, headaches, muscle tension, stomach and intestinal distress, palpitations, shortness of breath, anorexia, or overeating. Psychologically, the patient is vulnerable to unrealistic fears and obsessions with harmful ideas and compulsions. Patients may also try to self-medicate with multiple chemicals or substances in attempts to alleviate any of these symptoms. An anxiety disorder is identified by the persistence of these symptoms over a period of six months or more.

Medical conditions associated with depression

Patients experiencing depression have a greater tendency toward medical illnesses and vise versa. Underlying causes and links may be found in multiple areas of the assessment. Patients with cardiovascular disease, congestive heart failure, arrhythmias, and heart attacks are prone to a higher incidence of depression. Within the central nervous system cerebrovascular anoxia or accident, Huntington's disease, subdural hematoma, Alzheimer's disease and dementia, human immunodeficiency virus (HIV) infection, carotid stenosis, temporal lobe epilepsy, multiple sclerosis, postconcussion syndrome, myasthenia gravis, narcolepsy, and subarachnoid hemorrhage patients are at increased risk. Other causes can include rheumatoid arthritis, thyroid disease, diabetes, Cushing's disease, Addison's disease, anemia, lupus, liver disease, syphilis, encephalitis, alcoholism, and general malnutrition.

Health Maintenance

Hypertriglyceridemia

The main goal of any dietary changes should focus on weight loss because, in the absence of other causative diseases, it is often directly connected to the triglyceride level. A recommendation to limit total fat intake to 10% of the daily calorie consumption and to introduce exercise can often be made. Careful examination of the total LDL and HDL cholesterol levels will help with fine-tuning dietary and exercise recommendations. Testing should also be done to rule out metabolic syndrome. Medication supplements such as statins, fibrates, niacin, and fish oil can also assist in the preventative and recovery process. A referral to a lipidologist or endocrinologist may be needed.

Diet for phenylketonuria

Phenylketonuria (PKU) causes a buildup of the amino acid phenylalanine, found in protein-based foods, in the blood. Therefore, the main focus of diet recommendations for PKU is on restricting protein intake. General diet restrictions include avoiding milk, eggs, cheese, nuts, beans, soy, chicken, beef, pork, fish, peas, beer, chocolate, and foods containing aspartame. Limits on fruits, vegetables, and simple carbohydrates are also common. Diet, growth, and blood levels of phenylalanine will need to be frequently monitored in order to make adjustments in the individual patient's dietary needs.

Fecal impaction

Fecal impaction happens when it becomes impossible for a hard, dry portion of stool to pass through the rectum. This most often occurs in a patient experiencing chronic constipation who has been using laxatives for extended periods of time, then stops suddenly. The muscles of the intestines and colon have atrophied and can no longer move stool without assistance. Other risk factors include immobility and side effects from medications such as anticholinergics, antidiarrheal agents, and pain medications with methadone or codeine. Treatment options may include manual extraction, suppositories, or surgery. Preventative maintenance includes diet and activity modifications and setting specific parameters for laxative and stool softeners.

Common health screenings for adult females

Although clinical judgment should be used to decide how many, and which, screenings should be focused on for the individual patient, there are common health screenings that should be almost universally provided. Interview questions should include tobacco, alcohol, and recreational drug use; personal safety and abuse; mental health; and personal health beliefs and practices including any alternative health treatments the patient is pursuing. Physical and laboratory assessments should cover hypertension; vision; skin, colon, rectal, cervical and breast cancer screenings; cholesterol; and chlamydia and other sexually transmitted diseases.

Management options for gout

Treatment for acute episodes includes monitoring water and food intake and medications (pain reliever and anti-inflammatory agents). Gout can be exacerbated by obesity, high blood pressure, impaired kidney function, alcohol, fructose and corn syrup, dehydration, illness, and fever or injury. Long-term control depends on adequate hydration, weight loss, dietary restrictions (avoidance of alcohol, shellfish, organ and sweets), aerobic exercise, and medications (probenecid, sulfinpyrazone, allopurinol, and febuxostat) to help lower uric acid levels. When medication is being given to control uric acid, monitoring levels through blood testing is essential to find and maintain optimal treatment levels.

Diagnostic studies for suspected pulmonary embolism

While the best test may be the pulmonary angiogram, it carries more expense and risk than other options that may be considered first. X ray cannot diagnose pulmonary embolism, but it can rule out other disorders with similar symptoms. Lung scan measures blood flow in the lungs in the nonsmoker. Computerized tomography (CT) scan can provide great accuracy in visualizing the lung field. Magnetic resonance imaging (MRI) has even greater accuracy with a comparable raise in expense, but without the effects of the contrast dye used in the CT scan. Ultrasound pulses and echocardiogram may also be helpful, as well as a D-dimer blood test to detect the clot.

Somogyi effect

In the diabetic, the Somogyi effect is the body's tendency to overreact to low blood sugar levels. This overcompensation with glucagon and epinephrine to communicate to the liver to convert glycogen stores into readily available glucose creates a new spike in the blood sugar. This phenomenon most often occurs as a result of nighttime hypoglycemia that goes untreated. If a patient is consistently awakening with elevated blood glucose levels, they may need to wake up in the middle of the night in order to perform another blood sugar reading. Their evening intake and insulin dose can then be adjusted to prevent further episodes.

Modifiable and non-modifiable risk factors for cardiovascular disease

Risk factors that the patient and his or her healthcare provider can exercise some control over are identified as modifiable. These can include smoking; excess weight; alcohol use; cholesterol levels; blood pressure; and active management of diabetes, stress, and the amount of exercise the patient engages in. Risk factors beyond the patient's control include age, male sex, and genetic tendencies including race (Caucasian, black, or Native American) and family history. The greatest risk is to those who have already experienced a cardiovascular event, or have been previously diagnosed with a cardiac vascular disease such as peripheral vascular disease, aortic aneurysm, or carotid artery disease. Others with high risk include those who have at least two of the modifiable or nonmodifiable risk factors or type 2 diabetes.

Management and maintenance of major depression

Medication and therapy are normally needed in order to begin resolving major depression. It is important to note the differences in the amount of time it may take for these approaches to work, however. The patient, especially, needs to understand that their progress may seem slow. Selective serotonin reuptake inhibitors (SSRIs) take between two and six weeks to reach a therapeutic level and should not be adjusted until after that time. Tricyclic antidepressants (TCAs) can also take several weeks and carry an increased risk of adverse effects. Monoamine oxidase inhibitors (MAOIs) should not be combined with SSRIs. There should be a cleansing period of four to five weeks between administration of SSRI and MAOIs. Other treatments that may be considered include light therapy, transcranial magnetic stimulation (TMS), or electroconvulsive therapy (ECT). The patient should also be advised that alcohol and recreational drug use can feed the problem rather than provide the relief they are seeking.

ADC

The exact cause of AIDS dementia complex (ADC) is unknown, but it is a primary result of the disease process itself. Current theories suggest that the HIV infection stimulates an invasion of macrophages in the brain (microglia). These release cytokines that directly damage the nervous tissue by disrupting the neurotransmitter functions and causing encephalopathy. This condition affects as many as 15% of all AIDS patients. Prognosis is poor, and the disease is not reversible. However, retroviral drugs can delay its onset. Central nervous system HIV infections in children tend to have a more dramatic and pronounced effect than those occurring in adults. ADC is characterized by gradual memory loss, decreased concentration and cognition, as well as mood disorders. The patient may also experience physical symptoms of ataxia, incontinence, and seizures.

Osteoporosis

Osteoporosis describes bones that have become weak, brittle, and prone to fractures from even mild stress. Early signs and symptoms may include complaints of back pain, diminished height, hunched or stooped posture, and eventual fracture that occurs from what otherwise would have been considered a minor injury. Postmenopausal Caucasian and Asian women carry the greatest risk for developing osteoporosis. Diagnosis is made through measuring bone density with dual-energy x-ray absorptiometry (DXA). Therapy often includes the prescription of bisphosphonates (alendronate, risedronate, ibandronate, or zoledronic acid). Hormone replacement therapy (HRT) after menopause can help prevent osteoporosis. Prevention counseling might also include weight-bearing exercise, smoking cessation, minimal alcohol consumption, and guidance in safe environments and practices to avoid falls.

Kidney failure

When the kidneys become unable to function either short- or long-term, it is referred to as kidney failure. Causes for kidney failure may include toxins such as some medications, tumors, infections, diabetes, hypertension, and collagen vascular diseases such as lupus. When there is hope of restoring normal kidney function, peritoneal dialysis or hemodialysis as well as diuretics and the treatment of underlying causes such as hypertension can be used. Dietary treatments focus on managing the patient on a low-sodium, low-protein, and low-potassium diet. Dialysis, and its supplementary treatments, is also the treatment for chronic kidney failure. However, when there is no hope of return to normal kidney function, the patient faces the difficult decisions of whether or not to start, continue, or even stop the dialysis. These decisions will either prolong the patient's life or bring death within just a few days. As the disease progresses, it brings more pronounced complications in fluid and electrolyte balances, anemia, and uremia. At this point, the patient's treatment may turn to focus on comfort and medications rather than prolonged life by use of dialysis.

Education for patient with acute or chronic illnesses

Education for patients with acute or chronic illnesses should include the following:
- Diagnosis: Establish a basic understanding of the disease process, including areas of the body affected, causes, prognosis, and whether or not it is contagious.
- Complications: Clarify possible signs and symptoms, early warning signs, and signals to disease progression and healing.
- Management: Define what the patient can expect from his care and recovery, including treatments, diet, activity levels, and medications.
- Aggravating factors: Help the patient understand what behaviors or triggers may increase his symptoms and what can be done to avoid or control them.
- Prognosis: Patients need both an immediate idea of what to expect as well as a long-term picture of what to expect.
- Prevention: Establish self-care habits that can help prevent reoccurrence of the problem.
- Resources: Make sure the patient is informed of all available resources to help him on his healthcare journey.

Common health screenings for adult male

Though clinical judgment should be used to decide how much and which screenings should be focused on for the individual patient, there are common health screenings that should be almost universally provided. Interview questions should include tobacco, alcohol and recreational drug use, personal safety, mental health, and personal health beliefs and practices including any alternative health treatments the patient is pursuing. Physical and laboratory assessments should cover hypertension, vision, skin, colon, rectal, prostate and testicular cancer screenings, cholesterol, and chlamydia and other sexually transmitted diseases.

Childhood immunizations

Childhood immunizations should be administered at the following ages:
- Birth: Hepatitis B (Hep B)
- 1-2 Months: Hep B; rotavirus vaccine (RV); diphtheria, tetanus, pertussis (DTaP); *Haemophilus Influenzae* type B (Hib); pneumococcal conjugate vaccine (PCV); inactivated polio vaccine (IPV)
- 4 Months: RV, DTaP, Hib, PCV, IPV
- 6 Months: Hep B, RV, DTaP, Hib, PCV, IPV
- 12-18 Months: Hep B; DTaP; Hib; PVC; IPV; measles, mumps, rubella (MMR); varicella; hepatitis A (Hep A)
- 4-6 Years: DTaP, IPV, MMR, varicella
- 11-12 Years: DTaP, human papillomavirus (HPV), meningococcal conjugate vaccine (MCV4)

Environmental factors that can affect the severity of asthma

Common environmental triggers for asthma exacerbation include seasonal allergies created by pollen, weather patterns, mold spores, animal dander, smoke, smog, other odors such as perfumes, and household and cleaning chemicals. Exposure to things such as dust mites during infancy can even be a key factor in the initial development of asthma. Other factors to consider include hormone fluctuations, exercise, foods, and medications used for other conditions (NSAIDs and beta-blockers). Any effort made to control or remove known triggers creates positive results for overall lung heath as well as the number of acute asthma attacks.

Impacts of stress on health

Excessive stress occurs when the body's natural "fight-or-flight" instinct becomes overstimulated. This creates an overload of adrenaline, cortisol, and glucose in the system and reduces the function of body systems not needed for immediate response to a crisis. Stress alters the immune, cardiac, digestive, and reproductive systems. It increases the patient's risk for heart disease, sleep disorders, skin disorders, digestive problems, altered thought processes including memory and emotion, tobacco, alcohol and drug abuse, obesity, and autoimmune disorders as well as exacerbating these conditions once they exist.

Signs of abuse and/or neglect

Regular screening for domestic violence in a healthcare setting is a helpful and inoffensive method of identifying victims. Watch for injuries that do not seem to match the story given. Overbearing or overprotective partners who answer for or dominate your interview with the patient, frequent nonspecific complaints such as headache, stomach, neck and back pain, insecurity, stammering or avoidance in giving responses to simple questions, intestinal complaints, and sexually transmitted disease. In the abused adolescent female tobacco, alcohol and drug use, decreased school attendance, isolation, and bulimia are more common.

National Environmental Public Health Tracking program

The National Environmental Public Health Tracking (EPHT) program was designed by the Centers for Disease Control (CDC) in response to a need for a way to accurately record and analyze the correlations between environmental factors and health trends to help in finding ways to prevent diseases such as poisoning, birth defects, developmental disabilities, cancer, and neurologic and respiratory diseases. Information is gathered through biomonitoring (measurements of how much of various chemicals are actually absorbed into the body) from local, state, and federal agencies as well as academic institutions and other nongovernment organizations. The collected data can be accessed through the CDC.

Clinical Intervention

Sick sinus syndrome

Sick sinus syndrome is most common in the patient older than age 50. It is represented by a pattern of irregular sinus bradycardia with long pauses in conduction. There may also be an accelerated atrial rate or a pattern of bradycardia–tachycardia as the heart tries to correct its rhythm. There are often no clear symptoms, but vague complaints that could mimic other disorders may be seen. These might include angina or a feeling of fluttering or "wrongness" in the chest, a change in mental status, altered consciousness, dizziness, fatigue, and shortness of breath with exertion. Diagnosis is made by ECG (possibly with a Holter monitor) Treatment may not be needed if the patient is nonsymptomatic. Permanent treatment is provided by an internal pacemaker, and the associated surgical risks should be discussed with the patient. Complications include syncope, bradycardia, heart failure, Afib, and thrombus/embolus.

Thrombotic thrombocytopenic purpura

Thrombotic thrombocytopenic purpura is classified as a blood disorder with the formation of multiple blood clots and a low platelet count. Signs and symptoms include thrombocytopenia, fever, abnormal kidney function, neurologic symptoms, and hemolytic anemia. Diagnosis consists of the following:
- CBC will show low platelets and RBCs.
- Blood smear will show broken and torn RBCs.
- Coag studies, BUN creatinine, serum bilirubin, and lactate dehydrogenase.

The first line of treatment is plasma exchange, in which the patient's own plasma is removed and replaced with healthy plasma from a matching donor through transfusion. If the disease remains unresponsive to this treatment, immunosuppressive medications may be prescribed and a splenectomy can be anticipated. Neurological symptoms may continue even after treatment, and stroke and kidney impairment are additional possible complications.

Treatment options for seizures

The treatment of epilepsy attempts to find a balance for the patient between controlling seizures, maintaining a high quality of life, and managing side effects. Because of this antiepileptic medications are usually not neccesary after a single seizure and will only be used for patients who have risk for recurrent seizures. Selecting the antiepileptic drug should take into account type of seizures, possible adverse effects of medication, other medical conditions, if the patient wishes to have children, and other lifestyle and patient factors. Broad spectrum seizure medication control all seizure types: valproate, zonisamide, clobazam, lamotrigine, levetiracetam, torpiramate. Narrow spectrum seizure medications usually work on specific types of seizures: carbamazepine, vigabatrin, ezogabine, gabapentin, phenobarbitol, phenytoin, pregabalin, primidone. A ketogenic diet, a strict diet intended to induce a long-term starvation effect in order to burn ketones, may be tried in the child whose seizures aren't easily controlled by medication. This diet is high in fat and low in carbohydrates and requires careful monitoring. Alternative medicine includes biofeedback, melatonin, and folic acid supplements. Surgery is effective for some medication refractory focal seizures. Complications include a high risk of mortality due to injury and MVAs with seizures and the risk of seizures recurring when meds are tapered/stopped.

Cryptococcosis

Cryptococcosis is a result of a respiratory fungal infection by *Cryptococcus neoformans*. This condition is most often found among those with compromised immune systems. Healthy patients may be asymptomatic. Immunocompromised patients may experience angina, ha, nausea, confusion, bruising and bleeding, abdominal pain, nerve pain, night sweats and double vision. Diagnosis includes microscopic analysis or serology for Cryptococcus and may be done by CSF, tissue, or blood. Sputum cultures are only accurate 20% of the time and confirmation of cryptococcus of the lung requires antigen detection in the pleural fluid or culture of lung tissue. CSF by lumbar puncture can be done so cryptococcus meningitis can be ruled out. Mild cases may only require monitoring to ensure that the infection does not spread. In more advanced cases, the infection is treated with antifungal medications such as amphotericin B, flucytosine, and fluconazole. The patient should also be monitored for central nervous system infection and significant side effects caused by the medications. Complications include cryptococcal meningitis, which can lead to encephalitis; damage to the optic nerve; and brain damage.

Cryptorchidism

An undescended testicle (cryptorchidism) is a common occurrence in preterm infants. If the testicle hasn't descended by the time the child is one year old, it should be evaluated and watched. Some testicles will descend and then temporarily retract again. This condition is not true cryptorchidism. Cryptorchidism is linked with decreased fertility and cancer (of both testicles). Injections with the hormone beta human chorionic gonadotropin (B-hCG) or testosterone may help the testicle descend. If this does not work, surgery is the next option.

Pancreatic cancer

Tumor growth may begin without any symptoms and therefore go undetected for an extended period of time. The earliest symptoms include dark urine, clay-colored stools, weakness, fatigue, jaundice, changes in appetite, weight loss, epigastric pain, hepatomegaly, and pain in the stomach. Physical exam may show a positive Courvoisier sign: the presence of a palpable head tumor that can feel like an enlarged gallbladder. Diagnostic testing includes an abdominal ultrasound, computed tomography (CT) scan of the abdomen, ERCP, and tumor marker CA 19-9. Biopsy can confirm the diagnosis. The Whipple procedure (pancreaticoduodenectomy) and chemoradiation are used for treatment. However, the median survival rate is only 9 to 12 months. Complications include bowel obstruction, pain, weight loss, and death.

Trichomoniasis

Trichomoniasis is a sexually transmitted disease that presents with large amounts of foul-smelling, yellow-green vaginal discharge. This discharge is often described as foamy or frothy. The patient may complain of mild itching or irritation. Men are often asymptatic. A wet-mount microscopic specimen will show protozoan flagellate motile organisms. The treatment of choice for the patient with trichomoniasis, and all sexual partners, is with a single 2 gram dose of metronidazole. Clotrimazole 1% vaginally daily for seven days may be substituted when the disease presents in the first trimester of pregnancy, however metronidazole is preferred. Of note, many clinicians do not treat asymptomatic trichomoniasis until the patient is full term to prevent preterm deliver. Screen for other STIs and test partners. Complications include urethritis, cystitis, cervical neoplasia, PID, infertility, and preterm birth. It also increases susceptibility to HIV.

Health belief model

The health belief model is a theory framework that helps define how likely an individual is to make or maintain positive health choices. Adherence to any treatment regime is based on the patient's belief that their disease is serious and threatening to their well-being. Action is determined by cues to action, perceived benefits of action, and reduced barriers to action. In order to promote change, the individual, or group's, core motivations and beliefs must be identified and promoted. It is not a system of negative reinforcement or scare tactics but a way to promote positive internal attitude changes toward positive health outcomes.

Initial prenatal consultation

Routine information to gather during a prenatal visit includes weight and blood pressure, urinalysis for occult blood, glucose and bacteria, fundal height, and fetal heart tones after 10 weeks' gestation. Blood work should include type and antibody screening, complete blood count (CBC), rapid plasma reagin, hepatitis B antigen, HIV, and rubella. After 14 weeks, a maternal serum alpha-fetoprotein level can also be obtained. Pap smear and screening for sexually transmitted diseases are also performed. Feelings and expectations regarding pregnancy are explored, and careful questions regarding personal safety and abuse may be proposed. Smoking, alcohol, and recreational drug use should also be addressed.

Maternal care should be started by ten weeks. The major components of of early prenatal care include identifying patients who are at risk for certain complications; anticipating problems and intervening when able; educating and communicating with the patient; getting early, repeated, and accurate measures of gestational age; and doing ongoing evaluations of the status of the fetus and mom.

Treatment options and goals for hypertension in diabetic patient

Because of the higher risk for nephropathy, myocardial infarction, and stroke associated with diabetes, it is highly important to adequately treat hypertension. The believed contributors to hypertension in diabetes are diabetic neuropathy, hyperinsulinemia, arterial stiffness, and expansion of extracellular fluid. Antihypertensives in the diabetic patient prevents the progression of kidney disease, lowers risk of MI, stroke, and heart failure, and lowers risk for mortality. The first line of defense is angiotensin-converting enzyme (ACE) inhibitors; the next choice would be angiotensin II receptor blockers (ARBs), although multiple antihypertensives may be needed. Diuretics are often needed as well. The 8th Joint National Committee suggests that blood pressure in diabetics be kept less than 140/90.

Outside of medication, the diabetic patient should be encouraged to keep their blood sugar levels under tight control, lose weight as needed, exercise, and quit smoking. All of these will help mitigate the patient's increased risk for atherosclerosis and high blood pressure.

Smoking cessation options

Nicotine dependence is the most common addiction in the United States. The first intervention is simply to begin a conversation with the patient and assess their interest and history of quitting attempts. Counseling, behavioral modification therapy, and one-on-one support can be offered from various sources, but medication may be needed. Nicotine replacement therapy is safe for most patients. Over-the-counter options include nicotine patch, gum, and candy. Prescription options include nicotine inhalers and nasal spray. Non-nicotine medications that may also be helpful include bupropion SR and varenicline. Buproprion is contraindicated in patients with a history of seizures. Counseling must include the possibility of weight gain and advice about diet and exercise. Clonidine and nortriptyline may be considered but are not currently FDA approved and carry many more side effects. The Public Health Service recommends the 4-A's approach to aid patients with smoking cessation:
- Asking – about smoking.
- Advice – how to approach quitting and setting a date to quit.
- Assistance – with counseling as well as pharmacologic aids.
- Arranging – a follow-up appointment 2 to 4 weeks after the date set for quitting.

The combination of counseling and support groups with drug therapy has a smoking cessation success rate of about 50%.

HDL, LDL, and triglyceride levels

Hyperlipidemia is defined as an elevation of serum lipid levels. Diagnosis is made by performing a screening lipid profile. A fasting lipid profile is most accurate and should be routinely performed in men over 35 years of age and women over 45 years of age. Patients with other risk factors for cardiovascular disease or with a significant family history of cardiovascular disease should be screened at a younger age. Levels at which to begin treatment depend on individual patient characteristics, including gender, age, and presence of other risk factors for coronary artery disease. In general, optimal levels are considered to be:
- LDL <100 mg/dL
- HDL >60 mg/dL
- Triglycerides <150 mg/dL
- Total cholesterol <200 mg/dL
- Cholesterol/HDL ratio <4

Low-density lipoprotein (LDL) represents the "bad" cholesterol that is responsible for atherosclerosis. LDL increases heart disease risk. High-density lipoprotein (HDL) represents "good" cholesterol that helps to remove buildup from the vessel walls. Higher levels of HDL can help reduce the risk of heart disease. Triglyceride level correlation is still unclear, but elevated levels are linked with an increased risk of heart disease, especially in conjunction with elevated LDL levels.

Skin lesions

The following are types of skin lesions:
- Papule—small, solid, raised lesion no larger than 1 cm. Coloring may be brown, purple, red, or pink.
- Macule—small (less than 1 cm) discolored spot that is neither raised nor depressed against the surrounding skin. A macule also does not affect the skin texture.

- Vesicle—small (5 to 10 mm), elevated, fluid-filled, circular lesion that generally ruptures easily then dries to a yellow crust.
- Plaque—wide, large, well-demarcated, plateaulike, elevated lesion that appears red with silvery scaling. Often associated with psoriasis.
- Bulla—large (greater than 5 mm), elevated, clear fluid-filled, circular lesion.

Universal precautions

Universal precautions are designed to promote a reasonable amount of safety for the patient and provider in any caregiving situation. It emphasizes the belief that every patient is a carrier of an infectious agent such as hepatitis B or HIV. Universal precaution requires protective barriers (gloves, gowns, mask, and/or goggles) when there is any chance of coming in contact with blood; semen; and vaginal, synovial, spinal, pleural, peritoneal, amniotic, and pericardial fluids.

Contact precautions

Airborne precautions apply to tuberculosis, chicken pox, shingles, and measles. Doors must remain closed, respirators must be worn at all times within the room, and strict hand-washing procedure is observed. Contact and enteric precautions apply to cases of antibiotic-resistant infections [methicillin-resistant *Staphylococcus aureus* (MRSA) and vancomycin-resistant enterococci (VRE)], respiratory syncytial virus (RSV), diphtheria, herpes, impetigo, abscesses and skin ulcerations, pediculosis, scabies, staphylococcal furunculosis, zoster, *Clostridium difficile,* and *Escherichia coli.* Gown and gloves are required within the room as well as strict hand-washing procedure. Droplet precautions apply to meningitis, pneumonia, epiglottitis, pneumonia, bacteremia, group A streptococcal pharyngitis, influenza, scarlet fever, adenovirus, mumps, rubella, and parvovirus B19. This requires a simple mask and strict hand-washing procedure.

Compromised sterile field

A sterile field does not extend below the table or platform it is set up on. Contamination can occur if anything below this level comes in contact with the field (such as the sterile gown below the waist level or a portion of the sterile drape folding over the edge of the table touches the field), hands dropped below the level of the table, arms three inches above the wrist, and the back of the sterile gown are also considered contaminated. Sneezing or coughing over the field is contaminating as is replacing an implement in the field that has been transported out of the field or dropped. Fields that are established on a moist surface are considered contaminated. So is a field that is left unattended, uncovered, or has been completely turned away from during a procedure.

Discharge planning

Discharge planning is a formal process that allows care providers to coordinate the individual needs of the patient extending beyond their time in a hospital or long-term-care setting. This assessment process examines how to provide the appropriate provider care once they no longer meet criteria for hospitalization. Also considered is an understanding of the patient's insurance and benefit coverage to ensure that needed services will be available without unreasonable financial burden. The patient must receive clear and accurate teaching about their condition and self-care as well as community resources that will be available to them.

Heartburn

Occasional heartburn may be normal, but sometimes heartburn is a symptom of GERD (gastroesophageal reflux disease). The diagnosis of GERD can be made on clinical assessment information alone, or in combination with endoscopy. In some patients endoscopy will be needed to rule out other conditions. Burning feeling in the chest that seems worse after eating or when lying down. It is exacerbated by bending over. Nausea, vomiting, and difficulty swallowing are also common symptoms. Medication options include antacids (Maalox, Mylanta, Rolaids, and Tums) to neutralize stomach acid; however, long-term use can result in changes in bowel habits. H_2-receptor blockers (Tagamet HB, Pepcid AC, Zantac, and Axid AR) are meant to reduce the stomach's production of acid. Relief isn't as instant as with antacids, but it will last longer. Proton pump inhibitors (Prevacid 24HR and Prilosec) can both reduce acid production and heal the trauma caused to the esophagus. Patient counseling should include weight loss, if needed; avoidance of tight clothing; specific trigger foods; eating smaller, more frequent meals; smoking cessation; and remaining upright after eating. Complications include erosive esophagitis, esophageal bleeding, esophageal cancer, ulcers, and Barrett's esophagus.

Cancer treatment

There are three main types of cancer treatment available: surgery, radiation, and chemotherapy. These may be used alone or in combination. Surgery attempts to remove the entire tumor as well as surrounding tissues that may have been affected in order to produce a curative/cancer-free state in the patient. When this is not possible, surgery can be used as a palliative effort to remove as much of the tumor as possible in order to lessen the associated pain and symptoms for the patient. Radiation therapy provides localized cancer treatment focusing on the removal of cancer cells before they produce clinical symptoms. Radiation can also be palliative, or used in the treatment of medical emergencies such as spinal cord compression or superior vena cava syndrome. Chemotherapy uses medications to target and help destroy cancer cells. This therapy can be used alone but it is often combined with other treatments for either a curative objective or palliative focus on symptom and pain control.

Complementary and alternative medicine

The following are the five main types of complementary and alternative medicine as defined by the National Center for Complementary and Alternative Medicine (NCCAM):
- Biologically based practice: Focuses on the use of naturally occurring substances and diet for health promotion.
- Energy medicine: Asian-based energy and magnetic and biofield beliefs such as Reiki and Qi Gong.
- Manipulative and body-based practice: The practice of manipulating body parts or systems as a way to improve or manipulate their performance, such as chiropractic, message, and reflexology.
- Mind–body medicine: Focuses on the way mental outlook and belief systems affect health, promoting relaxation and meditation techniques.
- Whole medical systems: More conventional medicine working in conjunction and harmony with a specific cultural belief system such as traditional Chinese medicine.

Interpersonal and communication skills

The interpersonal and communication skills that are important for quality patient care are:
- The ability to establish a therapeutic relationship with appropriate boundaries.
- Effective and tolerant listening skills as well as the ability to correctly interpret nonverbal cues.
- An understanding of open-ended and guided questions and interview skills.
- Clear and concise writing and documentation skills.
- Comfort and confidence in communicating with individuals from all walks of life.
- Appropriately accommodate messages to optimize understanding in the recipient.
- Remain level-headed and emotionally stable, even in disruptive or contentious situations.
- Able to maintain strict patient confidentiality.

Status epilepticus

Status epilepticus is a seizure lasting longer than five minutes, or the state of repeated seizures without a subsequent return to consciousness, or return of normal brain function, between each separate episode. Most common etiologies include noncompliance with antiepileptic drug therapy, drug withdrawal, metabolic dysfunction and acute brain injury. Each type of seizure has characteristic movements, but general signs are jerking movements, decreased LOC, and tonic posturing. Diagnosis is made by clinical assessment. An EEG should be assessed later to check for less obvious forms of status epilepticus. Treatment for status epilepticus focuses on maintaining a clear airway, protecting the patient from eminent harm, and administering medication in an attempt to resolve the episodes. Assess for adequate patient perfusion, give a glucose solution, evaluate the electrolytes, and administer IV benzodiazepines followed by IV phenytoin. Lorazepam is generally the first line of defense; however, if the seizure does not respond to treatment within the first five to seven minutes, phenytoin or fosphenytoin should be added. In extreme cases, barbiturates, anesthesia, neuromuscular blocks, and propofol may be needed to control seizure activity. Complications include death, cerebral anoxia, neurologic damage, possible long term injuries as result of syncope/convulsions, cardiac arrhythmias, aspiration pneumonitis, respiratory failure and cardiac injury.

Successful lifestyle and health changes

Change begins with the patient making a firm, concrete commitment to a goal or positive outcome. No change can be achieved without a decision to pursue that change. Goals that are measurable, gradual, and within the realistic reach for the patient must be established. A clear path needs to be visualized. A realistic view of negative life events and relapses must be established that allows the patient to be forgiving of their perceived failures and maintain long-term resolve toward the change. The patient must receive support and encouragement from outside sources that they trust and value.

Facilitating better collaboration and coordination

Tools developed for this specific purpose in a healthcare setting include practice guidelines to help define each participant's role in care and clinical protocol or pathway to focus care and clarify procedure and strategies to be followed. The goal is to create a team in which the members understand their own, and each other's, role within the group; understand the goals of the team; share responsibility; reach collective decisions; and actively include the patient and his family in the care process. An effective collaboration effort includes all stages of care, from assessment of needs, action, communication, and evaluation of goals upon completion. A primary key is streamlined communication and respect for each individual's unique contribution.

Subacute care facilities

The four types of subacute care facilities that might be available for the patient who faces hospital discharge but is still too ill for home or nursing home care are as follows:
- General—patients discharged to this level of care are stable and healing well but still require skilled care for such things as long-term intravenous treatments.
- Chronic—chronic care facilities are for terminal and end-of-life patients that cannot be cared for in an at-home setting because of choice or complexity of care such as ventilator dependency.
- Transitional—at this level, the patient still needs complex medical and nursing care, such as deep-wound management.
- Long-term transitional—identifies a need for continued complex medical care that is expected to have an extended treatment time.

Pulmonary embolism

Pulmonary embolism is the second leading cause of sudden death. Immediate recognition and treatment for pulmonary embolism is crucial to the patient's chances of survival. Symptoms can be vague and nonspecific but might include chest pain, dyspnea, tachypnea, cough, abnormal lung sounds, low blood pressure, or even just a sense of impending doom or nonspecific agitation. Computed tomography pulmonary angiography is used to make a positive diagnosis. However, using pulmonary embolus risk assessments like the Wells score can help the clinician make decisions, especially if the patient in not stable. Bedside echo is sometimes used in an unstable patient to justify giving certain medications. Priority care is given to basic life functions, including monitoring oxygen saturation levels and administering oxygen as needed. Anticoagulants and thrombolytics may be used to dissolve the clot, or it may need to be surgically removed. A vena cava filter may also be inserted to prevent further clots from reaching the lungs. Complications include recurrent thromboembolism, pulmonary hypertension, and death.

Common non-pain complaints with terminal illnesses

Patients with cancer often express fatigue and anorexia as the top two reasons for emotional and physical distress. Nausea, constipation, states of delirium or other alterations of mental status, and dyspnea are also frequent. Fatigue encompasses symptoms of tiredness, a lack of energy not related to the amount of rest the patient is getting, diminished mental capacity, and weakness. These symptoms interfere with the ability to perform activities of daily living and are often underdiagnosed or downplayed by the patient as inevitable. Anorexia and cachexia are associated with the general wasting of many terminal illnesses and requires careful nutritional management. Nausea and constipation are often related to medications and other treatments but are easily treated if assessed and planned for. Palliative treatments are helpful for altered mental states and dyspnea as well if they are assessed and planned for.

Pharmaceutical Therapeutics

Nystatin

Nystatin (Mycostatin, Nadostine, Nilstat, Nystex) can be used to treat oral candidiasis (thrush) in children and adults as an oral suspension or lozenges at a dose of 200,000 to 600,000 units four times a day for up to two weeks. For treatment of intestinal candidiasis as oral tablets 400,000 to 600,000 units of nystatin is given, up to three times a day. For treatment of vaginal candidiasis, nystatin in the form of vaginal suppositories or tablets of 100,000 units is given up to twice a day for two weeks. Adverse reactions might include nausea, vomiting, stomach discomfort, diarrhea, rash, or vaginal irritation.

Colchicine

Colchicine (Colcrys) is prescribed for gout. Its function is to counteract the swelling and pain from uric acid build up. The normal dosage level is 0.5 to 0.6 mg daily. For acute attacks, an initial dose of up to 1.2 mg can be given, followed by 0.5 to 1.2 mg up to every hour until relief is reached. The intravenous dosage is 2 mg then 0.5 mg every 6 hours with a maximum 24-hour dose of 4 mg. Nausea, vomiting, stomach discomfort, and diarrhea are common reactions. Vitamin B_{12}, alcohol, and grapefruit can interfere with the action of colchicine.

Combantrin

Combantrin (pyrantel pamoate) is an anthelmintic used for treatment of infections caused by parasitic worms such as roundworm and pinworm. Normal dosage is 11 mg/kg (maximum of 1 g) orally, followed by a second dose after two weeks. It is important to treat all family members and others who have close contact with the infected individual and emphasize fastidious personal hygiene habits. Piperazine salts should not be used during the time of treatment, and caution should be used when treatment in needed in patients will severe malnutrition, anemia, or liver impairment.

Minoxidil

Oral minoxidil (Loniten): Loniten is an antihypertensive used in adult patients with severe high blood pressure. Therapeutic dosages must be built up to and usually range from 10 to 40 mg a day. It may cause edema, tachycardia, or other cardiac side effects. Loniten should not be used with NSAIDs or the herb ma huang because they interfere with its action.
Topical minoxidil (Rogaine): Rogaine is a hair growth stimulant available in 2% and 5% topical solutions. These solutions can be applied to areas of thinning hair up to twice a day. Patients should be educated about the possibility of skin irritation and what to expect for results. About 40% of patients will begin to see moderate hair growth after four months of use.

Opiate abuse and withdrawal symptoms

Opioid analgesic therapy is a widely used method of chronic pain control. The severity of symptoms is dependent on the amount and duration of use. Common side effects of abuse may mimic the flu and include increased respirations, diarrhea, runny nose, sweating, coughing, lacrimation, muscle twitching, and increased temperature and blood pressure. Withdrawal symptoms will overlap with abuse symptoms and become worse. Agitation, anxiety, nausea and vomiting, chronic goose bumps, and dilated pupils are also present.

Overdose is treated with naloxone. Withdrawal symptoms can be eased with methadone.

Acetaminophen

Acetaminophen is a non-narcotic analgesic for mild to moderate pain and fever. This pain relief effect can be enhanced when combined with caffeine. Likewise, when acetaminophen is combined with narcotics, it can enhance the pain relief quality of the narcotic. Acetaminophen has no effect on inflammation. It can be safely used in children. It also does not affect blood clotting time. Those with a history of heavy alcohol use should use it cautiously because the combination of the two has a greater chance of creating damage to the liver.

Aspirin

Aspirin is a salicylate analgesic for mild to moderate pain and fever reduction. Use in children is not recommended because of an increased risk of Reye syndrome. Aspirin is also often used as a prophylactic to reduce the risk of myocardial infarction, stroke, and transient ischemic attacks (TIAs) because of its blood thinning quality. It is beneficial in treating inflammation. However, aspirin can also decrease the reabsorption of uric acid, increase gastric irritation, and increase risk of occult blood loss.

Methyldopa

Methyldopa (Aldomet, Aldopren, Dopamet) is an antihypertensive that can be administered orally or by IV. IV dosing is 250 to 500 mg every 6 hours. Oral maintenance dose is 500 mg to 2 g in two or four equal doses. In long-term use, it is often recommended that this medication be taken at bedtime because of its tendency to cause sedation. Other common side effects are headache, orthostatic hypotension, nasal congestion, and dry mouth. Use cautiously with amphetamines, beta-blockers, norepinephrine, phenothiazines, tricyclic antidepressants, anesthesia, barbiturates, haloperidol, levodopa, lithium, MAO inhibitors, and tolbutamide. Monitor blood pressure and liver function closely.

Potassium-sparing diuretics

Potassium-sparing diuretics include amiloride, triamterene, spironolactone, and eplerenone. They are used to prevent sodium reabsorption and potassium secretion in the collection tubules while still promoting urinary excretion of excess fluid. Potassium-sparing diuretics are often used in conjunction with antihypertensive medications to manage high blood pressure or congestive heart failure. Although this class of medications can help prevent hypokalemia, potassium levels still need to be monitored and they should not be used at the same time as potassium supplements.

Occupational health hazards

The most common accidents to occur in the workplace involve system and mechanical failures. Musculoskeletal complaints such as back pain accompany heavy lifting and repetitive activities. Injuries can be to large muscles (such as the back) or smaller muscle groups (wrists, neck, ankles). Hearing loss is common in construction and manufacturing industries. Chemical and biological agents that can cause liver damage, reproductive disorders, and cancer are most common in professions that have constant exposure to pesticides, heavy metal, and corrosive substances. Healthcare workers are particularly vulnerable to HIV, tuberculosis, and hepatitis B and C.

Pharmaceutical treatments for mild to moderate acne

Over-the-counter options include lotions containing benzoyl peroxide, sulfur, resorcinol, or salicylic acid. These products are best for mild cases of acne. For more severe cases, the strength of the lotions can be increased through the prescription of tretinoin, adapalene or tazarotene. Beyond topical agents, antibiotics (tetracycline or clindamycin) can be considered as well as oral contraceptives. Chemical peels, microdermabrasion, and laser and light therapy can also be useful. Isotretinoin (Amnesteem, Claravis, Sotret) is an extremely powerful medication, which, while highly effective for scarring cystic acne, carries many risks and side effects and should be considered as a last resort.

Treatment options for COPD

Chronic obstructive pulmonary disease (COPD) cannot be cured, but it can be controlled with medication. Inhalers can be coupled with anti-inflammatory medications. The first line of defense is usually recommended as ipratropium and albuterol (beta-2-adrenergics and anticholinergics), the second-line option is albuterol, and the third choice would be methylprednisolone sodium succinate, followed by theophylline. Acute flare-ups may also require assistance from steroids, nebulizers with bronchodilators, oxygen therapy, and breathing assistance through aids such as a BiPAP portable ventilator. Other recommendations for the patient might include weight management, pulmonary rehabilitation, and reducing triggers in their environment such as smoke or perfumes. Surgery to remove severely damaged lung tissue may also be considered.

Initial dosing of levothyroxine sodium

Considerations for dosing must include patient age, duration and severity of hypothyroidism, and presence of any preexisting cardiac disease such as angina. There is a high level of sensitivity to thyroid medications, so the initial dose should begin at a very low level, generally 25 mcg a day, increasing as needed every one to two months in order to reach therapeutic levels. Adults older than age 60 will require less medication than a younger adult. Levothyroxine increases cardiac workload and elevates heart rate—the patient should inform you of any chest pain, palpitations, sweating, anxiety, or shortness of breath.

Chronic, stable angina

Initial medication choices include beta-blockers such as metoprolol in order to lower the heart rate, blood pressure, and oxygen requirements of the heart. Long-acting nitrates including isosorbide dinitrate may be considered if beta-blockers prove ineffective, but there is a tendency to develop a tolerance to these medications. Ranolazine is also a good choice. Angiotensin-converting enzyme (ACE) inhibitors lower blood pressure. Calcium-channel blockers help the heart relax to reduce workload and blood pressure. Preventive measures against myocardial infarction may also be considered using aspirin, clopidogrel, or prasugrel.

Cystitis

Cystitis is most often caused by *Escherichia coli* (*E. coli*). The patient presents with urinary frequency, urgency, and pain, and there may also be a pain response to light pressure on the suprapubic area. Urinalysis will show white and red blood cells. Because of the increase in strains of *E. coli* that are resistant to trimethoprim-sulfamethoxazole, a three-day course of fluoroquinolones such as ciprofloxacin has now become the standard treatment of choice. These recommendations change frequently according to the mutations of the bacterial strains and should be frequently revalidated in a dependable resource such as *The Sanford Guide to Antimicrobial Therapy*.

Warfarin and heparin

Warfarin (Coumadin) is an anticoagulant normally given in oral form (2 to 10 mg a day) as long-term therapy for those patients needing blood thinners. This requires both baseline and frequent prothrombin time (PT) and international normalized ratio (INR) levels to maintain a therapeutic level. The patient should also be monitored for unusual bruising and bleeding as well as cautioned against aspirin use and other over-the-counter supplements that affect bleeding times. Heparin sodium is an injectable anticoagulant that can be given intravenously or subcutaneously for more acute illnesses such as deep vein thrombosis, myocardial infarction, and pulmonary embolism. Partial thromboplastin time (PTT), PT, and INR will be monitored frequently. Heparin sodium is used cautiously in the patient who has/or will be undergoing surgery.

Hypertensive patients with heart failure and reduced cardiac output

Optimal treatment goals for the hypertensive patient with heart failure is to reach a stable blood pressure of less than 130/80 mmHg. This usually requires more than one medication. An angiotensin-converting enzyme (ACE) inhibitor with thiazide diuretic therapy slows cardiac remodeling, improves cardiac function, and reduces further cardiovascular events after a myocardial infarction. Beta-blockers are also commonly added. Other medications that might be considered are dihydropyridine calcium antagonists, angiotensin receptor blockers (ARBs), aldosterone inhibitors, and isosorbide dinitrate/hydralazine.

Opioid rotation

Opioid rotation is a process of systematically switching a patient's prescribed opioid when they no longer seem to be receiving effective pain relief on their current medication, rather than increasing the dosage. Changing from one opioid to another, or altering the delivery method, may become necessary under the assumption that incomplete cross-tolerance among opioids occurs. Changing analgesics or the method of delivery may result in a decreased drug requirement. When altering opioid delivery regimes, use morphine equivalents as the common factor for all dose conversions. This method will help reduce medication errors.

Spasmolytics

Spasmolytics for the bladder include flavoxate hydrochloride (Urispas), oxybutynin chloride (Ditropan, Oxytrol), phenazopyridine hydrochloride (AZO-Standard, Geridium, Pyridium, Urodine), and tolterodine tartrate (Detrol). These are used to offer relief to patients with urinary disorders such as urinary frequency, urgency, nocturia, incontinence, pain, and bladder spasms. Carisoprodol, cyclobenzaprine, metaxalone, and methocarbamol are used in conjunction with rest and physical therapy to treat acute/painful musculoskeletal conditions causing muscle spasms. These conditions frequently include fibromyalgia, tension headaches, and myofascial pain syndrome. These are contraindicated in neurological conditions such as cerebral palsy and multiple sclerosis.

Antiarrhythmic drugs

Antiarrhythmic drugs include sodium-channel blockers, beta-blockers, potassium-channel blockers, calcium-channel blocker, adenosine, digitalis, atropine, and even electrolyte supplements when given for the express purpose of helping to correct a cardiac rhythm anomaly. It is important to understand the action of each medication and match it carefully to the individual patient's needs. Antiarrhythmics are always given with caution because they not only stabilize cardiac excitability or depression, but they could also cause a secondary arrhythmia or other unwanted cardiac complication such as hypotension.

Antibiotic choice for otitis media

The current recommendation by the American Academy of Pediatrics is a 10-day course of amoxicillin. Secondary choices are erythromycin or sulfonamide. It is important to note that some cases of otitis media are viral in origin and require no antibiotic. These ear infections will resolve on their own. Treatment with antibiotics may be delayed by 48 to 72 hours in the child between the ages of 6 months to 2 years to avoid overuse of antibiotics if the cause may be viral in origin.

ACE inhibitors

Angiotensin-converting enzyme (ACE) inhibitors are used to lower blood pressure by promoting vasodilation as well as acting as a diuretic. This is a recommended treatment option for heart failure patients and those recovering from myocardial infarction. ACE inhibitors are identified by the ending "pril": benazepril, captopril, enalapril, fosinopril, lisinopril, moexipril, quinapril, and ramipril. Side effects are rare, but the patient may experience some dizziness or lightheadedness when therapy begins. ACE inhibitors should not be taken during pregnancy or when breastfeeding.

Beta-blockers

Beta-blockers (β-blockers) block norepinephrine and epinephrine from binding with their receptors to slow the heartbeat and lower blood pressure. These include acebutolol, bisoprolol, esmolol, propranolol, atenolol, labetalol, carvedilol, and metoprolol. Note the identifying ending of "lol." β-blockers are recommended for the diabetic patient, cardiac arrhythmias, heart failure, myocardial infarction recovery, and angina pectoris. β-blockers are generally not used in combination with calcium-channel blockers. Side effects are rare, but β-blockers are able to cross the blood–brain barrier, and this may result in central nervous system (CNS) symptoms such as headache or dizziness. β-blockers may also mask symptoms of hypoglycemia and exacerbate asthma. Gradual tapering over one to two weeks is advisable. Abrupt cessation can lead to rebound hypertension, tachycardia, sweating, unstable angina, myocardial infarction, and possibly death.

Calcium-channel blockers

Calcium-channel blockers (amlodipine, felodipine, diltiazem, verapamil, nifedipine, nicardipine, nisoldipine, and bepridil) relax blood vessels and reduce cardiac workload by preventing calcium from entering the cardiac tissue. This lowers pulse and blood pressure. They may be prescribed for cardiac disease, coronary spasms or angina, arrhythmias, hypertrophic cardiomyopathy, or right-sided heart failure. Patients should be educated not to eat or drink grapefruit or consume alcohol while on this medication. Dosages may need to be lowered in older adults because they are more prone to side effects.

Parkinson's disease

A combination of levodopa and carbidopa (Sinemet, Parcopa) is the treatment of choice for Parkinson's disease. Levodopa acts to reduce tremor, rigidity, bradykinesia, and postural inability, but it cannot slow or halt disease progression. Carbidopa facilitates the ability of levodopa to reach the brain in optimal amounts. When it is working well, mobility is improved; however, the patient can experience dyskinesia. There is also a varied cycle of effectiveness with prolonged use. When the medication is less effective, motor symptoms become more spasmodic and unpredictable. Possible interactions may be experienced when the patient is also taking antacids, antiseizure medications, antihypertensives, antidepressants, and a high-protein consumption.

Impetigo

Impetigo is a common bacterial skin infection caused by streptococcus, staphylococcus, or methicillin-resistant *Staphylococcus aureus* (MRSA) that enters through a break in the skin. Impetigo appears as a single or multiple blisters filled with clear, yellow fluid that burst easily. These leave behind a red, raw area of irritation. The rash is most common on the face and lips but may spread to other areas. It is contagious. Mupirocin ointment is recommended for treatment, but oral antibiotics may be needed for severe cases.

Constipation

Before medication is considered, review the patient's fiber and fluid intake, as well as his or her activity level. Encourage dietary modifications, exercise, and bowel training activities before a prescription is issued. Medication choices fall into four categories, listed by order of choice: bulk laxatives, stool softeners, osmotic laxatives, and stimulant laxatives. Bulk laxatives (methylcellulose, polycarbophil, and psyllium) are dietary fiber supplements taken when the patient's normal consumption is still inadequate. Stool softeners, also called emollient laxatives, (docusate calcium, docusate sodium) encourage water to enter into the bowel. Osmotic laxatives (lactulose, magnesium citrate, magnesium hydroxide, polyethylene glycol, sodium biphosphate, and sorbitol) stimulate osmosis and create more available water in the intestine. Stimulant laxatives (bisacodyl, cascara sagrada, castor oil, and senna) encourage greater intestinal motility and increase water in the bowel.

Oral contraceptives

Hormone-based oral contraceptives are the most common choice among women for birth control. But this method is not recommended for women older than age 35 with a history of smoking, high blood pressure, or thrombosis. The most common types of oral contraceptives are often a combination of both estrogen and progestin; these are preferable and most effective when used with accuracy. Effectiveness may be altered by rifampin and antiepileptics, phenytoin, and carbamazepine. The patient must also be aware that oral contraceptives do not prevent the spread of HIV or STDs. Oral contraceptives may also be prescribed to stabilize symptoms of premenstrual syndrome (PMS) or help treat acne. Progesterone-only contraceptives are recommended for the breastfeeding patient.

Antipsychotics

First-generation antipsychotics include haloperidol, chlorpromazine, perphenazine, and fluphenazine. They are used to treat schizophrenia and related disorders. These antipsychotics can produce Parkinson-like symptoms such as akinesia, bradykinesia, stoic facial expression, tremor, cogwheel rigidity, postural abnormalities, and tardive dyskinesia.

Second-generation (atypical) antipsychotics include clozapine, risperidone, olanzapine, quetiapine, ziprasidone, aripiprazole and paliperidone. Special care must be taken when prescribing clozapine to monitor the patient's white blood cell count. Other medications should be considered before clozapine. Atypical antipsychotics often cause weight gain.

NSAIDs for rheumatoid arthritis

NSAIDs (naproxen) can be used to treat symptoms and pain related to diseases such as rheumatoid arthritis, but they cannot slow or halt disease progression. Patients may benefit from NSAID use through its anti-inflammatory, analgesic, and antipyretic properties. NSAIDs tend to be the first line of defense against pain caused by inflammatory conditions. They may also be used in conjunction with opioid therapy to reduce the amount of opioid needed. Adversely, gastrointestinal bleeding or ulceration, decreased renal function, and impaired platelet aggregation may occur. Studies have also indicated that the therapeutic effects of NSAIDs may not extend beyond six to twelve months of use. Short-term memory loss may occur in older patients. There may be an increased cardiovascular risk with prolonged use. Patients allergic to sulfa drugs can also experience a cross-sensitivity to some types of NSAIDs.

Triptans

Triptans (sumatriptan, eletriptan, almotriptan, frovatriptan, rizatriptan, zolmitriptan) are serotonin receptor agonists that help relieve pain from acute migraine attacks by causing vasoconstriction of the intracranial blood vessels and relieving swelling. Sensitivity to light and noise, nausea and vomiting also associated with migraines will be quickly resolved as well. Combining triptans with acetaminophen or naproxen can boost its effectiveness even further. They can cause irritation at the point of administration (injection or nasal spray) and may cause some dizziness, drowsiness, or lightheadedness. Triptans cannot be used in patients with cerebrovascular disease. Patients should also be educated about rebound headaches.

Emergency contraception

Emergency contraception can be provided to women who have a fear that they may have been unintentionally impregnated. This may occur because of sexual assault or rape, protective device failure (condom breakage or dislodged diaphragm), or when no birth control was used at all (including forgetting to regularly take prescribed birth control pills). Two emergency contraceptive pills are available without a prescription: Plan B One-Step and Next Choice. Ulipristal requires a prescription. Any of these methods can be taken up to five days after the unprotected sex occurs.

Metronidazole

Oral metronidazole (Flagyl) is an antibiotic used to treat infections of the reproductive system or gastrointestinal tract such as pelvic inflammatory disease (PID), trichomoniasis, and *Clostridium difficile* (C-diff). Nausea and headache are common side effects. Flagyl may also be given intravenously. Topical cream metronidazole is applied to the skin once a day for the treatment of rosacea. It does not, however, cure the disease process. It may also be used as vaginal treatment for bacterial infections (two times a day for five days). Either application has the potential to cause skin irritation.

Adverse side effects and allergic reactions to medication

Although adverse side effects can be, at times, very severe, the body does not form antibodies against the medication. A true allergic reaction means that the body's immune system has created antibodies against the foreign substance it perceives as a threat. These antibodies cause an anaphylaxis reaction with hives, facial and throat swelling, wheezing, light-headedness, vomiting, and even shock. These reactions are almost immediate, occurring in under an hour, although there may be a delay of several hours.

Permethrin cream

Over-the-counter permethrin 1% cream can be used to treat lice. Permethrin 5% (Elimite) cream can be prescribed as treatment for scabies. The patient should be instructed to wash and dry their entire body, then apply the cream to every exposed surface, paying particular attention to the creases and folds. Permethrin 5% cream needs to remain on the skin for at least 8 to 14 hours. Then the patient should again wash and dry thoroughly and put on clean clothing. Patients should be aware that the itching will ease somewhat within the first 24 hours but may not be completely relieved for up to 4 weeks after treatment. It may also cause temporary redness of the skin as well. Permethrin is safe for use in infants after 2 months of age through the elderly.

Health risks associated with obesity

Obesity is defined as a body mass index (BMI) of 30 or greater. Children and adults who are obese are at a greater risk for developing gallstones, diabetes, high blood pressure, high cholesterol and triglyceride levels, coronary artery disease, stroke, and sleep apnea. If the distribution of fat is more toward a lower, pear-shaped body frame, it carries a slightly lower risk than those who carry a more central, stomach-fat distribution. Likewise, those who are able to lose weight and maintain a healthy lifestyle can reduce the chance of these health risks.

Panic attacks

Long-term treatment and prevention of panic attacks can often be treated by antidepressants. Selective serotonin reuptake inhibitors (SSRIs) such as fluoxetine (Prozac), paroxetine (Paxil), citalopram (Celexa), escitalopram (Lexapro), and sertraline (Zoloft) are the initial choices. The next choice is selective serotonin and norepinephrine reuptake inhibitors (SSNRIs). Treatment of an acute attack requires a sedative such as Xanax, Klonopin, Valium, or Ativan. In addition to medication, psychotherapy, cognitive-behavioral therapy, relaxation, and meditation training should also be considered.

Upper respiratory infections

Upper respiratory infections are the most common cause of doctor visits. An upper respiratory infection involves the sinuses, nasal passages, pharynx, and larynx. There is typically inflammation of these areas that causes pain, congestion, and cough. The patient may also complain of difficulty breathing and fatigue. These types of illnesses are most common during the fall and winter months. The virus is contagious through respiratory droplets that are inhaled or transferred by touch. The risk of contracting an upper respiratory infection is highest among those who spend long hours in close quarters with many other people, those with poor hand-washing habits, smokers, immunocompromised individuals, and those working in health-care settings. It is not caused by a bacterial infection and cannot be relieved through the use of antibiotics.

ADHD

Attention-deficit hyperactivity disorder (ADHD) must be properly diagnosed in order for prescribed medications to have the desired effect. The most common classification of medication used is psychostimulants: amphetamine-dextroamphetamine (Adderall), dexmethylphenidate (Focalin), dextroamphetamine (Dexedrine), lisdexamfetamine (Vyvanse), and methylphenidate (Ritalin). In true ADHD, these drugs have a calming effect on the patient rather than a stimulating effect. The nonstimulant atomoxetine (Strattera) may also be considered. The first line of choice for treatment in a newly diagnosed younger child is behavioral therapy. Medication should be prescribed only after prudent consideration and continued close patient contact to monitor its effects.

Gentamicin

Gentamicin is an antibiotic used to treat bacterial infections. In its injectable form, it is often used to treat serious infections such as *Pseudomonas*, *Escherichia coli*, and *Staphylococcus*. Standard dosing is 1 mg/kg every 8 hours. Common side effects include nausea, vomiting, and loss of appetite. When given as an intramuscular injection, patients often complain of pain and irritation at the injection site. Gentamicin in this form also carries a high risk of renal and ototoxicity. Gentamicin can also be prescribed in a solution for use as eyedrops to treat infections such as conjunctivitis.

Back pain

Depending on the source, amount, and consistency of the pain, treatment options can vary greatly. Treatment options include: physical therapy, mild anti-inflammatory medications, chiropractic referrals, transcutaneous electrical nerve stimulation (TENS) or intradiscal electrothermal therapy (IDET) units, injections, and surgical interventions. Any intervention is aimed at reducing pain and recovering movement. For an acute episode, an ice pack and anti-inflammatory agent may be sufficient. Long-term bed rest is not recommended. For more chronic needs, treatment options should progress from the most noninvasive that is needed for the patient to receive relief.

Doxorubicin

Doxorubicin is an antineoplastic drug common in the treatment of breast, bladder, ovarian, and endometrial cancers. It may also be used in certain types of lymphoma and leukemia, thyroid, and skin cancers. Injections are provided every 21 to 28 days. Common side effects include nausea, vomiting, mouth and throat lesions, changes in appetite, fatigue, and weight loss. Long-term monitoring of the heart should also be planned for because doxorubicin can have a damaging effect on cardiac health.

Salicylic acid

Salicylic acid is a popular medication used for treatment of various skin disorders such as psoriasis, ichthyoses, dandruff, corns, calluses, and warts. It works by reducing swelling, redness, and irritation while unclogging pores in the treatment of acne. For other conditions, it loosens and softens areas of thickened or calloused skin until it falls off naturally or can be easily removed. Mild concentrations are used for most conditions. Solutions of 2% to 10% concentration are used for treatment of corns and up to 17% for warts. However, salicylic acid should not be used to treat warts on the face, mouth or nose; any wart with a hair follicle; genital warts; moles; or birthmarks.

Antihistamines

Antihistamines are chemically designed to block histamines that are triggered by allergies in order to calm the body's reaction to the invasive organism. Not every antihistamine works for every symptom that may be experienced. The most marked side effect of first-generation antihistamines (diphenhydramine, clemastine) is a greater risk of sedation than second-generation antihistamines (loratadine, fexofenadine, desloratadine). All of these medications can also cause patient complaints of dry mouth and mucous membranes, dizziness, restlessness or change in mood, and occasionally nausea and vomiting.

Insulin

Rapid-acting insulin (Humalog, NovoLog, Apidra) is designed to act on the body's needs for insulin during meal consumption. Its peak is within 30 minutes to 1 ½ hours, and its full duration of action is between 1 to 5 hours. Short-acting insulin (regular Humulin, Velosulin) is used when a meal is anticipated within 30 minutes to an hour. Peak action is 2 to 5 hours, and the duration is 2 to 8 hours. Intermediate-acting insulin (NPH, Lente) covers an extended period such as the time when the patient is asleep, and their need will be steady. Peak action is anywhere from 3 to 12 hours, and the full duration is 18 to 24 hours. Long-acting insulin (Ultralente, Lantus, Levemir) gives coverage for a full 24 hours. Peaks are very gentle or nonexistent, and the duration is 24 to 36 hours. Combinations of insulin with different durations can be premixed to provide a more complex level of coverage. Premixed insulins include Humulin 70/30, Novolin 70/30, NovoLog 70/30, Humulin 50/50, and Humalog mix 75/25.

Addiction and pseudoaddiction

Addiction is a primary and constant neurobiologic disease with genetic, psychosocial, and environmental factors that create an obsessive and irrational need or preoccupation with a substance. Addictive behaviors include unrestricted, continued cravings, and compulsive and persistent use of a drug despite harmful experiences and side effect. Pseudoaddiction is an assumption that the patient is addicted to a substance, when in actuality the patient is not experiencing relief from the medication. It is prolonged, unrelieved pain that may be the result of undertreatment. This situation may lead the patient to become more aggressive in seeking medicated relief, thus resulting in the inappropriate "drug-seeker" label.

Physical dependence, tolerance, and pseudotolerance

Physical dependence is a condition of bodily adaptation to the presence of a specific drug or chemical. Abrupt removal or a rapid reduction of dosage will result in withdrawal symptoms. The patient does not present with the psychological and environmental dependence that are evident in addictions, such as an obsessive and irrational need or preoccupation with a substance, unrestricted, continued cravings, and compulsive and persistent use of a drug despite harmful experiences and side effects. Tolerance is the adaptation of the body to continued exposure to a drug or chemical. The effects of the drug at the same level of exposure are minimized over time. Additional dosing is required to maintain the same outcomes. Pseudotolerance is the misguided perception of the caregiver that a patient's need for increasing doses of a drug is due to the development of tolerance, when in reality disease progression or other factors are responsible for the increase in dosing needs.

Applying Basic Science Concepts

Dystocia

Dystocia is defined as an abnormal or difficult childbirth. This is a condition that occurs in approximately 20% of pregnancies. Complications can range from uncoordinated uterine contractions, abnormal fetal presentation, or cephalopelvic disproportion. The form of dystocia most often referred to is shoulder dystocia, in which the infant's shoulder presents into the birth canal first, making it impossible for the labor and delivery to progress naturally. Those women whose pregnancies occur too close together or too far apart, primigravida, and multiparous pregnancies are most often affected.

G6PD deficiency

Glucose-6-phosphate dehydrogenase deficiency (G6PD) is a genetic disorder in which the red blood cells undergo hemolysis. This disease process causes hemolytic anemia. The patient may present with pale skin, jaundice, dark urine, complaints of extreme fatigue, difficulty breathing, and an increased heart rate. This condition is not constant. Many people will not ever experience symptoms and complications from the disorder. Hemolysis may result from infection, medication, or allergen triggers (most often fava bean). G6PD is more common in males than females.

Normal heart sounds

Heart sounds are actually created by the noise of the blood pushing through the heart valves. S1, or the "lub" sound, is created by the mitral and tricuspid valves. S2, or the "dub" sound, is created by the aortic and pulmonary valves. During youth, a third benign heart sound, S3, or gallop, may also be present after S2. In the adult, this is an indication of cardiac disease. Abnormal sounds that might be observed occur when these valves do not close at the proper times or do not close completely.

Abnormal breathing patterns

The following are abnormal breathing patterns:
- Cheyne-Stokes: respiratory depression caused by heart failure and uremia.
- Kussmaul: deep, rapid, labored breathing related to acidosis.
- Obstructive: obstructive lung disease, or COPD, causing prolonged expiration due to narrowed airways and increased resistance.
- Ataxic: unpredictable irregularity, both shallow and deep breaths, apnea, from brain damage and respiratory depression.
- Tachypnea: rapid shallow breathing, with multiple causes.

Hypovolemia

Hypovolemia is a state of decreased blood plasma volume. Common causes of hypovolemia are dehydration, bleeding, vomiting, and burns. Dehydration can be a cause, but is not interchangeable with the term hypovolemia. Dehydration is a decrease in the available water within the body. A specific loss of blood plasma (hypovolemia) also includes a marked depletion in sodium levels as well. If the loss is greater than 10% to 20% of the body's total volume, the patient can begin to exhibit symptoms such as tachycardia, hypotension, pale skin, dizziness, change in mental status,

Copyright © Mometrix Media. You have been licensed one copy of this document for personal use only. Any other reproduction or redistribution is strictly prohibited. All rights reserved.

nausea, and excessive thirst. Hypovolemia shock can also result. If needed, treatment involves both fluid and blood plasma replacement.

Frank-Starling law of the heart

Frank–Starling law (also known as Starling's law or Maestrini heart's law) describes the correlation between cardiac blood volume and stroke volume. End diastolic volume is directly proportional to stroke volume. The greater the amount of fluid within the ventricles during diastole, the greater the amount of force that will be exerted during the systolic contraction. This process is independent from any neural or hormonal influences. When the heart's ability to contract is compromised, heart failure may be suspect. The heart will resort to the law of Laplace to try and compensate, and S3 may be detected.

Law of Laplace

The Frank–Starling law describes the correlation between cardiac blood volume and stroke volume. End diastolic volume is directly proportional to stroke volume. The greater the amount of fluid within the ventricles during diastole, the greater the amount of force will be exerted during the systolic contraction. If there is a reduced surface tension and the amount of blood being circulated becomes unstable, amphipathic phospholipid-based pulmonary surfactant allows alveoli to remain open in an attempt to increase the oxygenation to the circulating blood volume. If this process remains unchecked, an aneurysm can result.

Poiseuille's law/equation

Poiseuille's law explains the relationship between pressure and resistance that affects blood or air flow. The longer the length and smaller the size of a lumen creates greater resistance, making an increased pressure need that raises blood pressure and decreases oxygenation. The equation is as follows: (volume flow rate) is equal to (pi divided by eight) times (the pressure difference between the ends of the tube) times (the radius of the tube to the fourth power) divided by (the viscosity, or thickness, of the fluid) divided by (the length of the tube).

Sodium-glucose transport proteins

Sodium-glucose linked transporters (SGLTs) are found in the mucous membranes of the small intestines. Their role is to help with renal glucose reabsorption because sodium and glucose transport across membranes in the same direction. In cases where blood glucose levels have become too high, SGLT allows glucose to be excreted in the urine by creating a sodium gradient for the glucose to follow. This knowledge is currently being explored for its usefulness in treating type 2 diabetes mellitus.

Purine metabolism

Purine and xanthine are nucleotides involved in both DNA and RNA formation as well as energy transference and nitrogen disposal. The purine family includes adenine, guanine, caffeine, xanthine, uric acid, and others. Purine is metabolized by hypoxanthine-guanine phosphoribosyltransferase (HPRT). Disruptions in this process can cause DNA genetic disorders that are hereditary. Health problems such as Lesch–Nyhan syndrome, gout, anemia, epilepsy, developmental delays, deafness, kidney disease, and immune disorders as well as many others can be caused by the resulting disruptions in the purine metabolism that in turn cause DNA disruptions. The action of allopurinol inhibits the conversion of xanthine into uric acid, making it an effective treatment for gout.

SA node

The cells of the sinoatrial (SA) node are specialized to act automatically, regardless of the electrical impulses in the surrounding cardiac tissue. This allows it to act as the pacemaker for the heart. The impulses travel from the SA node to the atrioventricular (AV) node, through it to the bundle of His and Perkinje fibers to the rest of the cardiac tissues causing coordinated contractions. The SA node's natural rhythm is a steady 60 to 70 beats per minute. If there is a greater oxygen demand by the cells of the body, this message is relayed to the SA node, which responds by sending out more rapid impulses to increase blood circulation through the heart and lungs to the body. If there is a malfunction of the SA node, the AV node will act as a fail-safe and take over the regulation of the heart at a slightly slower rhythm.

Condyloma acuminata

Condyloma acuminata (genital warts) are caused by a contact infection with any one of more than 100 types of human papillomavirus (HPV). The most common types are types 6 and 11. The risk is highest between the ages of 17 and 33 among those who begin sexual activity at an early age, smoke, use oral contraceptives, have a previous history of a sexually transmitted disease (STD), have a compromised immune system, and have multiple sexual partners of both sexes. It may be difficult to pinpoint the origin of the infection if multiple partners are involved because the initial stages have no discernible symptoms. Lesions generally develop up to three months after contact. Identification of genital warts during pregnancy is important because the virus can also be passed to the infant during birth. Genital warts also increase the patient's risk for later developing cancer.

AIDS

AIDS is a progression of infection with human immunodeficiency virus. Because there is such a wide range of AIDS defining conditions, the patient may present with many types of symptoms, depending upon the diagnosis, but more than half of AIDS patients exhibit fever, lymphadenopathy, pharyngitis, rash, and myalgia/arthralgia. AIDS is diagnosed when the following criteria are met:
- HIV infection
- CD4 count less than 200 cells/mm3
- AIDS defining condition, such as opportunistic infections (cytomegalovirus, tuberculosis), wasting syndrome, neoplasms (Kaposi sarcoma), or AIDS dementia complex.

It is important to review the following:
- CD4 counts, to determine immune status.
- WBC and differential for signs of infection.
- Cultures to help identify any infective agents.
- CBC to evaluate for signs of bleeding or thrombocytopenia.

Treatment aims to cure or manage opportunistic conditions and control underlying HIV infection through highly active anti-retroviral therapy (HAART), 3 or more drugs used concurrently. Complications include:

- Opportunistic infections
- Dementia
- Neoplasms
- Wasting
- Death.

Organic Areas

Cardiovascular System

Dilated cardiomyopathy

Dilated cardiomyopathy will cause patients to feel short of breath, and paroxysmal nocturnal dyspnea may be present with complaints of fatigue. As the ejection fraction decreases, symptoms of CHF may be present, such as rales, edema, a systolic murmur, and an increase in jugular venous distention (JVD). The murmur heard with dilated cardiomyopathy should decrease when patients are standing or performing Valsalva maneuvers. An EKG will show ST-T wave changes with left ventricular hypertrophy and possible conduction abnormalities. A chest x-ray will show cardiomegaly and possible pulmonary congestion and effusions. An echocardiogram will assess valvular function and estimate the ejection fraction. If there is an autoimmune or infective process present, a myocardial biopsy will be done to identify the causative factor. A cardiac catheterization can be done to determine the extent of CAD present, and lab work will be done to identify if there is an endocrine abnormality. Finally, a urine or serum drug screen will identify if illicit drug use is the cause of the heart disease. Treatment includes ACE inhibitors to slow LV enlargement. Idiopathic dilated cardiomyopathy is highly familial, so when a new diagnosis is made, family screening should be done.

Cardiomyopathy

Dilated cardiomyopathy is the most common type of cardiomyopathy. It results in a reduction in strength of the ventricular contraction, which causes dilation of the left ventricle and a decreased ejection fraction. Most common causes are alcohol abuse, cocaine abuse, CAD, thyroid disease, and pheochromocytoma, but it can also be due to an autoimmune or infective process. Infective myocarditis due to the coxsackievirus can lead to dilated cardiomyopathy. Restrictive cardiomyopathy occurs due to some type of infiltrative process that results in decreased elasticity of the ventricles and heart failure. It can be idiopathic in nature or due to conditions that result in endomyocardial fibrosis, such as sarcoidosis or amyloidosis. Hypertrophic cardiomyopathy causes a significant enlargement of the left ventricle, especially the septum, which results in obstruction of the left ventricle. This is most often genetic in etiology and can be seen in young athletes. Hypertension may also contribute to development of this type of cardiomyopathy.

Hypertrophic cardiomyopathy

Hypertrophic cardiomyopathy may not give any warning signs to patients and is frequently the cause of sudden cardiac arrest in the young athlete. If symptomatic, patients may complain of dyspnea on exertion, angina, palpitations, fatigue, or episodes of syncope. A systolic murmur can be heard with hypertrophic cardiomyopathy, but unlike the other types of cardiomyopathy, the intensity of the murmur will not change when patients are standing or performing Valsalva maneuvers. EKG changes seen with hypertrophic cardiomyopathy include ST-T wave changes, left ventricular hypertrophy, and deep Q waves. An echocardiogram will be done to assess valvular function and the estimated EF. Increased thickness noted anywhere in the LV walls that isn't attributed to another disease process is confirmation of the diagnosis. Because hypertrophic cardiomyopathy tends to be a genetic condition, patients' families should undergo a thorough cardiac evaluation. Treatment focuses on controlling heart failure symptoms, maintaining euvolemia, controlling any arrhythmias. Complications include left ventricular outflow tract obstruction, endocarditis, and thrombus.

Restrictive cardiomyopathy

Restrictive cardiomyopathy may also cause dyspnea and fatigue with paroxysmal nocturnal dyspnea. Edema, rales, and an increase in jugular venous distention may also be present. A heart murmur may be auscultated, and patients may have chronic atrial fibrillation. The murmur heard with restrictive cardiomyopathy should decrease when patients are standing or performing Valsalva maneuvers. This is a diagnosis of exclusion, as this physiology can be seen in many other disorders and can also be secondary to heart disease. Echo may show bilateral atrial enlargement, small LV (but often have a normal LV function), and a restrictive pattern of filling. Though this can be idiopathic in etiology, a myocardial biopsy will be done to determine the cause. It would be expected that evidence of sarcoidosis or amyloidosis would be present on biopsy if either of these is the cause. Collagen deposits may also be present when collagen disease is the cause of the restrictive cardiomyopathy. BNP >400 could help differentiate between cardiomyopathy and pericardititis (though not helpful if renal failure present). Treatment includes decreasing vascular congestion by heart rate control, decreasing CVP, electrolyte balance, and correcting any arrythmias. Heart transplant will be indicated for patients who are eligible as heart failure advances. Symptomatic restrictive cardiomyopathy has a poor prognosis.

Atrial flutter

Atrial flutter on EKG results in a regular rhythm with an atrial rate up to 300 bpm. The P waves will follow a "sawtooth" pattern two or more times followed by a narrow QRS. A bundle branch block may be present, and this can result in a widened QRS. Etiology: Commonly occurs when the atrial focus is irritated, resulting in multiple firings. The AV node will block some of these impulses from being sent to the ventricles. This can cause abnormal ventricular rhythm. For patients who do not spontaneously convert to sinus rhythm with a new onset atrial flutter, cardioversion is the treatment of choice. If stable, the patient should be fasting, and electrolyte/dig levels should be WNL prior to procedure, and moderate to deep sedation. Pharmacologic conversion of atrial flutter if the patient is unable to undergo moderate sedation for cardioversion using ibutilide, amiodarone, flecainide, propafenone, or dofetilide. For patients with >48 hours (or unknown length) of atrial flutter, check TEE and give anticoagulation for at least three weeks prior to cardioversion. Radiofrequency catheter ablation is a permanent treatment option for atrial fibrillation. Atrial fibrillation places the patient at high risk for embolism. Patients should be evaluated after cardioversion, and if their risk level meets criteria, they should be placed on anticoagulant therapy for the recommended time as related to their risk. If the heart rate is >150 and patients are unstable, immediate synchronized cardioversion should be performed.

Atrial fibrillation

Atrial fibrillation on EKG results in an irregularly irregular rhythm with no visible P waves. The QRS complex is usually ≤ 0.12 seconds. With atrial fibrillation, there are multiple sites within the atria that are initiating electrical impulses for cardiac contraction. The AHA classifies Afib as paroxysmal (terminates within 7 days of onset), persistent (does not terminate within 7 days), long-standing persistent (occurring >12 mon), or permanent. Diagnosis: Assess causes, associated diseases, and complete cv evaluation. Some patients are asymptomatic. Common complaints include weakness, dizziness, dyspnea, and palpitations. Check TSH and T4. Diagnosis confirmed through ECG. Treatment: For rate control diltiazem, verapamil or beta-blockers can be used. Chemical cardioversion can be performed by administering ibutilide, dofetilide, flecainide, propafenone, or amiodarone. Dig should only be used as a first line agent in patients with Afib due to HF. For new onset Afib with low risk for embolism, cardioversion can be performed. For those with >48 hr onset Afib, anticoagulation therapy should be given for 3 weeks before cardioversion attempted. If patients are stable, but time of Afib unknown, anticoagulation should be performed and a TEE should be done to assess for atrial thrombus before chemical or electrical cardioversion is performed. If >150 bpm and patients are unstable, immediate synchronized cardioversion should be done to normalize the rate. Complications include reduced cardiac output and thrombus formation.

EKG changes present with two types of 2nd-degree AV block

Second-degree AV block can be categorized as type 1 or type 2. Type 1 2nd-degree AV block occurs when the time it takes for the electrical impulse to travel from the SA node to the AV node increases in length until a ventricular beat is finally skipped. On the EKG, this will look like a gradually increasing PR interval until a QRS is dropped. This can be treated with atropine if it results in symptomatic bradycardia or pacing can normalize the rate.
Type 2 2nd-degree AV block occurs when the electrical impulse signal travels from the SA node to the AV node, but the signal does not always continue onto the ventricles to cause a contraction. On EKG, this results in a normal PR interval and QRS or a normal PR interval and absent QRS. This is treated with pacing, and transcutaneous pacing may be necessary if patients are clinically unstable. Reversible causes should be investigated, and if none are found, this patient should get a permanent pacemaker, as they have a high likelihood of becoming symptomatic or progressing to complete heart block.

EKG changes present with 1st-degree AV block

1st-degree AV block occurs when there is a delay in the transmission of the electrical impulse in the heart from the SA node to the AV node. Diagnosis is made by EKG. Usually no change in the heart rate, but the EKG will exhibit a lengthened PR interval to >0.2 seconds. There should be regular P waves followed by a QRS complex and the rhythm should be regular. The rest of the EKG should be normal, and patients should be in normal sinus rhythm. 1st-degree AV block does not cause symptoms in patients, and no treatment is necessary. If patients have an underlying condition that could be contributing to the 1st-degree AV block, such as hypoxia, MI, or dehydration, then those conditions should be treated appropriately. The most likely cause for 1st-degree AV block is an electrical problem in the AV node itself, and it is more likely to develop in the elderly. There are usually no complications from 1st degree AV block. A few patients will progress to 2nd degree AV block.

EKG changes present with premature atrial contractions

With a premature atrial contraction (PAC), also known as an atrial premature beat (APB), there is an area within the atria that is irritated and is triggering delivery of sporadic impulses. This results in the atria contracting at a time out of sync with the regular rhythm of the atria. For diagnosis, per EKG, P waves may be present, but extra P waves may be hidden within the QRS complex or T waves. The QRS is usually narrow unless a bundle branch block that causes it to be widened is present. A holter monitor may be worn to assess the frequency of PACs and an echo may be ordered to assess cardiac structure and function. Premature atrial contractions are generally not symptomatic and not considered dangerous. Some patients may feel a palpitation in their chest when premature atrial contractions occur. Treatment is not required unless there is an underlying problem that needs to be managed (usually found in patients with frequent PACs). PACS are found in both the young and elderly and in those with and without heart disease. There are some known PAC precipitants, and these should be minimized- smoking, caffeine, stress, and alcohol. If the patient has ongoing symptomatic PACs, beta blockers or catheter ablation may be used. PAC may trigger other dysrhythmias, especially Afib.

EKG changes present with 3rd-degree AV block

Third degree AV block is considered complete heart block. The SA node continues to send its electrical impulse to the AV node, but the AV node is not transmitting this signal onto the ventricles. The ventricles are contracting, but this contraction is due to stimulation of the ventricular fibers so the heart rate is usually decreased to <40 bpm. Diagnosed by EKG, this results in regularly-occurring P waves and regularly-occurring QRS complexes that are completely independently of each other. The atrial rate is normal at 60-100 bpm, but the ventricular rate will be bradycardic. The QRS complexes may appear wide. Some causes include idiopathic conduction disease, drugs that depress AV conduction, increased vagal tone and myocardial infarction. Myocardial infarction, resulting in cardiac hypoxia, can cause a disruption in the electrical system of the heart by damaging the AV node so the impulse cannot be transmitted from the SA node to the ventricles. Signs and symptoms include dizziness, angina, syncope, and exacerbation of HF symptoms. This condition requires transcutaneous pacing until permanent pacing can be established. Patients should be closely monitored for a change in symptoms. Complications include asystole, Vfib/Vtach, and death.

EKG changes present with paroxysmal supraventricular tachycardia

Paroxysmal supraventricular tachycardia (PSVT) is an elevated heart rate that originates within the atria. The rate is so fast that the underlying rhythm cannot be diagnosed. The heart rate is usually >150 bpm and regular. On EKG, P waves are usually not present, or they are buried behind the QRS complex. The PR interval cannot be determined because of the absence of P wave, and QRS complex is usually very narrow. Signs and symptoms vary depending on rate, but include dizziness, syncope, shortness of breath, chest pain, and palpitations. If patients have a heart rate >150 but are clinically stable, vagal maneuvers can sometimes help to convert the rate to sinus rhythm. Adenosine 6 mg IV rapid push followed by a rapid flush can be given. If this does not work, this can be followed by adenosine 12 mg rapid IVP followed by rapid IV flush. If a central line is in place, the dose may be reduced to 3mg rapid IVP and flush. If the underlying rhythm can be determined, that can be treated appropriately. Determine if there are any underlying causes. If patients have a rate of >150 bpm and is unstable, immediate electrical synchronized cardioversion is necessary to attempt to return to sinus rhythm. If untreated, cardiac arrest can occur.

EKG changes present with bundle branch block

A bundle branch block (BBB) can occur within the left or right ventricle. It is usually due to an area of muscle damage. As the electrical impulse travels from the atria to the ventricles, the undamaged ventricle will transmit the signal normally. The damaged ventricle, however, will be delayed in transmitting the signal and this will result in two QRS complexes on EKG. Signs and symptoms are most often asympomatic. The patient presenting with a new onset BBB should have a complete cardiac workup performed. A quick way to diagnose a patient with a bundle branch block is to look at the V1, V2, V5, and V6 leads. With a right BBB, the V1 and V2 leads will exhibit an abnormal QRS complex with a "rabbit ears" appearance. With a left BBB, leads V5 and V6 will exhibit a widened QRS complex with a notched appearance. Ventricular rhythms, Brugada syndrome and ventricular pacing should be ruled out. A left or right chronic bundle branch block does not require treatment.

A pacemaker would only be indicated with syncope. It is important to remember, however, that a patient with clinical symptoms representing an acute MI cannot be diagnosed with an MI by EKG alone if a bundle branch block is present. Prognosis is tied to underlying heart disease, for example, a right bundle branch block associated with an MI is associated with increased mortality.

EKG changes present with ventricular tachycardia

Ventricular tachycardia occurs when the ventricles repeatedly contract without the atria contracting. This can be a deadly arrhythmia and is considered a cardiac emergency. On EKG, all that will be seen are tall, widened QRS complexes. The rate is usually regular at around 150 up to 250 bpm. No P waves are present. Signs and symptoms include syncope, palpitations, chest pain, SOB, dizziness. In treating V-tach, the first thing that should be assessed is whether or not the patient has a pulse. If the patient does not have a pulse, ACLS protocol should be started, making sure to defibrillate the patient as quickly as possible, as this increases likelihood of survival. If the patient does have a pulse, assess if patient is otherwise hemodynamically stable or unstable. If stable, antiarrhythmics, such as amiodarone, sotalol, or procainamide should be given to convert to sinus rhythm. If the patient is unstable, cardioversion is indicated (sedate if able). If the patient loses pulse, defibrillation is indicated. In patients with monomorphic Vtach, with structurally normal hearts, catheter ablation or medication is usual management. In patients with more complicated issues, an ICD should be placed, especially if there is a history of heart disease, to decrease risk of SCD.

EKG changes present with premature ventricular contractions

Premature ventricular contractions (PVCs) occur when there is an area of irritability within a ventricle, causing it to contract early. The heart rate can vary and will depend upon the underlying rhythm. PVCs generally cause an irregular heart rate, but there can be regularity present if bigeminy is present. This occurs when PVC is present after every regular ventricular beat. Trigeminy occurs when PVC occurs during every third ventricular beat. The cause of PVCs is often unknown, but can be due to electrolyte imbalance, medications, alcohol/drugs, adrenaline (caffiene, anxiety, etc), or myocardial injury. On EKG, the QRS will appear abnormal with a much-widened QRS complex. The pattern of bigeminy or trigeminy may be present. P waves are not present before the widened QRS. For differential diagnosis, check electrolytes and cardiac workup if indicated. Most are asymptomatic, but some experience palpitations. Treating the underlying cause, if it can be identitied. For example, discovering if there is myocardial damage of some sort, or an electrolyte imbalance. Oxygen may help to decrease the PVCs, beta blockers suppress PVCs in some patients but antiarrhythmic medications (Lidocaine, etc.) may be necessary if the PVCs are frequent to reduce the risk of ventricular tachycardia or ventricular fibrillation. Complications include increased risk of arrhythmias and increased risk of cardiomyopathy.

EKG changes present with ventricular flutter and torsades de pointes

Three types of ventricular tachycardia include ventricular flutter, torsades de pointes, and repetitive monomorphic ventricular tachycardia. Ventricular flutter is a type of rapid monomorphic ventricular tachycardia. The rate is often about 300 bpm. The ventricles will spasm without any discernible pattern of organized activity. On EKG, the heart rate will not be able to be determined because of the irregularity. No P waves will be discernible and no organized QRS complexes will be present. The rhythm can appear to be coarse or fine. Ventricular flutter can resemble artifact, so the leads must be placed correctly on patients, and patient pulse checked. A magnesium deficiency can cause a form of polymorphic ventricular tachycardia called *torsades de pointes.* The name means "twisting of points" because of the changing axis of this rhythm. This rhythm will appear as a series of widened QRS complexes that vary in height in a wave pattern. Magnesium sulfate (usually 2 gm over 2 minutes) should be given. Other causes include hypokalemia and other medications.

Repetitive monomorphic ventricular tachycardia is a recurring, monomorphic tachycardia. It is the most common type of idiopathic Vtach. It occurs in those without cardiac structural disease. On EKG, it may appear as prolific ventricular ectopy or alternating nonsustained Vtach with sinus rhythm.

EKG changes present with ventricular fibrillation

Ventricular fibrillation occurs when the ventricles are in a state of uncontrolled spasm, like quivering, without being able to complete a forceful contraction. This is considered a true cardiac arrest. On EKG, the heart rate will not be able to be determined because of the irregularity. No P waves will be discernible, and no organized QRS complexes will be present. The rhythm can appear to be coarse or fine. Vfib can resemble artifact so the leads must be placed correctly on patients, and pulse checked. ACLS protocol should be followed for treatment of vfib, including, high quality CPR, immediate unsynchronized defibrillation, epinephrine 1 mg every 3-5 minutes, amiodarone 300 mg bolus and 150 mg second dose. Patients should be well oxygenated and eventually intubated when able to ensure oxygen needs are being met. Look for causes, such as the 5 H's & 5 T's: Hypovolemia, Hypoxia, Hydrogen ions (acidosis), Hypo/Hyperkalemia, Hypothermia, Tension pneumo, Tamponade, Toxins, Thombosis (cardiac), Thrombosis (pulmonary). Prognosis is often related to time of onset of vfib and medical treatment. Anoxic encephalopathy and death may follow, even after initial successful resuscitation.

Coarctation of the aorta

Coarctation of the aorta is a congenital heart defect in which there is narrowing of the aorta distal to the left subclavian artery. This results in the development of collateral circulation through the intercostal arteries and the branches of the subclavian artery. It is most common in male children and is often associated with Turner's syndrome in females.

Clinically, the infant may exhibit hypertension with varying blood pressure between the upper and lower extremities. The pulses may also vary between the two sets of extremities. Symptoms of congestive heart failure may be present along with weak or absent femoral pulses. A systolic murmur will be heard predominantly over the back. Coarctation of the aorta is diagnosed using a chest x-ray in which rib notching will be evident due to the development of collateral vessels trying to pass over the coarctation. An EKG and echocardiogram will also be done. Diagnosis is confirmed using angiogram. Treatments include balloon angioplasty to attempt to widen the aorta. Resection, aortoplasty, bypass graft or prosthetic patch aortoplasty may need to be performed. If left untreated, coarctation of the aorta leads to high blood pressure, stroke, rupture of the aorta, cerebral aneurysm, coronary artery disease, and organ failure. Survival rates after repairs are better the younger the patient at the time of the first repair.

Atrial septal defect

An atrial septal defect (ASD) is a congenital heart defect in which there is an opening between the left and right atrium. This results in failure to thrive in the infant. The infant will exhibit dyspnea, clubbing of the nails, and excessive fatigue. On exam, a systolic murmur and a widely split and fixed S_2 will be heard. EKG findings will include atrial fibrillation, with a right bundle branch block and a right axis deviation. An atrial septal defect is diagnosed initially through a combination of exam findings and EKG changes. An echocardiogram and an angiogram will be done to confirm the diagnosis. This is not diagnosed *in utero* because of the presence of the patent foramen ovale. It is usually detected within a couple of days of birth. Treatment is now being done using cardiac catheterization techniques to patch the defect, though open-heart surgery is the most commonly-used form of treatment. A small ASD may close during childhood and never cause issue. Complications are often related to the size and can include heart failure, arrhythmias, stroke, and pulmonary hypertension.

Tetralogy of Fallot

Tetralogy of Fallot is a congenital heart defect that comprises four conditions: a ventricular septal defect, overriding of the aorta, right ventricular hypertrophy, and right ventricular outflow obstruction (pulmonary stenosis). This is the most common cyanotic infant heart disease and the least understood. There are likely genetic factors associated with the development of this condition. There may also be some medications taken by the mother during pregnancy that can result in Tetralogy of Fallot in the fetus. Clinically, the infant will be cyanotic with dyspnea and clubbing. A holosystolic murmur can be heard on exam. This condition can result in retarded growth in childhood. Tetralogy of Fallot can be diagnosed using EKG, echocardiogram, and angiogram. A CBC will show polycythemia. Surgery (called an intracardiac repair) is necessary, and usually done in the first year of life to treat Tetralogy of Fallot. Patients will always require endocarditis prophylaxis before all dental procedures and other invasive procedures throughout their lifetimes. Endocarditis is a common and serious complication. If untreated, this defect leads to disability and death by adulthood.

Patent ductus arteriosus

Patent ductus arteriosus is a congenital heart defect in which the ductus arteriosus fails to close after birth. The ductus arteriosus is an opening, present *in utero*, that serves as a shunt between the left pulmonary artery and the aorta. This opening can fail to close due to a rubella infection while *in utero*. Clinically, the infant will exhibit pulmonary hypertension and a failure to thrive. On exam, there will be a continuous machinery murmur heard. A thrill may be palpated over the chest wall and the back. A widened pulse pressure will also be present. Patent ductus arteriosus is diagnosed through a combination of exam findings, EKG, echocardiogram, and chest x-ray, but is confirmed by angiogram. It is diagnosed within a couple of days of birth. A small patent ductus arteriosus may not cause complications, but larger ones usually require treatment. Closure of the ductus arteriosus can usually be achieved using less invasive cardiac catheterization techniques, but open surgery may be necessary. Complications include pulmonary hypertention, heart failure, and endocarditis.

Essential, secondary, and malignant hypertension

Essential hypertension is the most common form of hypertension. The cause of this type of hypertension is unknown. Most patients are also unaware that they are suffering from hypertension with this type. It is diagnosed after patients have three separate episodes of blood pressure 140/90 or higher, not found to be due to some type of medical condition. Secondary hypertension only affects about 5% of the population of patients who have been diagnosed with hypertension. It is due to another medical condition, such as renal disease (most common), renal artery stenosis, aldosteronism, or pheochromocytoma. Moderate to severe hypertensive retinopathy (formerly malignant hypertension) is uncontrolled severe hypertension and can be life-threatening. It can be due to secondary causes (renal artery stenosis) or the cause may be unknown. The goal with malignant hypertension is to provide immediate treatment by decreasing the blood pressure slowly, no more than 10-15% over the first hour, and no more than 25% by the end of treatment day one. Nitroprusside, clevidipine, nicardipine, labetalol, and fenoldopam are the most common medications used to treat this condition.

Ventricular septal defect

A ventricular septal defect is a congenital heart defect in which there is an opening between the left and right ventricles. There is no known cause of this condition, but it probably occurs during development of the heart *in utero*. This condition can be associated with Eisenmenger's syndrome. Clinically, the infant will exhibit signs of pulmonary hypertension and congestive heart failure. Very rapid respirations may be present with sweating and pallor. The infant may have great difficulty eating because of the difficulty breathing, resulting in the failure to gain weight and failure to thrive. On exam, a holosystolic murmur can be heard, and a systolic thrill may be palpated over the chest wall and back. A ventricular septal defect is diagnosed using exam findings, echocardiogram, chest x-ray, and angiogram. An EKG will show a right bundle branch block. Small VSDs may not need treatment. Closure of the ventricular septal defect can be attempted using cardiac catheterization techniques, but open surgery may be necessary. Complications include arrhythmias, endocarditis, pulmonary hypertension.

Hypertension

Classifications
Standard classifications of hypertension in adults:

Classification	Systolic BP mm Hg	Diastolic BP mm Hgb
Normal	< 120	And < 80
Pre-hypertension	120 – 139	Or 80 – 89
Stage 1 hypertension	140-159	Or 90 – 99
Stage 2 hypertension	≥ 160	Or ≥ 100

Moderate to severe hypertensive retinopathy (previously malignant hypertension) is severe hypertension with retinal hemorrhages or papilledema. Hypertensive encephalopathy may be present as well. Hypertensive urgency- severe hypertension without target-organ damage found.

Hypertensive emergency- severe hypertension with acute target-organ damage.

Treatment
Beta-blockers: Beta-blockers help to lower blood pressure by decreasing the heart rate and the force that is exerted by the ventricles with each heartbeat. Beta-blockers work on beta-receptors, though not all beta-blockers are created to work just on cardiac beta-receptors. Some of these medications, especially the older medications, work on all the beta-receptors in the body. Beta-blockers are now thought to help extend life in patients with known CAD, those who have had an MI, and those patients with known CHF. Because beta-blockers reduce the heart rate, there is a risk that they can cause the bradycardia and hypotension. This can result in dizziness, confusion, and possibly even syncope. The most commonly reported side effects of beta blockers are sexual dysfunction, depression, and fatigue. Beta blockers should not be used in those with symptomatic bradycardia that is associated with sick sinus syndrome. Although beta blockers are a routine part of therapy for those with heart failure, in patients with acute decompensated heart failure, they may exacerbate heart failure symptoms. Sudden withdrawal from beta blockers can cause ischemic symptoms, especially those with coronary artery disease. Beta blockers are associated with

increased airway resistance in patients that already have lung disease. Some examples of beta-blockers include metoprolol (Lopressor®), atenolol (Tenormin®), and carvedilol (Coreg®).

ACE inhibitors: ACE inhibitors work on the arteries to cause dilation, which decreases the pressure within the arteries and leads to a decrease in blood pressure. Their effects also help patients with congestive heart failure by potentially preventing hospitalizations, decreasing the risk of a future MI, and decreasing the risk of death due to CHF. Because ACE inhibitors cause arterial dilation, they can, in rare cases, cause angioedema. This results when there is an excessive dilation in the arteries of the lips and face. Though rare, this type of allergic reaction is a medical emergency and should be treated immediately. The most common potential side effect of ACE inhibitors is a chronic, nonproductive cough (5-20% of patients). This can be very annoying to patients and may be a reason for noncompliance in those who develop the cough. ACE inhibitors may cause the kidneys to decrease excretion of potassium, so patients should be monitored for hyperkalemia. Hypotension, ARF, and issues with pregnancy are other related side effects. Some examples of ACE inhibitors include captopril (Capoten®), enalapril (Vasotec®), and quinapril (Accupril®).

Diuretics: Diuretics work on the kidneys to increase the amount of water and sodium that are excreted from the body through the urine. This helps to reduce the actual fluid volume in the body, thus decreasing the amount of pressure within the arteries and resulting in a lowered blood pressure. Because diuretics work on the kidneys, they may not be appropriate for all patients, especially those with renal disease. Along with the water and sodium that is increasingly excreted from the body, potassium is also depleted with some of the diuretics. This can result in hypokalemia in some patients, so a potassium supplement is often prescribed along with the diuretic. Eating foods high in potassium may also help patients prevent a decrease in potassium levels. An increase in urinary frequency is frequently seen, so patients should take diuretics in the morning to prevent having to get up frequently during the night. Examples of some diuretics include furosemide (Lasix®), hydrochlorothiazide, spironolactone (Aldactone®), and torsemide (Demadex®).

Calcium channel blockers: The older calcium channel blockers (CCBs) work in two different ways. They dilate the arteries, thus decreasing the pressure within the arteries, resulting in a decrease in blood pressure. They also decrease the heart rate and decrease the force of ventricular contractions. The new calcium channel blockers only work to cause arterial dilation. Previously, calcium channel blockers were the first line treatment for pulmonary hypertension, but currently CCB therapy for all patients with pulmonary hypertension is no longer indicated. Current research shows that calcium channel blockers usually benefit those patients who have positive reactivity to a vasodilator challenge (done with a short acting CCB in an intensive care setting). While this is a small group of patients, somewhere between 5-15%, they have been shown to benefit greatly from CCB therapy. The older calcium channel blockers that cause a decrease in ventricular force may worsen CHF in those patients who suffer from this illness. Nifedipine is associated with an increase in mortality in the acute period after an MI. 10-20% of patients will experience one of the following side effects while taking calcium channel blockers: headaches, flushing, dizziness and peripheral edema. Constipation is a specific adverse effect of the calcium channel blocker verapamil. Examples of older calcium channel blockers include diltiazem (Cardizem®) and verapamil (Calan®). New calcium channel blockers include amlodipine (Norvasc®) and felodipine (Plendil®).

Angiotensin-receptor blockers: Angiotensin-receptor blockers (ARBs) work the same as ACE inhibitors. They work on the arteries to cause dilation, which decreases the pressure within the arteries and leads to a decrease in blood pressure. Their effects also help patients with congestive heart failure by potentially preventing hospitalizations, decreasing the risk of a future MI, and decreasing the risk of death due to CHF. The reason that an ARB may be prescribed instead of an ACE inhibitor is because of a lesser risk of side effects. ARBs have a lower incidence of chronic cough and angioedema than ACE inhibitors. Shared side effects that have simliar rates between the two drugs include: hyperkalemia, renal dysfunction, syncope. ARBs have a higher rate of hypotensive symptoms that is found with ACE inhibitors. Examples of ARBs include losartan (Cozaar®), telmisartan (Micardis®), and valsartan (Diovan®).

Orthostatic hypotension: Orthostatic hypotension is a sudden drop in blood pressure that is symptomatic. It usually occurs when a patient stands up quickly or is rising from a lying to sitting or standing position. Medications are a common cause of orthostatic hypotension, including antihypertensives, antianxiety drugs, and diuretics. Hypovolemia or excessive alcohol use can also cause orthostatic hypotension. S/S: Patients will describe a sudden dizziness or light-headed sensation, syncope, or near syncope when moving too quickly, usually rising from sitting or lying down. Other symptoms are leg buckling, visual changes such as blurring, coat-hanger headache, and weakness/fatigue. Some patients may also experience these symptoms on exertion, after prolonged standing or after eating, as well.

Diagnosis: A 20 mmHg decrease in systolic pressure or a 10 mmHg decrease in diastolic pressure is noted within five minutes of standing after a five (or more) minute time of resting in the supine position. Treatment includes removing medications that could be responsible if able, correcting hypovolemia, using elastic stockings, and exercise. Advise rising slowly from a sitting or lying position. If severe symptoms remain after nonpharmacologic intervention, consider fludrocortisone and then midodrine if needed.

Complications include falls, strokes, and heart disease.

Cardiogenic shock

Cardiogenic shock is a condition in which the heart is not able to supply the body with the necessary blood, O_2, and nutrients that are necessary for proper functioning. It is most often secondary to MI damage that reduces the contractibility of the ventricles, interfering with the pumping mechanism of the heart, decreasing O_2 perfusion. Cardiogenic shock has 3 characteristics: Increased preload, increased afterload, and decreased contractibility. Together these result in a decreased cardiac output and an increase in SVR to compensate and protect vital organs. This results in an increase of afterload in the left ventricle with increased need for oxygen. As the cardiac output continues to decrease, tissue perfusion decreases, coronary artery perfusion decreases, fluid backs up and the left ventricle fails to adequately pump the blood, resulting in pulmonary edema and right ventricular failure. Decreasing O_2 consumption is a major initial goal of cardiogenic shock.

Symptoms include:
- Hypotension with systolic BP <90 mm Hg.
- Tachycardia > 100 beats/min with weak thready pulse and dysrhythmias.
- Decreased heart sounds.
- Chest pain.
- Tachypnea and basilar rales.
- Cool, moist skin, pallor.

Treatment includes:
- IV fluids.
- Inotropic agents.

- Anti-dysrhythmics.
- IABP or left ventricular assist device.

Acute myocardial infarction

Remember the mnemonic: MONA has great ABs. This stands for MI treatment with morphine, oxygen, nitrates, aspirin, ACE inhibitors, and beta-blockers. Fibrinolytic infusion is indicated for acute myocardial infarction under these conditions:
- Symptoms of MI, <6-12 hours since onset of symptoms.
- ≥1 mm elevation of ST in ≥2 contiguous leads.
- No contraindications and no cardiogenic shock.

These can have serious side effects and a careful assessment of patients' medical history should be done before considering these medications. Ideally, patients should be stabilized and taken for a cardiac catheterization within 90 minutes of presenting to the ER. Angioplasty can be performed during catheterization, if possible, to open the blocked coronary artery and restore blood flow to the heart muscle. The quicker that blood flow is restored to the heart muscle, the less the risk of permanent muscle damage. The decision to use PTCA versus CABG is based on multiple factors, including symptoms, severity of CAD, EF, comorbidities, number of blocked arteries, and degree of narrowing of arteries. This procedure is done to increase circulation to the myocardium by breaking through an atheroma if there is collateral circulation. A stint may need to be placed to prevent collapse and spasm of the coronary artery.

Acute myocardial infarction

Clinical manifestations of myocardial infarction may vary considerably, with males having the more "classic" symptom of sudden onset of crushing chest pain and females and those under 55 often presenting with atypical symptoms. Diabetic patients may have reduced sensation of pain because of neuropathy and may complain primarily of weakness. Elderly patients may also have neuropathic changes that reduce sensation of pain. More than half of all patients present with acute MIs with no prior symptoms of cardiovascular disease. Patients may complain of a crushing pressure throughout the chest, radiating into the neck or left arm. They may also have epigastric pain or a feeling of weakness or anxiety. Elderly patients and diabetics may not have any of the classic symptoms of an acute MI. Objectively, patients may be pale and diaphoretic. They may appear restless or lethargic. On exam, an S_4 gallop may be heard. Blood pressure may be high or low. Acute symptoms of CHF may be seen. EKG may show ST elevation, though depression can also be seen. Cardiac enzymes should be drawn every 8 hours x 3. Troponin 1 is usually the first enzyme that is elevated, followed by CKMB. Evaluate the CKMB percentage to ensure there is an elevation. A 5-10% elevation in the CKMB most likely indicates ischemia. Higher elevations are indicative of an acute MI. An echocardiogram may show a decreased EF. Cardiac wall stiffness may be seen if there is an S_4 gallop.

Acute rheumatic fever

Acute rheumatic fever can occur approximately 2 weeks following a pharynx infection with β-hemolytic *Streptococcus*. It usually affects children 5 to 15 years old and is no longer common in the United States. Approximately 75% of cases will affect the mitral valve and 30% affect the aortic valve. For diagnosis, at least 2 of the Jones criteria must be present: carditis, erythema marginatum, subcutaneous nodules, Sydenham's chorea, or migratory arthritis of the large joints. Along with the Jones criteria, patients will have a fever. They may complain of polyarthralgia. An

EKG will show a prolonged PR interval. Abnormal lab tests will include an elevation in erythrocyte sedimentation rate (ESR) and throat cultures positive for Strep. Rheumatic fever can be deadly and lead to permanent heart disease, CHF, arrhythmias, and pericardial effusions. Treatment includes bed rest, penicillin, and steroids. Haldol may be given to control the movements of chorea. Complications include valve regurgitation and stenosis (usually mitral or aortic), heart dysfunction.

Angina

Angina is chest pain that is usually brought on by stress or exertion and relieved by rest and/or nitrate medications. It can be classified as stable, unstable, or Prinzmetal (variant) type. Stable angina lasts < 30 minutes. It is increased with activity and decreased with rest and/or nitrates. It is described as a clenching sensation over the chest and may be accompanied by pallor, diaphoresis, and hypertension. Unstable angina (also known as preinfarction or crescendo angina) is a progression of coronary artery disease and occurs when there is a change in the pattern of stable angina. The pain may increase, may not respond to a single nitroglycerin, and may persist for >5 minutes. Usually pain is more frequent, lasts longer, and may occur at rest. Unstable angina may indicate rupture of an atherosclerotic plaque and the beginning of thrombus formation so it should always be treated as a medical emergency as it may indicate a myocardial infarction. Variant angina (also known as Prinzmetal's angina) results from spasms of the coronary arteries, can be associated with or without atherosclerotic plaques, and is often related to smoking, alcohol, or illicit stimulants. Elevation of ST segments usually occurs with variant angina. Variant angina frequently occurs cyclically at the same time each day and often while the person is at rest. Nitroglycerin or calcium channel blockers are used for treatment.

Dissecting aortic aneurysm

A dissecting aortic aneurysm occurs when the wall of the aorta is torn and blood flows between the layers of the wall, dilating and weakening it until it risks rupture (which has 90% mortality). DeBakey classification uses anatomic location as the focal point:
- Type I begins in the ascending aorta but may spread to include the aortic arch and the descending aorta (60%). (AKA Stanford type A)
- Type II is restricted to the ascending aorta (10-15%). (AKA Stanford type A)
- Type III is restricted to the descending aorta (25-30%). (AKA Stanford type B)

Patients will describe a fairly sudden onset of mid-abdominal pain or back pain that is ripping or tearing in quality. This pain may be aggravated by taking a deep breath or by performing any activities. Hip pain may also be present if blood is pooling in the lower abdominal cavity. Clinically, a pulsatile mass may or may not be palpated. It is advised that no hard palpation be performed on the abdomen until an aneurysm is ruled out because of fear of causing sudden rupture if the dissection is advanced. Diagnosis: Immediate CT should be done to confirm the diagnosis. Treatment consists of emergency aortic resection for patients with acute presentation. However, in patients that present with chronic aortic dissection, medical management using beta blockers to control bp is sometimes chosen. Complications include death or organ failure.

Aortic aneurysm

An aortic aneurysm is a dilation of the aorta >3 cm. It is usually seen at a level below the renal arteries but can be common in the thoracic aorta in patients who have Marfan's syndrome. High risk for developing an aortic aneurysm are men >60-y/o who smoke and have hypertension. Most patients with an aortic aneurysm are asymptomatic unless dissection or rupture occurs. Patients may have complaints of vague back pain before dissection or rupture occurs. A pulsatile mass may be felt, or an abdominal bruit heard. If dissection or rupture occurs, there will be decreased pulses below the level of aneurysm. Ultrasound or CT/MRI will visualize the aneurysm. Angiography will confirm diagnosis. If a patient has a known aneurysm, an annual ultrasound should be done to monitor its growth. The risk of surgerical repair outweighs the risk of aneurysm rupture until the abdomninal aneurysm reaches 5.5 cm, except in special circumstances, so most treatment will be watchful waiting and monitoring until the aneurysm reaches this size. For thoracic aneurysm, the size before surgery is indicated varies based on location of the aneurysm: ascending aortic aneurysm 5-6 cm, descending aortic 6 to 7 cm. In the asymptomatic patient, medical management includes aggressive control of blood pressure with beta blockers, serial imaging, and patient education of signs of complications (sudden intense back or abd pain). Complications include thrombus/embolus, dissection, rupture, or death.

Peripheral arterial disease

Peripheral arterial disease occurs when there is obstruction or narrowing of an artery that interferes with blood flow. This can be due to atherosclerosis, trauma, or inflammation. Patients will frequently complain of pain in their legs or calves after walking a short distance. This pain is relieved with rest. Some male patients may complain about erectile dysfunction. Patients may also state they have numbing and tingling sensations in their extremities. Clinically, there may be obvious signs of obstructed blood flow, such as pallor, atrophic skin, and hair loss. The peripheral pulses may be decreased or absent if occlusion is present. In severe cases, arterial ulcers may be present with development of gangrene.

Diagnosis: Ankle-brachial index (ABI) is the most common test used to diagnosis PAD. Doppler ultrasound will identify decreased blood flow through the arteries. Angiography confirms the diagnosis by providing visualization of the narrowed vessels. Patients should also be assessed for CAD because, generally, all of the arteries in the body can be affected by this. Treatment includes quitting smoking, cholesterol control medications, antihypertensives, antiplatelet medications, blood glucose control. Cilostazol and pentoxifylline help treat symptoms of claudication. Angioplasty, thrombolytics or bypass surgery may be indicated. Limb ischemia is a possible complication, which can lead to infections/amputations.

Arterial thrombosis and embolism

An arterial thrombosis is a blood clot located within an artery. This is a stationary clot that can grow large enough to cause occlusion of the vessel. An arterial embolism is the term used for the thrombus once it breaks free and begins moving through the vascular system. This embolism will eventually travel to an artery that is too small to accommodate its size. This results in occlusion of the artery with possible life-threatening results. Treatment of an arterial thrombus is centered on prevention, such as exercise and wearing compression stocks. Daily aspirin therapy (81 mg) can provide antiplatelet activity that prevents platelets from forming a clot. Other anticoagulant medications, such as Coumadin® and Plavix®, can be used to prevent platelet accumulation and help prevent clot formation. If an arterial thrombus does form and becomes an embolism, treatment is more of an emergency. For example, an arterial embolism is usually a fatal condition, but "clot buster" thrombolytic medications or even surgery to remove the clot may help improve patients' prognosis. Vena cava filters can be used in patient with high risk for embolus. Complications include pulmonary embolism, stroke, MI, ischemia to limbs, and postphlebitic syndrome.

Phlebitis and thrombophlebitis

Phlebitis is inflammation that is present in a vein. It is gradual in onset and develops into a reddened, often streaky area that follows the path of a vein. The area may be swollen, indurated, and warm. Patients will often complain of pain in the area. If the phlebitis is superficial, warm compresses, elevation of the affected limb, and compression can help to resolve the problem. If recurrent phlebitis is occurring in the deeper vessels, an anticoagulant may be prescribed to prevent formation of a blood clot. Thrombophlebitis occurs when a blood clot forms within the vein, causing inflammation. Patients complain of pain that may be gradual or sudden in onset. It is seen most often in more sedentary patients. The affected area may be red, swollen, or indurated. Patients may have a positive Homan's sign. Treatment consists of anticoagulants to prevent recurrence and to decrease the risk of embolism. Prevention is crucial in treatment with compression stockings, leg elevation, and decreasing the amount of time spent immobile.

Giant cell arteritis

Giant cell arteritis, or temporal arteritis, is an inflammatory process that affects the vessels, most commonly the temporal artery. This condition can lead to occlusion of the temporal artery, resulting in blindness, so diagnosis and treatment should be started quickly. The most common symptom with giant cell arteritis is a severe headache. This can be accompanied with a fever, generalized body aches, fatigue, or weight loss. Approximately 50% of patients who are diagnosed with giant cell arteritis will also have a diagnosis of polymyalgia rheumatica. Diagnosis consists of erythrocyte sedimentation rate, C-reactive protein, biopsy (this is the standard), MRI, PET, and Doppler. Because of the nature of the illness, treatment is started before the biopsy results are available. Treatment consists of prednisone, usually 40-60 mg per day. This should be continued for at least 1 month and then tapered. If symptoms return as the dose of prednisone is tapered, the dosage can be increased. Low dose aspirin is usually given to reduce chance or blindness, TIA, and stroke. Chest x-rays are done annually to assess for aortic aneurysm as a significant number of patients develop aortic aneurysm. Complications include blindness, stroke, increased risk of aortic aneurysm.

Aortic stenosis or insufficiency

Aortic stenosis is very common and is the worst valve disease. Most patients are asymptomatic until they reach middle age. Aortic calcifications are frequently seen in those >55-years-old. Aortic stenosis can be due to a congenital disorder of the valve or rheumatic fever. Patients may have syncopal episodes when aortic stenosis becomes symptomatic. They may complain of chest pain, fatigue, and shortness of breath with activity. Symptoms of CHF can be present when the disease is advanced and prognosis is usually poor by the time these symptoms are present. On exam, a systolic murmur that is crescendo/decrescendo in nature during the middle to late portion of the cardiac cycle can be heard. This murmur will radiate superiorly to the carotid arteries. There may also be an early systolic ejection click. *Pulsus parvus,* or a weakened pulse, may be palpated. Diagnosis consists of echocardiogram for initial diagnosis, and sometimes a transesophageal echo is needed. CT/MRI may be used to assess valves, arteries and the size of the aorta before treatment is decided upon. Medications can't reverse aortic stenosis, but they can decrease symptoms. Common meds used include antihypertensive meds, diuretics, and meds to help with heart rate control. To correct aortic stenosis, valvuloplasty, aortic repair/replacement is needed. Complications include arrhythmias, angina, syncope, heart failure, and cardiac arrest.

Varicose veins

Varicose veins occur due to faulty valves within the distal veins, leading to distention and stretching of the veins. Because the valves are not functioning properly, blood tends to pool in the extremities and cause further distention of the veins. Patients will complain of aching pain in the legs after standing or sitting for extended periods of time. They may also experience an itching sensation around the veins. If severe, venous stasis ulcers can develop in the lower extremities. The veins will be visibly distended, bulging, and contorted. The skin may appear darkly pigmented due to venous stasis. The best treatment of varicose veins is prevention. This includes avoiding standing for prolonged periods of time, exercising regularly to keep weight under control, and wearing compression stockings or maintaining leg elevation to promote venous return from the lower extremities. Medical treatments include sclerotherapy, laser vein ablation, vein stripping, or, in severe case, complete removal of the varicose veins.

Mitral stenosis

Mitral stenosis is characterized by blood flow being obstructed through the left atrium to ventricle by way of the mitral valve. It is fairly common, and symptoms will be much more pronounced in females during pregnancy. In many cases its etiology is rheumatic. Patients may complain of hoarseness that will not go away because of recurrent pressure being applied to the laryngeal nerve. Patients may have an annoying cough and may even have hemoptysis. On exam, a diastolic rumble can be heard along with an opening snap. Patients may also have a louder than normal S_1. Symptoms of CHF may be present with dyspnea, crackles, and rales heard in the lungs as well as fatigue. Atrial fibrillation may also be detected either palpably or on EKG. Symptoms are worse in females during pregnancy because of the increased blood volume and the strain this puts on the mitral valve. Diagnosis includes echocardiography, TEE, or cardiac catheterization. Conservative management, including diuretics and beta blockers are used to treat patients usually initially. Endocarditis prophylaxis is required. Anticoagulation should be used in patients who have had embolus or Afib. Mitral valve surgery is indicated in symptomatic patients or patients with severe stenosis (have a mitral valve area less than 1.5 cm^2.
Complications include Afib, heart failure, pulmonary hypertension, pulmonary edema, and thrombus/embolus.

Aortic insufficiency

Aortic insufficiency can have many causes, including hypertension, rheumatic heart disease, endocarditis, syphilis, and Marfan's syndrome. It can also be congenital in nature. Patients will complain of fatigue and shortness of breath with activity. The symptoms may be chronic or acute. On exam, a diastolic murmur will be heard, increasing when patients are sitting or holding their breath. A widened pulse pressure will also be detected. Corrigan's sign, a water hammer pulse, may be present. Quincke's pulse, an alternating erythema and paleness in the nail beds with each heartbeat, may also be seen. Musset's sign, patients visibly nodding the head with each heartbeat, may be evident. An Austin flint murmur may be present in severe cases. This murmur sounds like a mid-diastolic, low-pitched rumbling over the cardiac apex. Patients may have all or only a few of these findings. Diagnosis is made by echo, which can help classify the insufficiency as mild, moderate or severe. Treatment includes exercise, vasodilators, or valve replacement. Complications include heart failure and endocarditis

Mitral valve prolapse

Mitral valve prolapse is more common in females and is a condition in which the mitral valve leaflets are bulging into the atrium. It can be congenital in nature with Marfan's syndrome or connective tissue disorders, or may be due to CAD or cardiomyopathy. It is most likely due to congenital changes and is frequently seen in multiple members of a family. Patients may complain of chest pain and shortness of breath with activity. They will be fatigued and may feel palpitations at times. They may also be completely asymptomatic. On exam, a midsystolic ejection click can be head with a mid to late systolic murmur. On patient assessment, the auscultation of midsystolic ejection click and systolic murmur should prompt echo. Echo findings of leaflet displacement greater than or equal to 2 mm is the criterion for diagnosis. Complications include mitral valve regurgitation, arrhythmias, and endocarditis.

Mitral insufficiency

Mitral insufficiency occurs when the mitral valve begins to degenerate. It can be due to rheumatic fever, congenital disorders, endocarditis, or myxoma cardiac tumors. Dysfunction of the papillary muscles can also lead to mitral insufficiency as can coronary artery disease. The symptoms of mitral insufficiency may be acute or chronic. Patients may complain of shortness of breath with activity, fatigue, and weakness. A holosystolic murmur can be heard over the cardiac apex, and this murmur will radiate into the axilla area. An S_3 may also be heard. Patients may exhibit signs of CHF with rales, crackles, and dyspnea. Atrial fibrillation may be palpable or present on EKG. A chest x-ray and EKG can show the signs of CHF and left ventricular hypertrophy or cardiomegaly. Pulmonary edema may also be present. Diagnosis is made by echo. Cardiac catheterization may be used to evaluate certain echo findings. Treatment includes vasodilators, mitral valve repair or replacement, and anticoagulation for patients with atrial fibrillation or mitral annular calcification. If due to papillary muscle dysfunction, patients may present in cardiogenic shock if a papillary muscle has ruptured. This is a life-threatening emergency with a very poor prognosis.

Tricuspid insufficiency

Tricuspid insufficiency is more common than tricuspid stenosis. Each time the right ventricle contracts, there is blood flow backward through the tricuspid valve. It can occur due to muscle damage in the right ventricle from an acute MI. It may be due to right ventricular overload, endocarditis, or congenital anomalies. It can also occur due to mitral valve disease. A congenital condition called Ebstein's anomaly can result in an abnormally formed tricuspid valve, resulting in enlargement of the right atrium and congestive heart failure. Patients may complain of swelling in their extremities that is not completely relieved with elevation. They may feel fatigued and have shortness of breath with activity. On exam, the symptoms of right-sided CHF may be seen with pulmonary edema and right atrial enlargement on chest x-ray. A harsh systolic murmur can be auscultated. If severe, there may be symptoms of hepatomegaly, and patients may complain of abdominal discomfort. Some complain of a pulsating feeling in the neck. While chest x-ray and ECG may show ventricular enlargement if present, echo is the diagnostic tool of choice. It also helps to evaluate severity. Treatment includes diuretics to remove fluid, treatment of pulmonary hypertension, exercise, and valve repair/replacement. Heart failure is a possible complication.

Tricuspid stenosis

Stenosis of the tricuspid valve is frequently due to carcinoid tumors, rheumatic fever, or endocarditis. It is not very common and can result in right atrial enlargement. The right ventricle may appear smaller than normal because of the decreased amount of blood entering the chamber. Patients with tricuspid stenosis may be fatigued and frequently feel cold. They may notice a fluttering sensation in the neck or palpitations. If the condition is advanced, they may feel abdominal pain and bloating due to hepatomegaly. On exam, symptoms of right-sided CHF may be seen, including pitting edema. A bounding pulse may be palpated in the neck over the carotid arteries. A diastolic rumble can be auscultated. Chest x-ray will show right atrial enlargement with right ventricular shrinkage. An echocardiogram can measure the amount of blood flow through the valves and determine if the flow through the tricuspid valve is decreased. Treatment includes diuretics, ACE inhibitors, and balloon valvotomy. Very rarely, the valve is damaged badly enough that surgery is required to repair or replace it. Tricuspid valve stenosis is usually found in conjuction with mitral stenosis. Right atrial enlargment is a complication.

Pulmonary insufficiency

Pulmonary insufficiency can occur in patients who suffer from pulmonary hypertension. It can also be due to endocarditis, rheumatic heart disease, congenital abnormalities, or carcinoid syndrome. Patients may complain of fatigue, chest pain, and shortness of breath with activity. There are usually no symptoms with this condition until it becomes advanced. Patients can have syncopal episodes if symptoms become severe. On exam, a low-pitched murmur, which may increase with breathing, may be heard. When pressure rises in the pulmonary artery with advanced disease, a Graham-Steel murmur, which is a high-pitched blowing decrescendo murmur, can be heard. There will be a widely split S_2, and a right-sided S_3 or S_4 may be heard during breathing. On EKG, right ventricular hypertrophy will be seen along with a right bundle branch block. Diagnosis is made per echo. Usually the symptoms are not severe enough to warrant treatment with replacement of the pulmonary valve, but surgery can be done if patients are extremely symptomatic. Most treatment will focus on correcting the underlying problem, such as pulmonary hypertension.

Pulmonary stenosis

Pulmonary stenosis is most often due to congenital abnormalities and is frequently seen along with other cardiac abnormalities. It can also occur as a result of rheumatic fever or endocarditis. Patients may complain of fatigue and shortness of breath with activity. They may have episodes of chest pain, especially with activity, and may have even had syncopal episodes. They may have cyanosis due to decreased flow of blood to the lungs for oxygenation, though this is usually only present in very advanced stages. A mid-systolic murmur will be present that tends to increase with breathing. A wide split S_2 can be present with a right ventricular heave. Symptoms of right-sided CHF may be present with edema and right atrial enlargement on chest x-ray. Infants may exhibit failure to thrive and poor weight gain. Diagnosis is made per echo to assess the valve's anatomy, location of stenosis, and to check right ventricle. Surgery is often necessary to repair the valve. A valvotomy can be performed in children and adults, though not infants. Valvotomy involves stretching the valve with a balloon in order to widen the opening. Complications include endocarditis and arrhythmias.

Bacterial endocarditis

A patient with heart disease affecting the valves is at risk for developing endocarditis. This includes those with congenital heart disease or valvular disease and those who have prosthetic valves. IV drug abusers and those who have had a prior infection are also at risk. Endocarditis can also be acquired through contamination during invasive procedures or surgery. Almost all patients with endocarditis will have a new, regurgitant-type murmur. They may complain of fatigue. Splinter hemorrhages may be evident in the nail beds with Osler nodes and Janeway lesions present in the fingers. Roth spots may be evident on funduscopic exam and patients may show signs of emboli being present, such as hematuria and renal dysfunction. Anemia may be present with leukocytosis. Appropriate antibiotic therapy based on culture and sensitivity results should be used for treatment. For acutely ill patients, while waiting on blood cultures, Vancomycin 15-20 mg/kg every 8-12 hours is used. These patients will require prophylactic antibiotics for future invasive procedures. Treatment includes amoxicillin 2 g one hour before the procedure. If people have penicillin allergy, clindamycin 600 mg or azithromycin 500 mg is given one hour before the procedure. Complications include infection, sepsis, heart failure, stroke, or organ damage.

Endocarditis

The modified Duke criteria states a patient must have 2 major criteria, 1 major and 3 minor criteria, or 5 minor criteria in order to have a definite diagnosed with endocarditis. The major criteria are two positive blood cultures that indicate which organism is causing the infection and evidence of endocardial involvement on an echocardiogram or the presence of a new regurgitant murmur. The minor criteria are risk factors, a fever >100.4°F, vascular features such as emboli, immunologic features such as glomerulonephritis, a positive blood culture that does not meet a major criteria, and changes on an echocardiogram that do not meet the major criteria. The blood cultures should be drawn three times with the samples taken 1 hour apart. The most likely organism to cause endocarditis is *Streptococcus viridians* with *Staphylococcus aureus* the second most common. The echocardiogram will show vegetation on the valves in the heart, and a transesophageal echocardiogram may be necessary for accurate visualization.

Cardiac tamponade

Cardiac tamponade is an emergency condition in which fluid accumulates around the heart, leading to constriction that decreases venous return to the heart and prevents the ventricles from filling. It can occur with pericarditis, acute MI, a dissecting thoracic aortic aneurysm, or end-stage lung cancer. Patients who have undergone recent cardiac surgery are also at risk of developing a cardiac tamponade. The four types are acute, subacute, low pressure, and regional. A *pulsus paradoxus*, which is a >10 mm drop in systolic pressure during inspiration, can be present. The pulse pressure will be narrowed, and patients will be hypotensive. Patients will be tachypneic, experience angina and jugular venous distention will be present. A Swan line to measure pressure within the heart will reveal that all of the pressures are equal. In patients with suspected cardiac tamponade, perform echocardiogram, ECG, and chest x-ray. However, the diagnosis is confirmed through evaluating the response to the drainage of pericardial fluid. It is an emergency situation, and an immediate pericardiocentesis should be performed to withdraw the fluid off the heart. Use inotropes and IV fluids as needed to stabilize patient. Complications include death, shock, and pulmonary edema.

Acute pericarditis

Acute pericarditis occurs when the pericardial sac becomes inflamed. This can most commonly be due to a viral infection, but a bacterial or parasitic infection can also cause this condition. Connective tissue disorders, such as lupus or rheumatoid arthritis, can also cause pericarditis, as can metabolic disorders such as renal failure and gout. Patients with pericarditis will complain of pleuritic chest pain that is relieved by sitting up and leaning forward. They will have a nonproductive cough accompanied with dyspnea. They will also have pain through the trapezius muscle, either unilaterally or bilaterally. On exam, a pericardial rub may be heard and leukocytosis may be present. An EKG will show ST elevation and PR depression. An echocardiogram will indicate a pericardial effusion. Treatment is with NSAIDs, aspirin, and steroids to reduce the inflammation. If severe, a pericardial window may be created surgically to reduce the tension on the pericardial sac. In rare cases, the pericardial sac is completely removed to treat this condition. Complications include cardiac tamponade and death.

Pericardial effusion

A pericardial effusion occurs when >250 cc of fluid accumulates within the pericardial space. It can occur due to a viral infection, tuberculosis, radiation to the chest cavity, or trauma. A malignant tumor in the chest cavity can also cause a pericardial effusion. Patients with pericardial effusion do not always complain of chest pain. They will have a cough and appear dyspneic. If the cause is infection, they may have a fever. On exam, distant sounds with a pericardial rub will be heard. Chest-x-ray will show cardiomegaly with a globular shape. EKG changes will be non-specific and may show a low voltage QRS complex. Treatment may include NSAIDs and steroids to treat the inflammation, but surgery frequently needs to be done to drain off the fluid. In severe cases, the pericardial sac can be completely removed from around the heart. A pericardial biopsy may also need to be done to determine the cause of the effusion. Complications include cardiac tamponade and death.

Dermatologic System

Contact dermatitis

Contact dermatitis is an allergic response to an allergen. This can be caused by skin irritants, such as lotions and soaps or poison ivy and poison sumac. The skin rash associated with contact dermatitis often occurs quickly following exposure to the allergen. The symptom is an extremely pruritic rash. The skin will become red, and vesicular lesions that resemble a burn may be present. The skin can become red, dry, and cracked when exposed to irritants and may not develop the typical contact dermatitis lesions seen with exposure to an allergen. Diagnosis is made mostly per history/physical. Finding and eliminating the possible trigger(s) can also be diagnostic. For cases that don't easily resolve, patch testing may be effective. Treatment consists of discontinuing exposure to the causative substance. The skin should be kept clean and dry. Anti-itch medications or corticosteroid creams can be applied. Benadryl can be taken if the dermatitis is due to exposure to an allergen. This will help to decrease the release of histamine. If contact dermatitis is severe, oral steroids can be given to reduce the inflammation. Complications include neurodermatitis and infection.

Atopic dermatitis

Atopic dermatitis, or eczema, is a skin rash that is more prevalent in children than adults though it can occur at any time in life. The exact cause is not known, but it is thought to be immune-mediated. It is frequently seen along with asthma or hay fever. Stress can exacerbate symptoms. Patients will have reddish to dark-colored discolored areas on the skin and are extremely pruritic. This pruritus is worse at night and can be aggravated by temperature changes, hot showers or baths, or allergens such as cigarette smoke. Atopic dermatitis most often occurs over the antecubital fossa, behind the knees, and on the feet, though it can occur anywhere on the body. The areas may have small papules that can become fluid-filled and will crust over after opening.

Diagnosis consists pruritic skin plus three of the four following:
- Generally dry skin over the last year
- Symptoms beginning before age 2
- Skin creases involved in pruitic skin
- Dermatitis on flexural surfaces.

Lubricating creams and oils can be used in infants with eczema. Topical corticosteroid creams can also be used when prescribed. Avoiding irritants that trigger the outbreaks also helps to decrease the symptoms. Complications include neurodermatitis, skin infections, blepharitis, conjunctivitis, and sleep issues.

Nummular eczema

Nummular eczema is a form of eczema that causes coin-shaped patches on the skin. There is no definite known cause, but it does tend to be aggravated by strong soaps and detergents. Abrasive fabrics and extremes in temperature can also aggravate the condition. The lesions with nummular eczema are initially often confused with a drug allergy. They are very pruritic and tend to be dry and scaly. The rash can also resemble a fungal infection or ringworm, but it tends to occasionally re-occur. Diagnosis is made per H&P that shows round pruritic lesions in a patient that has very dry skin. Treatment is with strong corticosteroid creams or ointments to help control the symptoms. With a severe outbreak, short-term oral steroids may be necessary. Coal tar preparations can help with an outbreak, but they tend to stain clothing. A secondary skin infection may develop with persistent itching of the skin, and appropriate antibiotic therapy should be given if this occurs. Avoiding the triggers that cause flare-ups of the condition is necessary to decrease the severity and frequency of outbreaks. Complications include dermatitis and skin infections.

Diaper rash

Diaper rash is very common and occurs in babies wearing diapers or in adults who are incontinent. It is caused by exposure of the skin to the moisture of urine and waste material. If severe, the rash can develop into a bacterial or fungal infection. The skin that has the moisture against it will become very inflamed and red. There may be areas where the skin is broken or cracked. The area will be very tender. If a fungal infection develops because of the moisture, there may be small red papules surrounding the inflamed area. Diagnosis is made clinically. Often there is irritation in the convex surfaces of the infant's body. This irritation can be simple erythema, lesions, papules, or erosions. The goal of treating diaper rash is to keep the skin clean and dry. Leaving the skin open to air and avoiding a wet diaper against the skin will help to relieve the rash. Barrier creams and ointment containing zinc oxide can help to prevent further irritation of the skin. An antifungal or antibacterial cream may be necessary if a secondary infection occurs. Persistent fungal diaper rashes can be a sign of and underlying immune condition or type 1 diabetes. Complications include candidal or bacterial infections.

Lichen planus

Lichen planus is a skin condition that appears to be immune-mediated. The exact cause is not known, but it may be linked to a drug allergy. Patients with hepatitis C have shown an increased incidence of this condition, but a definite link cannot be confirmed. The lesions seen with lichen planus are flat-topped papules that usually form a row. It most commonly occurs around the ankles or the distal upper extremities. It can also become severe and form over the oral mucosa and the genitals, or any other part of the body. The lesions are very pruritic and may burn. Once the lesions fade, they may leave a darker pigmented scar on the skin. Diagnosis is made per clinical evaluation. On H&P note mediations that may induce disorder. A skin biopsy may be needed. Lichen planus usually resolves spontaneously within 1 year, but symptoms can be controlled with creams containing immunomodulating medications. If severe, oral steroids may be necessary. Antihistamines and UV light therapy may also be helpful in controlling the symptoms of lichen planus. Complications include infection, sexual dysfunction, and increased risk of skin cancer.

Dyshidrosis

Dyshidrosis, or dyshidrotic eczema, is a form of eczema that causes vesicular lesions to form on the palms and soles. This condition is more common in women than men, and the exact cause is not known. It seems to occur more frequently during stressful times, and may be linked to exposure to metal salts. There also seems to be an increased incidence of this condition in those patients who suffer from hay fever. Signs and symptoms include extremely pruritic vesicular lesions on the palms of the hands and soles of the feet. These will break open and can crust over. As the lesions are resolving, the skin becomes very dry and cracked, and this can be painful. Secondary skin infections can occur when there are breaks in the skin. Diagnosis is made upon clinical assessment: pruritis, reoccurrence, acute onset, deep seated bullae or vesicles on the soles and palms or the lateral finger. Dyshidrosis is a chronic condition, and there is no known cure. Corticosteroid creams or ointments can help with symptoms, and antihistamines may decrease the severity of the flare-ups. UV light therapy can also help to control the symptoms during an outbreak. Complications include limited use of hands and feet and skin infections.

Folliculitis

Folliculitis is an infection around the hair follicle. It can be mild and self-limiting or may be reoccurring and painful. The most common causes are frequent shaving, perspiration in the area of the infection, and chronic inflammatory conditions of the skin. It can also be linked to exposure of the skin to coal tar or pitch. Patients will have small erythematous pustules surrounding the hair. These pustules may break open and crust over. Lesions may be pruritic or tender. Folliculitis can occasionally involve a large area and cause swelling and extreme pain. Diagnosis is made upon clinical evaluation: clusters of raised red, pruritic lesions. They will have a diameter of less than 5 mm. Pustules may be seen. Warm compresses can help relieve the symptoms, and folliculitis will usually resolve spontaneously without medical treatment after a few days. If severe, or caused by *Staphylococcus* or MRSA, antibiotics may be necessary to treat the condition. The most common causative organism is *Staphylococcus*. If patients have excessive exposure to water on their skin, *Pseudomonas* may be the cause. Complications include infections, skin damage (spots and scarring), and permanent hair loss.

Stevens-Johnson syndrome

Stevens-Johnson syndrome, or erythema multiforme major, is a severe condition that usually occurs due to a medication reaction or illness. Antibiotics, NSAIDs, and anticonvulsant medications are most likely to cause this syndrome. Patients who are immunocompromised are more likely to develop this condition, and there may be a genetic link that causes some people to be more susceptible. Patients will have vague, flu-type symptoms for a few days followed by development of an erythematous to purple rash over the oral mucous membranes. This can form vesicles and swelling will spread over the skin. Usually the top-most layer of skin will slough off. There are not univeral accepted diagnostic standards, but the following features are often present: necrosis of the epidermis, acute onset fever, a history of drug exposure often 1-4 wks before symptoms, diffuse erythema that progresses to vesicles, positive Nikolsky sign. Hospitalization is necessary to treat Stevens-Johnson syndrome. Fluid replacement and wound care is needed, along with supportive therapy. If the syndrome is severe, immunoglobulin therapy may be necessary to control the symptoms. Skin grafting may be necessary if the skin loss is severe. It may take several months for patients to recover from this condition. Complications include skin infections, sepsis, organ damage, MODS, skin issues including scarring, discoloring, and permanent hair loss.

Melanoma

Melanoma is the most serious form of skin cancer and can be fatal. It develops in the melanin cells of the skin and can metastasize internally. It is more likely to occur in those who are fair skinned and those who have a positive family history of melanoma. It is caused by exposure to UV light. Melanoma can develop in a mole or may be a new lesion on the skin. The discolored skin will have asymmetrical borders, and the color will change over time. The lesion may be flat or appear as a bump. Melanoma lesions are usually at least ¼-inch in diameter and may become hard or bumpy. Diagnosis is made per histopathology. A sentinel lymph node biopsy may be needed to see if the cancer has spread to adjacent lymph nodes. Treatment consists of surgical excision to include a small amount of surrounding normal tissue. Radiation and chemotherapy are used when melanoma has spread or is causing pain. Diagnostic studies should be done to ensure there has not been any metastasis of the melanoma. Regular checks with a dermatologist and vigilant use of sunscreen are necessary. Skin should be shielded from the sun when outside.

Complications are as follows:
- Deep tissue damage.
- Spread to other parts of the body.
- Many symptoms from treatment.
- Death.

Basal cell carcinoma

Basal cell carcinoma is the most common and slowest-growing form of skin cancer. It is caused by excessive exposure to UV light. Patients who develop a basal cell lesion are very likely to have more in the future. The lesions with basal cell are usually pearly white to brown in color and may have a waxy appearance. They can be flat or scaly in appearance. These tend to bleed if picked at and will crust over and heal. There may be a depressed area in the center and superficial blood vessels may be visible on the lesion. Diagnosis starts by discovery on clinical exam. Diagnosis is then confirmed by histology. Treatment of basal cell carcinoma is with removal of the lesion. This can be surgically excised or removed with laser therapy, cryotherapy, or antineoplastic creams, such as 5-fluorouracil. Patients should be educated on the importance of protecting the skin from sun exposure. Sunscreen with a high SPF level should be used whenever patients are outside. Complications include increased risk for other types of skin cancer, disfigurement and spreading of cancer (rare).

Varicella-zoster infection

A varicella-zoster infection, or shingles, can be a very painful condition. It is caused by the same virus that causes chickenpox in children. The virus lies dormant in the nerve cells. Increased stress, an immunocompromised state, or other infections may cause the virus to be reactivated, resulting in shingles. Patients will complain of burning pain at the site of the lesions and may develop this sensation before the lesions appear. Lesions most frequently occur around the chest wall, following a dermatomal pattern, though they can occur anywhere on the body, including the face and eyes. The vesicular lesions will open and eventually crust over. Patients may be left with chronic pain, called post-herpetic neuralgia, after the lesions resolve. Diagnosis is usually made per clinical evaluation. If uncertain, polymerase chain reaction assay (PCR) is the most sensitive diagnostic test. Treatment is with antivirals, such as acyclovir, to help decrease the length and severity of the outbreak. Topical anesthetics, such as Lidocaine patches, can also help to decrease the pain. Anticonvulsants and antidepressants may help with the lasting pain of post-herpetic neuralgia. Complications are as follows:

- Especially in immunocompromised, cutaneous dissemination.
- May develop visceral organ involvement, which presents rapidly and includes encephalitis, hepatitis, and pneumonia.

Squamous cell carcinoma

Squamous cell carcinoma is a form of skin cancer that can spread to surrounding tissue, lymph nodes, and organs and can be fatal if left untreated. Though not as deadly as melanoma, squamous cell carcinoma is more likely to cause serious complications than basal cell carcinoma. Squamous cell carcinoma is caused by exposure to UV light and is more likely to occur in men than women, especially those who are fair-skinned. It is thought that smokers and those with human papilloma virus (HPV) infection are more likely to develop squamous cell lesions. Squamous cell carcinoma lesions are usually red and firm. These can occur anywhere on the body and the appearance may vary. They can be crusty or scaly and may appear white when forming on mucous membranes. Diagnosis is made per histopathology. Treatment consists of removal of the lesion. This can be accomplished with excision, laser therapy, or cryotherapy. The skin should always be protected from sun by shielding or applying sunscreen with a high SPF rating. For high risk lesions, a more aggressive approach may be used. Complications include metastasis to lymph nodes and organs.

EENT (Eye, Ear, Nose, and Throat)

Blowout fracture

A blowout fracture is a fracture of the orbital floor and involves the maxillary bone and the posterior medial floor of the orbit. It occurs due to excessive facial trauma. These patients will report trauma and complain of significant pain. Diplopia may be present because of restriction of the extraocular muscles. The eyelid may be edematous with crepitus present on palpation. A potential complication of a blowout fracture is possible entrapment of the orbital contents within the maxillary sinus. If this occurs, the eye may have a sunken appearance, or enophthalmos. Diagnosis is made per history and confirmed with imaging studies, usually CT scan. A blowout fracture will typically heal on its own with regular follow-up to ensure proper healing is occurring. Patients should be advised to avoid blowing their noses. Oral antibiotics may be given to decrease the risk of orbital infection. In some cases, such as with restrictive diplopia or enophthalmos, surgery may be necessary to repair the orbital wall. Complications include inferior rectus muscle entrapment leading to ischemia, nerve damage to the infraorbital nerve, and enophthalmos.

Sialadenitis

Sialadenitis is an infection of the salivary glands. It differs from parotitis, or mumps, in that it involves a blockage of the flow of saliva, causing bacteria to grow within the ducts. This leads to a bacterial infection, usually caused by *Staphylococcus aureus*. The most common salivary glands affected are the parotid gland in the cheek and the submandibular gland under the chin. Patients will complain of pain in the affected area. Purulent drainage may flow into the mouth, causing a foul-smelling and foul-tasting sensation. Patients may have a fever and headache. Diagnosis is usually made by clinical assesment, but CT may be useful if stones are suspected but not palpable. Treatment is usually accomplished with appropriate antibiotic therapy. If infection is severe, the gland may need to be drained with culture and sensitivity testing performed on the extracted pus. If a stone is causing a blockage of the ductwork leading from the salivary gland, this will need to be surgically removed. Patients may develop a chronic form of sialadenitis that causes recurrent flare-ups of the condition.

Blepharitis

Blepharitis is an inflammation or infection of the eyelid and eyelashes. There are two types, Staphylococcus *blepharitis* and *Seborrheic blepharitis*, with *seborrheic* being the most common. In addition to the eyelids and eyelashes, blepharitis can affect the eyebrows and scalp. Patients may complain of burning of the eyes and matting of the eyelashes. The eyes may be irritated with a gritty feeling. They can also appear red. Include questioning in the history regarding possibly allergens or use or retinoids. Note any history of eczema or acne. Diagnosis is made per clinical assessment, usually pink or reddened eyelid with crusting. Under otoscope, if a hard crusty material is visible in eyelashes this most often indicates staphylococcus blepharitis, whereas if the material in the eyelashes looks like oily flaky material, this is more compatible with seborrheic blepharitis. Treating blepharitis involves debriding the lid margin of the matted material, usually using a cotton applicator. Warm compresses may be helpful. Topical antibiotics may be given and should be applied in the morning and at bedtime to prevent blurred vision from interfering with activities. Antihistamine eye drops do not help to relieve the symptoms of blepharitis caused by *Seborrhea* or *Staphylococcus*. If the irritation is allergic in origin, then the drops will have an immediate effect. Lubricating eye drops will not help. Patients, especially in unilateral cases, need to be evaluated for sebaceous cell malignancy.

Conjunctivitis

Conjunctivitis ("pink eye") is an infection of the conjunctiva of one or both eyes. It can be caused by a bacteria or virus or can be allergic in nature. Patients will complain of a gritty, irritating, itching sensation in the eye, which is red from hemorrhage of small vessels. Vision is usually not affected. With bacterial conjunctivitis, there is a mucus discharge, and patients may have problems with the eye being matted closed in the morning. Viral and allergic conjunctivitis typically cause a watery discharge. This is a diagnosis of exclusion, based on clinical assesment. The following should be ruled out: stye, ulceration, or blepharitis. If bacterial conjunctivitis is suspected, treatment consists of erythromycin 5mg/gm ointment opthalmically 1.25 cm four times per day for 5 to seven days or trimethoprim-polymyxin B opthalmic 1-2 drops opthalmically four times daily for 5 to 7 days. If no response to antibiotic drops the patient should be referred to opthalmologist. Viral conjunctivitis only requires symptomatic relief. Patients should avoid rubbing the eye. Frequent hand washing can decrease transmission of the condition. Allergic conjunctivitis can be treated with ophthalmic antihistamines, but this condition may be chronic in patients who suffer from recurrent environmental allergies. Corneal injury may occur resulting in vision impairment.

Chalazion

A chalazion is caused by the inflammation of a sebaceous gland on the eyelid. It is not the same thing as a sty. A sty will also involve hair follicles and is more superficial appearing. It is commonly found in patients with rosacea or blepharitis. A chalazion usually occurs on the upper eyelid. There may be gradual swelling that increases over the course of a few days to a few weeks. The lesion may appear red and inflamed, and patients may complain of pain. Eventually, it becomes a painless nodular lesion. Diagnosis is made by clinical assessment. Warm compresses may help to relieve the pain and promote absorption of the oil that is trapped in the sebaceous gland. If a bacterial infection is superimposed on the chalazion, an ophthalmic antibiotic may be prescribed. An injection of triamcinolone (Kenalog®) directly into the mass may help to relieve the inflammation and promote healing. In rare cases, surgical incision of the mass may be necessary if it persists and is not resolving with more conservative treatments. If the patient experiences recurring chalazions, they should be assessed for carcinoma.

Dacryocystitis

Dacryocystitis is a condition in which the lacrimal sac becomes inflamed. This inflammation can be due to a blockage at some point in the tear drainage system or a stone that has formed within the lacrimal sac. Patients will complain of pain along the inside corner of the eye. The area will appear red and swollen and may extend from the inner canthus of the eye to the upper nose or nasal bridge. If the dacrocystitis is chronic in nature, tearing is the most prevalent complaint. Diagnosis is made by clinical assessment. CBC may show elevated WBCs, and occasionally CT scans are ordered to show anatomy and surrounding areas of lacrimal sac. To treat this inflammation and infection, antibiotics can be given. Depending upon the severity, patients may require hospitalization for IV antibiotic therapy. If severe, incision and drainage may be necessary to treat an abscess. Once the inflammation and infection have resolved, surgery may be necessary to correct the blockage. If a stone is present within the lacrimal sac, this will need to be surgically removed to prevent future blockages leading to abscess formation. Complications include cellulitis, sepsis, meningitis, fistula, and abscess.

Corneal abrasion

A corneal abrasion is caused by minor trauma to the surface of the eye, resulting in a scratching of the cornea. Patients will complain of pain and tearing of the eye, and may even complain of blurred vision. First rule out penetrating trauma, infection, and exclude the diagnosis of open globe before proceeding. To diagnose a corneal abrasion, topical anesthetics should be instilled in the eye. Fluorescein is then administered in the eye, and an UV light is used to examine the eye. The area of the cornea that is affected will brightly light up, indicating the area of abrasion. The eye should be gently irrigated to ensure there are no lingering foreign objects that can continue to cause damage. Topical antibiotics (most often erythromycin ointment 4 times a day for 3 to 5 days OR polymyxin B/trimethoprim 1 drop ophthalmically 4 times per day for 3 to 5 days) and cycloplegia are recommended. Patching is only recommended in patients with large abrasions. This condition should heal within a couple of days of treatment. Patients with contact lenses should be examined for corneal infiltrates or ulcers, and if found should be referred to ophthalmologist immediately. Contact wearers without infiltrate or ulcer should be treated with ofloxacin or ciprofloxacin drops 4 times a day to cover for pseudomonas. Complications include bacterial keratitis, corneal ulcer, and loss of vision.

Primary open angle glaucoma

To diagnose glaucoma, the angle at which fluid flows from the eye is measured. The pressure is measured within the eye to determine if it is increased. With primary open angle glaucoma, the angle is open with the presence of optic nerve damage and a loss of peripheral vision found on visual field testing. It is the most common form of glaucoma and is usually age-related. Treatment begins with ophthalmic eye drops. Ophthalmic beta-blockers, such as Timolol, can be used. Medications such as Pilocarpine that work on the muscarinic receptors of the eye to increase fluid flow may are also prescribed. There has been some controversy over whether to start with medical treatment or proceed with surgical treatment first for primary open angle glaucoma. Laser treatment and traditional surgical treatment are usually reserved for treatment once medical management has failed to produce adequate results in decreasing the ocular pressure.

Ectropion and entropion

An ectropion is a condition in which the lower eyelid turns outward. This usually occurs during the aging process due to laxity of the muscles within the eyelid. The ectropion causes dryness and irritation of the eye. A paralysis of the facial nerve can cause this to occur because of the loss of neuromuscular control of the facial muscles on the affected side. Scarring due to trauma or burns can also cause an ectropion. Repair of the ectropion is accomplished through surgery to tighten the muscles of the lower eyelid. An entropion is a condition in which the lower eyelid turns inward. This is most commonly caused by the aging process due to muscle laxity causing the lower eyelid to involute. Facial nerve palsy and scarring can also cause this condition. Patients will complain of irritation of the eye with tearing and the sensation of a foreign body being in the eye due to the eyelashes rubbing on the sclera. Treatment is by surgical correction.

Hordeolum

A hordeolum, or "stye," is a condition in which an eyelash follicle becomes infected. Patients may complain of tenderness around the area. The small abscess will appear red and swollen. It will eventually come to a head and purulent discharge may be expressed from the small infection. Treatment of a hordeolum generally consists of frequent application of warm compresses to draw the abscess to a head so that the infectious material can be expressed. The hordeolum may not drain and can resolve on its own. If the condition becomes severe, or if patients develop recurrent hordeola, tetracycline may be given to eradicate the infection. It is important to remember that children should not be given tetracycline because of alterations that can occur in tooth or bone development. Tetracycline should also not be given to females who are or may become pregnant because of the risk of birth anomalies.

Angle closure glaucoma

There are two types of angle closure glaucoma: primary and acute. Primary angle closure glaucoma affects approximately 10% of those patients who have glaucoma. The angle through which fluid drains from the eye is narrowed, resulting in an increase in ocular pressure. This is treated with surgery by creating an opening behind the iris through which the fluid can flow from the eye, resulting in a decrease in ocular pressure. Acute angle closure glaucoma results in the sudden onset of blurred vision with visual halos, pain, red eye, and possibly nausea and vomiting. This requires urgent treatment. The cornea may be edematous when examined, and ocular pressure readings are extremely elevated with this condition. Medications may be necessary at first to reduce the corneal edema. Ultimately, laser surgery is necessary to open the angle so that fluid can flow from the eye to cause a decrease in the ocular pressure.

Macular degeneration

Macular degeneration is the most common cause of blindness in the Caucasian population. It is rare in other races. There are two types of macular degeneration: dry and wet. The dry form is more common and occurs when drusen are deposited deep in the eye near the retina. It begins in middle age and progresses slowly, causing a loss of central vision not usually resulting in legal blindness. It can, however, develop into wet macular degeneration. Wet macular degeneration occurs when capillaries break through the retina and grow behind the macula of the eye. This form of the disease is more debilitating and can lead to legal blindness. Any vision loss that occurs over a period of weeks or days requires opthalmic evaluation. Drusen under the retina on eye exam. Center of vision deficits. There is no definitive cure for macular degeneration. Vitamin C, E, Zinc, Copper and beta-carotene may slow the process of dry macular degeneration. Medications (ranibizumab, aflibercept, or bevacizumab) and surgery may improve vision in wet macular degeneration. There is a genetic link with this disease and prevention is important. Eating leafy green vegetables high in carotenoids, quitting smoking, and protecting the eyes from UV light, can reduce risk. Dry macular degeneration can suddenly turn to wet macular degeneration. Vision loss can occur.

Hyphema

Hyphema is blood in the anterior chamber of the eye. It is most frequently caused by blunt trauma to the eye, but can also occur following eye surgery or certain medical disorders, such as sickle cell anemia. A hyphema is very obvious because blood will be visible underneath the cornea and cause the iris to be blocked. There may also be conjunctival hemorrhages present. Treatment involves strict activity restrictions with avoidance of all strenuous activities. Aspirin and other anticoagulant medications should be avoided to decrease the risk of additional bleeding. If the hyphema is managed on an outpatient basis, patients should be re-evaluated every couple of days to assess for rebleeding. Bleeding can reoccur 3-6 days following the initial eye trauma and may be worse than the initial bleeding that caused the hyphema. Once the hyphema has resolved, patients should continue to be evaluated annually because these patients are at risk for developing glaucoma later in life.

Pterygium

A pterygium is a triangular-shaped raised lesion that grows on the surface of the eye. It most commonly occurs on the nasal side of the cornea and may appear red. Patients usually seek treatment for this because of cosmetic appearances, but it can grow to obstruct the visual fields. This occurs if it extends over the cornea. Occasionally, it can be irritating to the eye. Diagnosis is made by clinical assessment. Care should be made to differentiate from any neoplastic conditions. Treatment involves surgical removal of the pterygium, though this is usually reserved for cases in which the lesion affects the visual fields or is irritating. Surgery may be necessary to replace a portion of the conjunctiva. An antimetabolite may also be applied during surgery to prevent recurrence of the lesion.
Almost one-half of patients who develop a pterygium will go on to develop the lesion again. There are usually no long-term effects of decreased visual acuity following surgery if the lesion is not encroaching upon the cornea.

Orbital cellulitis

Orbital cellulitis is an infection that results in cellulitis of the eyelids. It is a serious condition and must be managed urgently to prevent further complications. Patients will have a painfully swollen and red eye, sometimes severe enough to cause the eye to be swollen shut. Patients may have blurred or double vision along with a headache. They may be febrile if the infection is severe. On exam, the eye may be displaced anteriorly with a sluggish pupil reaction to light. The extraocular movements may also be restricted, depending on the amount of edema. A CT scan can be done to rule out the presence of a foreign body and to assess any damage to the optic nerve. Patients usually require hospitalization and treatment with IV antibiotics. *Staphylococcus* is the most common cause of bacterial infection, but immunocompromised patients may develop a fungal orbital cellulitis. Once the infection is controlled with IV antibiotics, patients can be discharged home on oral antibiotics with close follow-up. Complications include intracranial expansion, vision loss, and sinus thrombosis.

Tractional retinal detachment

A tractional retinal detachment occurs in conditions that cause scarring within the vitreous humor, such as diabetic retinopathy. The fibrous strands that make up a scar cause traction to be applied to the retina. This traction results in separation of the retina from the posterior eye. Some patients may have floaters or flashes of light in their vision, along with the curtain-type vision loss, as seen with rhegmatogenous retinal detachment. More commonly, there will be visual loss with a description of blind spots in the vision.
Treatment usually involves removing the vitreous humor, thereby removing the fibrous scar material. Gas or an oily substance may be injected into the eye to prevent recurrence of this condition. The best treatment is prevention by maintaining adequate control of blood sugar levels in diabetics to prevent the development of diabetic retinopathy. There is a chance of permanent visual loss with this condition, despite aggressive treatment.

Rhegmatogenous retinal detachment

Rhegmatogenous is the most common form of retinal detachment. Rhegmatogenous retinal detachment occurs when there is a tear in the retina, allowing the vitreous humor to enter the space behind the retina and causing a detachment of the retina from the posterior eye. The most common cause of this type of retinal detachment is the aging process, which leads to shrinkage of the vitreous humor. This causes pulling on the retina, leading to a tear or hole in the retina. Patients will describe floaters and flashes of light with an associated decrease in vision. The loss of vision will occur in a curtain-type fashion, where the vision seems to be blocked out momentarily and then returns. This occurs as the torn retina flaps down and then back up. Patients complaining of floaters who present with mono decreased visual fields should be referred to an ophthalmologist immediately. This condition is a surgical emergency and needs to be treated immediately. Delay of even one day can result in some degree of permanent visual loss after surgical repair.

Hypertensive retinopathy

Uncontrolled blood pressure is the cause of hypertensive retinopathy. As pressure rises within the body's arteries, the small arteries in the eye are also affected. This results in narrowing of the retinal arteries and a decrease in blood flow to the structures of the eye. Patients may or may not notice a decrease in their visual acuity. On exam, narrowed retinal arteries are visible, along with retinal hemorrhages and possibly some swelling. A swollen optic nerve can result with malignant hypertension, a condition in which the diastolic blood pressure is >120 mm Hg. This is a diagnosis of exclusion. If neurological signs ameliorate after hypertension is corrected, this is considered confirmation of the diagnosis. Treatment involves controlling the blood pressure with diet, exercise, and medications. Malignant hypertension is an emergency condition and should be treated immediately, but slowly.

Visual loss that results from hypertensive retinopathy may be permanent, but control of the blood pressure can prevent additional damage. Hypertensive encephalopathy, stroke, and hemorrhage are additional possible complications.

Exudative retinal detachment

An exudative retinal detachment occurs when fluid builds up behind the retina. This can occur with several medical conditions, including various collagen-vascular diseases, posterior scleritis, tumors affecting the eye, and congenital abnormalities. This results in visual loss with patients complaining of experiencing blind spots in their vision. They may also experience floaters or flashes of light in their vision. Surgery is not usually necessary to treat this condition. Treatment of the underlying condition is usually sufficient to prevent permanent visual loss. With chronic medical conditions that cause an exudative retinal detachment, achieving adequate medical control of the condition can result in reversal of the detachment as the fluid behind the retina dissipates. Urgent treatment of the cause of the retinal detachment is necessary to prevent permanent visual loss. Some patients may develop a chronic problem with this condition, and then surgery to prevent fluid accumulation behind the retina is necessary.

Strabismus

Strabismus is a condition in which the extraocular muscles are weakened, leading to a gaze deviation in one eye. It differs from a "lazy eye," or amblyopia, because there is no loss of visual acuity associated with a strabismus. The condition is labeled by the direction in which the gaze is affected:

- Hypertropia occurs when the gaze is diverted upward.
- Exotropia when the gaze is deviated outward.
- Esotropia when the gaze is deviated inward ("cross-eyes").
- Hypotropia when the gaze is deviated downward.

A wide, flattened nose with a skin fold at the inner canthus can cause the appearance of esotropia and is called pseudoesotropia. This usually resolves with age. Eye muscle strengthening can be performed to help straighten the gaze in mild cases of strabismus. If this fails or if the strabismus is severe, surgery may be necessary to draw the affected muscles tighter in order to straighten the gaze.

Diabetic retinopathy

Diabetic retinopathy is the leading cause of blindness in the US in diabetics <65-years-old. It begins as tiny microaneurysms in the retina. Exudates form in the retina as these aneurysms rupture. Patients frequently have no visual loss at this stage. As retinopathy progresses, the exudates become larger and the rupturing aneurysms can lead to swelling of the macula. Patients may or may not have a decrease in visual acuity. Focal laser photocoagulation is done at this stage to decrease the macular edema by cauterizing the leaking microaneurysms. The final stages of diabetic retinopathy occur when new vessels are developed around the optic nerve. These vessels are very fragile and are easily ruptured, which leads to bleeding within the retina and vitreous humor. As scar tissue forms, the fibrous strands of the scar may cause a tractional retinal detachment. Focal laser photocoagulation can be performed to decrease the rupture of these new vessels, but visual loss is common with this condition, and blindness frequently occurs.

Mastoiditis

Mastoiditis is an infection of the mastoid bone of the skull and usually occurs following otitis media. In the past, mastoiditis was relatively common and the leading common cause of death in children. Since the advent of antibiotics and prompt treatment of otitis media infections, the incidence of mastoiditis has greatly declined. Patients, if old enough, may complain of severe pain in the ear and behind the ear. There may be swelling in the area that causes the affected ear to stick out from the head. Patients may have a high fever and headache. A skull x-ray or CT of the head will show a honeycomb appearance of the mastoid bone due to the infection. Treatment includes aggressive IV antibiotics in order to penetrate the bone tissue and treat the infection. If IV antibiotics are effective, patients will continue on oral antibiotics to completely eradicate the infection. Myringotomy may be needed to remove fluid and ventilate the ear. If medical treatment is not effective, a mastoidectomy may be performed. Complications include hearing loss, brain absess, and meningitis.

Otitis media

Otitis media is an infection of the middle ear. It is most commonly bacterial or viral and affects children more often than adults because of the straight anatomic structure of the auditory canal and eustachian tube, which promotes the accumulation of fluid behind the tympanic membrane. The most common cause of otitis media in children is infection with *Streptococcus, Pneumoniae,* or *H. influenzae.* The incidence of infection with these organisms is on the decline, however, because of immunizations now available to help prevent infection. *M. catarrhalis* can also cause otitis media. In immunocompromised individuals, fungal infections can lead to otitis media. Signs and symptoms include ear pain and fever. Symptoms of an upper respiratory infection may also be present. On exam, a bulging tympanic membrane with purulent effusion may be evident. There should be decreased movement of the membrane with insufflation. Diagnosis is most often by clinical assessment by otoscope. Amoxicillin is the drug of choice for uncomplicated OM without penicillin allergy, due to its low cost, long history, and the organisms that it is active against. The most common dose is 500 mg every 12 hours. Drug resistance varies across the US, so current guidelines for any specific area should be followed. Complications include mastoiditis, labyrinthitis, and hearing loss.

Labyrinthitis

Labyrinthitis is an inflammatory condition affecting the labyrinth of the inner ear. It usually occurs following a viral infection, such as a cold or the flu. Bacterial infections of the upper respiratory system can also cause labyrinthitis. Trauma to the head or ear, along with benign tumors of the ear, can also cause this condition. Vertigo is the main symptom that patients will experience. This can be quite severe with nausea and vomiting, along with a complete loss of balance. Patients may have a headache and may experience tinnitus with the condition. The symptoms can be positional or may occur at rest. Diagnosis is made by clinical assessment, using imaging to rule out other disorders if needed. Labyrinthitis is usually treated with anti-vertigo medications, such as Antivert®. Viral labyrinthitis is often treated with a tapering dose of corticosteroids, most often prednisone, beginning at 60 mg. Rarely, antibiotics will be given if it is suspected the condition is caused by a bacterial infection. Small stones within the labyrinth can occasionally cause this condition, and the Epley maneuver can be used to change the position of the stones. For symptom relief, antihistamines, antiemetics, and benzodiazepines are commonly used, but should be used short term. Complications are not usually common, but include tinnitis and hearing loss.

Ménière's disease

Ménière's disease is a condition affecting the labyrinth of the ear. The labyrinth is made up of bony and membranous portions. The membranous portion contains a fluid called endolymph. It is thought that Ménière's disease results when the membranous portion of the labyrinth ruptures, causing the endolymph to mix with perilymph, a fluid separating the membranous portion from the bony portion. Signs and symptoms include tinnitus, vertigo, and loss of hearing. Some patients experience a feeling of pressure within the affected ear(s). These symptoms are often not constant, but rather occur intermittently. Diagnosis is made by clinical assessment. Sensorineural hearing loss, tinnitus, and at least two episodes of rotational vertigo are the usual qualifiers for a diagnosis. Other diagnoses should be ruled out. There is no cure of Ménière's disease. The symptoms can be decreased, though, with the dietary restriction of sodium, caffeine, and alcohol. Quitting smoking may help decrease the severity of symptoms. Gentamicin eardrops may help decrease the vertigo. With severe cases, the labyrinth can be surgically removed, but this will result in a loss of hearing in the ear. Benzodiazepines, antihistamines, and antiemetics are often used for acute episodes of symptoms. Complications include intractable vertigo and hearing loss.

Sinusitis

Sinusitis, is inflammation of the nasal passages and paranasal sinuses that is symptomatic. Mucus cannot drain because of the edematous sinuses, producing an excellent environment in which bacteria can thrive, leading to a sinus infection. Most often this presents after a cold. Signs and symptoms include cold symptoms that are present or resolving and headache, generally over the frontal, ethmoid, or maxillary sinuses. Complaints of positional increases in the headache, a full feeling, or pressure within the head, a stuffy nose, fever, and aching in the teeth may also be present. Diagnosis is made per clinical assessment. It is important to attempt to distinguish bacterial from viral sinusitis. Sinusitis is likely bacterial if the patient presents with sinusitis symptoms which have gone on for more than 10 days, severe symptoms with high fever and facial pain, or 5-6 days following a viral infection which was improving and then suddenly presents with worsening symptoms. Treatment will be decided based on whether the sinusitis is of bacterial of viral origin. For both viral and bacterial sinusitis, symptoms can be improved with analgesia, mucolytics, decongestants, glucocorticoids, nasal irrigation, and antihistamines. However, this does not shorten the course of illness, whether viral or bacterial. The recommended antimicrobial is amoxicillin-clavulanate 875mg/125mg PO BID. Drug resistance varies across the US, so clinicians should be aware of local resistance trends when necessary.

Otitis externa

Otitis externa is an infection of the external ear canal. It is usually caused by *Pseudomonas* bacteria, but can also be due to *Staphylococcus* or *Streptococcus* infections. Rarely, the infection can be due to a fungal infection. This is often referred to as "swimmer's ear" because of the prevalence in those who spend a lot of time in the water. Significant ear pain that is exacerbated with movement of the external ear is the main symptom. Patients may have enlargement of the preauricular lymph nodes. Exam of the ear canal will reveal edema, erythema of the ear canal, possibly with purulent discharge. Diagnosis is made by clinical assessment and history. The mainstays of treatment with otitis externa involve cleaning the ear, treating the inflammation, controlling pain, and avoiding contributing factors. After cleaning the ear, the ear is treated with topical antibiotics, antiseptics, glucocorticoids, or acidifying agents. For drops, tilt head towards opposite shoulder, pull superior part of auricle up and instill drops. The patient should side lie for 5 minutes or use a cottonball in the ear. For some topical agents, a wick is placed in the ear canal to facilitate installation of an acidic solution. Aminoglycoside eardrops can also be used, but care should be taken to ensure the tympanic membrane is intact because of the risk of ototoxicity with these medications. Complications include malignant external otitis and periauricular cellulitis.

Pharyngitis

Pharyngitis is an inflammation of the pharynx, causing a sore throat. It is most commonly caused by a viral infection. The most common bacterial cause of pharyngitis is Group A *Streptococcus* (GAS). Patients will complain of a very sore throat that may or may not have been accompanied with other cold symptoms. Cold symptoms are usually present with viral forms of pharyngitis. A fever and headache may also be present. Children with *Streptococcal* pharyngitis may have some nausea and vomiting with the illness. On exam, cervical and tonsillar lymph nodes will be enlarged, the oropharynx will appear edematous/erythematous, possibly with white exudates present. Centor criteria are symptoms that may be present and are used to guide the clinician: tonsillar exudates, absence of cough, fever (may be by history), and tender anterior cervical adenopathy. For patients that have 3 or more Centor criteria, use a rapid antigen detection test to diagnosis GAS. Those with < three Centor criteria, unless with a high risk for infection, are usually treated as viral pharyngitis. Culture confirms diagnosis but as RADT is very sensitive, it is not often ordered. Viral pharyngitis is supportive with warm salt water, antipyretics, and analgesics. GAS pharyngitis most often treated with penicillin V in adults and amoicillin in children. Complications include glomerulonephritis, rheumatic fever, scarlet fever, toxic shock syndrome, otitis media, sinusitis, and cellulitis.

Allergic rhinitis

Allergic rhinitis affects the nose and eyes. It occurs in those individuals with allergies to environmental irritants, such as pollen, animal dander, trees, and dust. The symptoms due to exposure from these irritants can vary from minor symptoms to hives and throat constriction. The onset of symptoms can usually be associated with exposure to an environmental irritant. Signs and symptoms include runny nose, itchy and watery eyes, mild cough, sneezing, facial itching, and sore throat. Patients may complain of a headache, possibly over the sinuses, with a feeling of pressure in the head. This is due to increased mucus production through the sinuses and nasal passages. Fatigue, irritability, reduced performance and depression are also side effects. Diagnosis is made by clinical assessment, history, and findings. Allergy skin testing is not necessary but can be useful. Treatment includes avoiding known allergens when possible. Intranasal glucocorticoid sprays are the most effective maintenance therapy. Antihistamines can be given to decrease the release of histamine and suppress the allergic symptoms; however, they have sedative and impairing side effects. If antihistamines are used second generation agents are usually preferred. Complications include sinusitis, otitis media, and asthma.

Dental abscess

A dental abscess is an infection that forms around the roots of a tooth, or teeth, or in the gum tissue. Infection within the dental pulp is more common in children while an abscess in the surrounding tissue is more common in adults. Patients will develop severe pain in an isolated area of the mouth. The check will appear red and swollen, and lymph nodes in the neck on the affected side will be enlarged. A fever may be present as well as a headache. The abscess may rupture, resulting in a sudden rush of warm, foul-tasting and foul-smelling fluid in the mouth. The pain will subside after the abscess ruptures, but treatment is still necessary. Diagnosis is made per clinical assessment. Treatment includes drainage of the abscess if it has not drained on its own. Antibiotics will be given to eradicate the infection after drainage. Antibiotic treatment of this infection is very important to prevent spread of the infection systemically. Referral to oral surgeon if needed. Complications include deep tissue infection, osteomyeltitis, and increased cardiovascular problems.

Aphthous ulcers

Aphthous ulcers, or canker sores, occur within the oral cavity. They can appear on the lips, oral mucosa, gums, or tongue. Canker sores are not contagious and always occur on the soft tissues of the mouth. They have no definite known cause, but irritants in the oral cavity, such as strongly acidic foods or candies, may contribute to aphthous ulcers. Patients will complain of a painful area in the oral cavity with some swelling in the area. Exam will reveal a shallow, white or yellowish ulcer, usually less than 1 cm in width. There is usually no bleeding noticed, but there may be some edema and erythema of the surrounding tissue present. Diagnosis is made per clinical assessment and history. Treatment includes avoiding acidic foods and drinks that irritate the ulcer. Smoking can also irritate the ulcer, as can very rough foods. Warm salt-water swish and swallow may be soothing to the lesion. Over-the-counter topical numbing medications may be helpful in decreasing the pain. Aphthous ulcers generally resolve spontaneously within a few days. Complications are uncommon.

Oral leukoplakia

Oral leukoplakia is a white patchy lesion found in the oral cavity. It is caused by tobacco use, either smoking or chewing, and is considered a premalignant form of oral cancer. Another form of the condition is hairy leukoplakia, which is seen in HIV-positive patients or others with suppressed immune systems and is probably caused by the Epstein-Barr virus. Patients will complain of a white patch in their mouths. This patch can be on the oral mucosa, the tongue, or gums. It is a painless, slightly raised, rough patch that is white or grayish in color. There may occasionally be leukoplakia lesions that appear pink or red in color. Eventually the lesion can become painful or sensitive to heat, cold, or spicy foods.
Diagnosis is made by clinical assessment and confirmation by biopsy. Treatment includes surgical excision of the lesion. There is a chance that patients can develop these lesions again, especially if they continue to smoke or use smokeless tobacco. Quitting smoking is the best treatment for prevention of future lesions. Oral cancer is a possible complication.

Oral candidiasis

Oral candidiasis, or oral thrush, is a fungal infection affecting the oral mucosa. It is not contagious. It commonly occurs in those who wear dentures. It can also occur in diabetics, patients who take steroids (especially inhalation steroids), immunocompromised patients, and those taking antibiotics that affect the natural flora of the mouth. Radiation to the head and neck can also cause thrush. Patients will have white plaques over the oral mucosa. The plaques can be scraped off with a tongue depressor to reveal red, raw areas. The lesions may or may not be painful to patients. Foul-smelling breath and alteration in taste are also common symptoms. Diagnosis is most often made by clinical assessment, however if confirmation is needed, cultures can be taken. An antifungal swish and swallow solution is used to treat oral candidiasis. Impregnated swabs can also be used in those who are unable to swish the solution in their mouth before swallowing. Patients should be reminded to clean their dentures thoroughly daily. Patients using inhaled steroids should completely rinse their mouths after each treatment. There are usually no complications in the immunocompetent, but in the immunocompromised, candidiasis can spread to the blood stream, GI tract, heart valves, etc. It can lead to malnutrition if eating becomes difficult.

Mumps

Mumps is a viral infection of the salivary glands. It generally affects the parotid salivary glands, which are the largest. Mumps is a viral infection that is transmitted through airborne respiratory particles. It generally affects children more than adults, but there is an immunization available to prevent contraction of the disease. Patients may complain of facial pain with a fever and headache. The affected side of the face will appear swollen, like "chipmunk cheeks." Parotitis can become systemic and affect the testes in boys and may lead to infertility. Treatment is supportive. Ice or heat applied to the cheeks may help with pain relief, as can acetaminophen or ibuprofen for pain and fever relief. Chewing may be painful, so soft foods should be given with plenty of fluids. Boys should be frequently assessed for the formation of a lump or mass in the scrotum. Aseptic meningitis is a possible complication.

Peritonsillar abscess

A peritonsillar abscess can occur as a complication of bacterial tonsillitis. The causative organism is usually grouping A-beta hemolytic *Streptococcus*. An abscess can develop in the soft tissue surrounding the tonsil and lead to a severe infection. Patients will have severe throat pain with enlarged lymph nodes on the affected side. Signs and symptoms include fever, headache, difficulty swallowing, muffled voice, difficulty closing the mouth, drooling, neck swelling, ipsilateral ear pain, and trismus. Trismus occurs in around 65% of patients and can help distinguish abscess from tonsillitis. Diagnosis is made by clinical assessment- deviation of the uvula and tonsil displacement. Culture of the fluid drained can later confirm diagnosis. The abscess should be drained, and culture and sensitivity testing should be done on the extracted pus. Treatment is usually with IV antibiotics, for adults, ampicillin-sulbactam 3 g every six hours IV or clindamycin 600 mg every six hours IV. As always, local patterns of susceptibility should be taken into consideration. If MRSA is common, use clindamycin or vancomycin, if severe or not responding. Patients may require future surgery to remove the tonsils and prevent recurrence of this infection. Complications include airway obstruction, sepsis, aspiration pneumonia, carotid artery rupture, thrombophlebitis (of the jugular vein), mediastinitis, and necrotizing fasciitis.

Endocrine System

Hyperparathyroidism and hypoparathyroidism

Most patients with calcium levels <12 are asymptomatic. Symptoms usually begin as the calcium level rises above 12, and the symptoms will worsen as the calcium level continues to rise. Initially, patients may complain of nausea and vomiting with a loss of appetite. They may feel muscle weakness and fatigue. Constipation may be present. As the calcium level rises, they may become confused and lethargic. Polyuria can occur with renal failure. Cardiac arrhythmias can occur and even coma. As calcium levels drop, patients may become confused or lethargic with mental status changes. Muscular changes with hypoparathyroidism will be the opposite of those with hyperparathyroidism. Patients will show signs of neuromuscular irritability with carpopedal spasm, laryngeal spasm, and facial grimacing. A positive Chvostek's sign, which will involve unilateral spasm of the facial muscles when the facial nerve is tapped, may be present. Patients may have seizures or cardiac arrhythmias when calcium levels are dangerously low.

Adrenal insufficiency

Adrenal insufficiency can be primary or secondary, and chronic or acute. Primary, or Addison's disease, is due to autoimmune factors, infections, or disease within the adrenal gland. This causes a decrease in cortisol secretion. Secondary factors include a pituitary adenoma or discontinuation of steroid use. Adrenal crisis is a life threatening emergency of acute adrenal insufficiency. Patients may complain of fatigue, weakness, lightheadedness. They may have orthostatic hypotension, weight loss, nausea and vomiting. The skin may become hyperpigmented with a tan or bronzed appearance. The oral mucosa may have bluish-black patches present. Secretion of the adrenal androgens will also be decreased, sometimes causing a decrease in libido. For initial diagnosis in chronic adrenal insufficiency do an 8 AM serum cortisol and plasma ACTH along with an ACTH stimulation test (should be high dose). Addison's disease should be treated with cortisol replacement therapy. Patients may also require androgen replacement therapy. With secondary adrenal insufficiency, the cause should be the focus of treatment. This could entail resection of a pituitary adenoma. Patients going off steroid therapy should be slowly weaned off the medication to prevent adrenal insufficiency. Complications include Addisonian crisis, shock, seizure, and coma.

Hypopituitary dwarfism

Hypopituitary dwarfism occurs in children who suffer from decreased production of growth hormone. Growth hormone secretion can be decreased in adults, resulting in increased fat and decreased muscle mass, but this will not affect bone growth. Children who have decreased secretion of human growth hormone, or dwarfism, will be very short in stature because of inadequate bone development. Dwarfism is categorized as a person less than 4'10" tall. These patients are more susceptible to developing sleep apnea and obesity. They may also develop arthritis, decreased flexibility of the joints, scoliosis of the spine, and bowed legs. There are no intellectual deficits associated with dwarfism. Serial measurements >2.5 deviations belows the normal mean should prompt growth hormone evaluation. Rule out other causes. Diagnosis can be confirmed by low levels of insulin-like growth factor-1 and insulin-like growth factor binding protein-3. If dwarfism is due to decreased human growth hormone, and not due to a primary skeletal disorder, the child can be treated with human growth hormone treatments to try and stimulate normal growth. Surgery may be necessary to remove a pituitary adenoma if that is the cause of the dwarfism. Complications include poorly developed organs including the heart, impaired sexual maturation, kyphosis, arthritis, sleep apnea, spinal stenosis, motor delays, ear infections, and hearing loss.

Type 2 diabetes mellitus

Diabetes mellitus is a disease of carbohydrate metabolism dysfunction. It results in impaired secretion and response to insulin. Many patients are asymptomatic. After diagnosis they may retrospectively report polyuria, polydipsia, blurred vision or weight loss. Patients with type 2 diabetes are usually obese. Often times, patients become diagnosed with type 2 diabetes after developing some of the conditions that accompany this condition, such as peripheral vascular disease, peripheral neuropathy, and retinopathy.
In a patient presenting with classic symptoms and a random blood glucose over 200 mg/dL the diagnosis can be made. In an asymptomatic patient, with fasting blood glucose >125 mg/dL, two hour glucose challenge values >200 mg/dL, and hemoglobin A1C level >6.5. Treatment includes

preventive monitoring: eye exams, foot exams, screening for coronary artery disease, screening for albumin in urine. Dietary modification, weight reduction, and exercise are the steps to slowing the progression and improving glycemic control in diabetics. Metformin therapy should be started with previously mentioned lifestyle changes at diagnosis. A1C should be rechecked at least every three months at first. If regimen is unsuccessful, add another oral or injectable medication or change to insulin. Consult endocrinologist. Complications include cardiovascular disease, neuropathy, diabetic retinopathy, nephropathy, and infections (especially of the foot).

Types of cholesterol and guidelines for lipid control

The following are types of cholesterol and guidelines for lipid control:
- Chylomicrons are the least dense particles and are rich in triglycerides.
- Very low-density lipoproteins (VLDL) are made in the liver and are rich in triglycerides.
- Low-density lipoproteins (LDL) are rich in cholesterol and are the most arthrogenic.
- High-density lipoproteins (HDL) are rich in cholesterol and are the smallest.
- Treatment goals for hyperlipidemia are based upon CAD risk. They are as follows:
- Low risk (0-1 risk factors): LDL goal is <160. Lifestyle changes should begin with LDL ≥160. Medications should be started with LDL ≥190.
- Moderate risk (2+ risk factors with 10-year risk <10%): LDL goal is <130. Lifestyle changes should begin with LDL ≥130. Medications should be started with LDL ≥160.
- Moderately high risk (2+ risk factors with 10-year risk 10-20%): LDL goal is <130. Lifestyle changes should begin with LDL ≥130. Medication should be started with LDL ≥130.
- High risk (10-year risk >20%): LDL goal is <100. Lifestyle changes should begin with LDL ≥100. Medications should be started with LDL ≥100.

Parathyroid hormone and hyperparathyroidism and hypoparathyroidism

Parathyroid hormone, or PTH, is secreted by the parathyroid glands, which set posterior to the thyroid gland. Release of PTH is controlled by the pituitary gland's secretion of parathyroid stimulating hormone. The function of PTH is to control the body's calcium and phosphorus balance. When the calcium levels are low, PTH secretion is increased; when calcium levels rise, PTH secretion is suppressed. PTH causes calcium to be released from bones into the circulating blood stream. Most commonly, an adenoma on the parathyroid glands can cause increased amounts of PTH to be released. With some types of cancer, there can be ectopic sources of parathyroid tissue that will secrete excess PTH. Multiple endocrine neoplasia syndromes can affect multiple endocrine glands, including the parathyroids, and lead to hyperparathyroidism. Accidental removal of the parathyroid glands during thyroid surgery can cause hypoparathyroidism. Hypomagnesemia can also cause there to be a decreased amount of PTH secreted by the glands. Rarely, there can be genetic causes of deficiencies in PTH secretion.

Hashimoto's thyroiditis

Hashimoto's thyroiditis is an autoimmune-mediated form of hypothyroidism. The body's immune system attacks the thyroid tissue, preventing the normal secretion of thyroid hormones. Patients may complain of symptoms of hypothyroidism, including fatigue, cold intolerance, weight gain with a decreased appetite, forgetfulness, dry skin, and a puffy face. Patients may have a goiter. Female patients may also have increased menstrual flow. Thyroid hormone levels may be normal early in the disease. The TSH level will be elevated, though, and the thyroid hormone levels will begin to decrease as the disease progresses. Anti-thyroid antibodies can also be tested to determine if this is autoimmune in etiology. Treatment includes thyroid replacement hormone therapy. TSH levels are regularly performed (measured six weeks after initiation and any changes in doing until normal levels are achieved) to measure the thyroid hormone levels and ensure that patients have reached a therapeutic dose of hormone replacement therapy. Treatment should be continued through pregnancy. Complications include Hashimoto encephalopathy, goiter, heart failure, depression, decreased libido, and myxedema.

Graves' disease

Graves' disease is an autoimmune disease with its most common feature being hyperthyroidism. Exophthalmos and pretibial myxedema are usually present with Graves' disease whereas these two symptoms are not seen with regular hyperthyroidism. Along with those symptoms, patients may complain of irritability and nervousness, heat intolerance with increased sweating, and weight loss with an increase in appetite. Patients may be tachycardic and hypertensive and atrial fibrillation is not uncommon, especially in elderly patients. Hyperreflexia may be present and patients may have a fine tremor. Alopecia may occur, or the hair may be finer in texture. A goiter may be evident. Low TSH, with high T3 and T4 confirms hyperthyroidism, but with Graves' disease usually only the T3 is elevated. The cardiac symptoms of Graves' disease can be treated with beta-blockers. Most often atenolol 25-50 mg PO QD is the starting dose, and it can be increased up to 200 mg PO QD if the blood pressure tolerates. To treat Graves's disease antithyroid drugs, radioactive iodine and thyroidectomy are all used depending on the patient. Methimazole may be given; starting dose for mild hyperthyroidism is 10 mg PO QD. Complications include dysrhythmias, osteoporosis, thyroid storm, CHF, pregnancy issues including miscarriage.

Hypothyroidism

Hypothyroidism is most commonly due to autoimmune factors, such as with Hashimoto's thyroiditis. Outside the US, a primary iodine deficiency is the most common cause of hypothyroidism. Pituitary tumors can also cause a decrease in TSH secretion, which will lead to secondary hypothyroidism. Patients may complain of fatigue and weakness with weight gain and a decreased appetite. The skin may be dry and coarse and patients may have edema of the face, hands, and feet (myxedema). There will be cold intolerance and a hoarse voice, hypertension and bradycardia, and reduced concentration and memory. Patients may describe paresthesias in the hands in a median nerve distribution. Lab results with hypothyroidism will show an elevated TSH as the pituitary gland tries to stimulate more production of the thyroid hormones. T3 and T4, the primary thyroid hormones, will be decreased. With Hashimoto's thyroiditis, thyroid antibodies will be present. Treatment includes thyroid replacement hormone and careful monitoring of the thyroid hormone levels to reach therapeutic dosage. Complications include goiter, depression, weight gain, infertility, myxedema, birth defects, neuropathy, high cholesterol, and heart failure.

Thyroid storm

A thyroid storm is very rare, but can be life-threatening. It is a situation in which the thyroid secretes a massive amount of thyroid hormones at one time, causing an acute state of hyperthyroidism. This can be due to a tumor, excessive manipulation during surgery, infection or trauma. Those who take excessive doses of thyroid hormone can also have symptoms of thyroid storm. Signs and symptoms include CHF, cardiac arrhythmias, or hyperthermia. On a milder level, patients may develop a fever, vomiting and diarrhea, or disorientation and delirium. This can progress to the point of seizures or coma. A patient presenting with symptoms of thyroid storm should have a thyroid panel done. The degree of the hyperthyroidism in patients is normally comparable to a patient with hyperthyroidism without major complications, therefore lab levels and clinical picture are considered. Beta-blockers should be given to treat increased adrenergic tone, thionamide to stop new thyroid hormones from being made, iodine to stop the release of thyroid hormone, radioactive iodine to stop the conversion of T4 to T3, bile acid sequestrants to slow liver recycling of hormones, and glucocorticoids to decrease T4 to T3 conversion (this also assists with adrenal insufficiency). Complications include hypotension, shock, coma, and death.

Cushing's syndrome

Cushing's syndrome results when cortisol levels are increased. Most commonly, this is due to steroid treatment with prednisone. A pituitary adenoma that causes excess amounts of adrenocorticotropic hormone (ACTH) will lead to elevated cortisol. A primary tumor of the adrenal gland may cause Cushing's due to increased cortisol secretion. Other forms of cancer can present with ectopic sources of ACTH secretion. Patients will develop proximal muscle weakness and atrophy with an obtunded abdomen. Purple striae will develop across the abdomen. The face will be rounded ("moon face"), and fat deposition can occur across the upper back ("buffalo hump"). Patients will bruise easily and may have non-healing sores. Osteoporosis can occur, as can pathologic fractures. Glucose levels can be elevated, and patients may require insulin. For diagnosis a patient should have at least two abnormal test results of the following: daily urinary cortisol excretion, low dose dexamethasone suppression tests, late evening salivary cortisol, late evening serum cortisol. Discover and treat the cause. Patients should be weaned off prednisone if possible. Removal of a pituitary adenoma can decrease ACTH production. Removal of an adrenal adenoma or other ectopic source of hormone secretion can decrease cortisol levels.

Subacute thyroiditis

Most commonly, subacute thyroiditis is caused by a viral infection with coxsackie, mumps, influenza, or adenovirus. Patients will have a painful, tender, asymmetrically enlarged thyroid gland. They may remember having symptoms of an upper respiratory infection before the thyroid symptoms began. In addition to the localized tenderness, patients may describe symptoms of either hyper- or hypothyroidism. Usually, patients are initially in a hyperthyroid state, followed by a period of hypothyroidism, and then returning to a euthyroid state. Lab tests will show an elevated WBC and sedimentation rate. Thyroid antibodies will be negative with this condition because it is not immune-mediated. A thyroid panel and a thyroid biopsy may be done. Patients are treated with NSAIDs, aspirin, or steroids to decrease the inflammation within the thyroid gland. Antibiotics do not have a role here because of the condition's viral etiology. The TSH and T4 levels should be monitored for resolution of subacute thyroiditis as this can take several months. Around 95% of cases will resolve on their own without complication in a year and a half. In the other cases, hypothyroidism will be permanent.

Acromegaly

Acromegaly occurs in adults who suffer from excessive production of human growth hormone, usually due to a pituitary adenoma. It can also occur in athletes who treat themselves with high doses of the hormone. In children, human growth hormone helps with bone growth and development. In adulthood, the epiphyseal plates are closed and the bones are no longer able to grow. With excess human growth hormone, more calcium is laid down on the bone, causing enlargement of the bones. GH and IGF-I are helpful in diagnosis. Growth hormone supresion testing for definitive diagnosis. MRI is used to check for pituitary tumors. Signs and symptoms include prominent forehead and jawbones, large hands and feet, and arthritis in the spine. Patients may develop left ventricular hypertrophy, CHF, hypertension, and cardiac arrhythmias. Treatment is aimed at treating the cause. Removal of a pituitary adenoma will decrease or stop the production of human growth hormone. Athletes who use human growth hormone should be urged to discontinue use because of the potential health risks. Complications include diabetes, hypertension, cardiomyopathy, osteoarthritis, sleep apnea, carpal tunnel syndrome, spinal cord compression, uterine fibroids, and polyps in the colon.

Diabetes insipidus

Diabetes insipidus (DI) results from resistance to the effects of ADH by the kidney. DI can occur because of increased levels of ADH, or vasopressin, damage to the hypothalamus gland where ADH is produced, damage to the pituitary gland where ADH is stored, or primary kidney damage that prevents the kidneys from functioning properly. Signs and symptoms include increased urinary output with poorly concentrated urine, along with extreme thirst. The patient presents with dehydration, hypernatremia, and low levels of ADH. After clinical assessment leads to suspicions of DI, diagnosis is confirmed by water restriction testing. If water restriction testing results are uncertain, give exogenous ADH if plasma osmolality or sodium indicate it. In infants and patients on long term lithium, test for a lack of response to desmopressin instead of water restriction testing. A low solute diet and DDAVP (intranasally 5-20 mcg QD or 0.1 to 0.8 mg PO QD) are treatments of choice for central diabetes insipidus. Hypothalamic tumors can be surgically removed or debulked, if possible. With primary kidney disease, medications should be given to decrease urinary output and prevention dehydration. High-dose anti-inflammatory drugs and diuretics, such as HCTZ, may be helpful. Electrolyte imbalances and dehydration may cause many symptoms including hypotension, tachycardia, and dysrhythmias.

Types of insulin to control glucose levels with type 1 diabetes mellitus

The different types of insulin available for controlling glucose levels with type 1 diabetes mellitus are explained below:
- Rapid-acting (Lispro®/Aspart®)
  - Onset of Action: 5-15 minutes
  - Peak Action: 1-2 hours
  - Duration of Action: 4-6 hours
- Short-acting (Regular insulin)
  - Onset of Action: 30-60 minutes
  - Peak Action: 2-4 hours
  - Duration of Action: 4-10 hours
- Intermediate-acting (NPH insulin)
  - Onset of Action: 1-2 hours
  - Peak Action: 4-8 hours
  - Duration of Action: 10-20 hours
- Long-acting (Glargine®)
  - Onset of Action: 1-2 hours
  - Peak Action: No peak
  - Duration of Action: Approx. 24 hours

Type 1 diabetes mellitus

Type 1, insulin-dependent, diabetes mellitus is autoimmune in nature with effects in the islet cells in the pancreas, which cause decreased insulin production. Diabetes mellitus is usually diagnosed early in life, before age 30, and symptoms may come on fairly suddenly. There is <20% chance of family history with this form of diabetes, but a concordance rate in twins. Patients with type 1 diabetes mellitus will, classically, have symptoms of polyuria and polydipsia. Children may develop bedwetting. There will be weight loss even though patients are eating more, and patients will complain of weakness and fatigue. Diagnosis may be made when patients presents with ketoacidosis or some of the retinal, neurologic, or vascular conditions that accompany diabetes. Diagnosis is made when fasting blood glucose levels are >126 on two separate occasions, when a 2-hour GTT is >200 on two separate occasions, or when random blood glucose levels are >200 on two separate occasions and symptoms of diabetes are present.

Oral medications to control glucose levels with type 2 diabetes mellitus

There are a number of medications to control glucose levels for type 2 diabetes mellitus:
- Insulin secretagogues – This class of drugs is best utilized in patients who were diagnosed within the last few years. They can decrease the Hgb A1C level by 1-2 points. They should be avoided in renal failure. Side effects include weight gain and hypoglycemia.
- Metformin – This medication is best used in obese patients with insulin resistance. It can decrease the Hgb A1C by 1-2 points. It should be avoided in liver or renal disease, in those with CHF, and before receiving IV contrast. Side effects include nausea, vomiting, diarrhea, and lactic acidosis.
- Glitazones – This class of drugs is best used in obese patients with insulin resistance. It can decrease the Hgb A1C by 0.5-1.5 points. It should be avoided in liver disease and CHF. Side effects include edema, weight gain, anemia, and hepatotoxicity.
- A-glucosidase inhibitors – This class of drugs is best given after meals when glucose levels are highest. It can decrease the Hgb A1C by 0.5-1 points. It should be avoided in intestinal or liver disease. Side effects include flatulence.

Treatments to control cholesterol levels

There are a number of medical treatments available to control cholesterol levels:
- Niacin can decrease LDL by 15-25%, can increase HDL by 25-35%, and is very effective at decreasing triglycerides. Side effects include flushing, itching, gout, and peptic ulcers.
- Bile acid-binding resins can decrease LDL by 15-25%, can increase HDL by 5%, and may or may not be helpful with decreasing triglycerides. Side effects include constipation, gas, and decreased fat-soluble vitamin and drug absorption.
- Statins can decrease LDL by 25-50%, increase HDL by 5-15%, and may be quite helpful at decreasing triglycerides. Side effects include myalgias, myositis, and increased liver enzymes.
- Fibrates can decrease LDL by 10-15%, can increase HDL by 15-20%, and are very effective at decreasing triglycerides. Side effects include myalgias, myositis, hepatitis, and gall stones.
- Ezetimibe can decrease LDL by 20%, can increase HDL by 5%, and may or may not be helpful with decreasing triglycerides. Side effects include increased liver enzymes when used in conjunction with a statin.

Gastrointestinal System/Nutrition

Esophagitis

When the lower esophageal sphincter becomes lax and does not remain closed properly, the stomach acids can reflux into the esophagus. This causes inflammation in the esophagus, known as esophagitis, eventually leading to ulceration of the mucous membranes lining the esophagus. Patients will complain of GERD-type symptoms with a burning or bad taste in the throat, pain over the chest into the throat, and possibly a mild cough. They may experience nausea and vomiting. If esophageal ulceration occurs, patients will have severe pain over the chest, worsening with eating. If the ulcer is bleeding, vomiting of blood may occur or the stools may become very dark and tarry. If severe, patients may become anemic due to blood loss. Treatment involves lifestyle modifications. These include diet changes to avoid spicy foods, fried foods, and caffeine. Alcohol should be avoided. If patients smoke, they should quit. A histamine 2 receptor agonist or proton pump inhibitor (depending on severity and if the esophagitis is erosive) is given to decrease the acid production in the stomach. Erosive esophagitis leading to bleeding is a possible complication.

Esophageal stricture

Damage to the lower esophageal sphincter, either from gastric reflux or some cancers, can cause scarring of the tissue. This scarring can cause the sphincter to be narrowed, which prevents food and fluids from passing into the stomach appropriately. Patients will complain of difficulty swallowing and a sensation that food is "stuck" in their throat. They may have chest pain and a full feeling. Vomiting can occur if food will not pass into the stomach, especially larger pieces of food. Treatment of an esophageal stricture involves dilating the sphincter to widen it. This can be accomplished during an EGD by passing dilators, which gradually increase in diameter, through the sphincter. A balloon procedure can also be performed during EGD to widen the sphincter. A risk with both of these procedures is tearing of the esophagus, requiring surgical repair. If these treatments fail to relieve the symptoms, surgery may be needed to correct the sphincter.

Mallory-Weiss tear

A Mallory-Weiss tear is a laceration of the esophageal mucosa that occurs in the distal portion of the esophagus, near where the esophagus meets the stomach. The tear can be caused by forceful, long-term vomiting or coughing. Patients will describe an episode of forceful vomiting or coughing followed by vomiting of bright red blood. If this has been going on for a period of time, they may have experienced bloody stools. A past history of a Mallory-Weiss tear may cause a patient to have recurrent incidents of this condition.
Most tears do not need to be surgically corrected. An esophagogastroduodenoscopy (EGD) will be done to confirm diagnosis, and cauterization may be performed if the bleeding has gone on for more than a few hours. Antacids can be given to prevent further irritation of the tear. If there has been significant blood loss, a transfusion may be necessary to correct a volume-depletion anemia.

Esophageal varices

Esophageal varices almost always occur along with cirrhosis of the liver, but any form of liver disease can lead to their development. With liver disease, blood flow through the organ is obstructed and slowed. This causes portal hypertension, which leads to pressure building in the vessels leading to the organ, and can affect vessels in the esophagus, causing swelling and the formation of varicose veins surrounding the esophagus. Patients are usually asymptomatic from the esophageal varices themselves but will show signs of liver disease. They may have a history of alcoholism, though not all forms of cirrhosis are caused by alcohol. Other known liver disease may also be present. Antihypertensives may be given to prevent rupture of the varices, a usually-fatal situation. Anticoagulant medications can be injected into the varices and rubber bands can also be placed around them to prevent rupture. Once rupture occurs, emergency surgery can be performed to try and cauterize the bleeding, but this is usually a futile effort.

Peptic ulcer disease

Peptic ulcer disease occurs in the stomach or duodenum and has several causes. Infection with *H. pylori* bacteria can lead to ulcers. Excessive acid production in the stomach due to a tumor can also break down the gastric mucosa and cause ulcers. The most common cause of peptic ulcer disease is the use of anti-inflammatory medications, like ibuprofen and naproxen. Aspirin use can be caustic to the stomach and cause ulcers. Patients will complain of abdominal pain. The pain may be relieved with eating as food coats the stomach, though spicy foods can aggravate the pain. Patients may feel bloated and have nausea and vomiting. With bleeding of the ulcer, stools may be tarry, and there may be blood in vomitus. Treatment is focused on treating the cause. NSAIDs should be stopped if this is the cause. Infection with *H. pylori* should be treated with a combination of antibiotics and an antacid. Dietary changes to reduce acid secretion are recommended. Surgery is necessary if the ulcer has perforated.

Gastric cancer

Gastric cancer can be caused by infection with the *H. pylori* bacteria. This infection causes chronic inflammation in the gastric mucosa, leading to development of cancerous cells in the stomach lining. Eating a diet high in smoked and pickled foods that are high in nitrates may also cause changes in the gastric lining, leading to cancer. Smoking and alcohol use may also play a role in the development of gastric cancer. Most patients are not aware they have stomach cancer until the disease has progressed to an advanced stage. Most symptoms are similar to GERD-type symptoms and treated at home with antacids. Other symptoms include abdominal pain not relieved by antacids, unintentional weight loss, chronic feeling of fullness, and tarry stools if bleeding is occurring. Patients may develop a blockage within the stomach with a large tumor that prevents them from eating. Treatment is with surgical removal of the malignant tissue. Radiation and chemotherapy may be necessary.

Cholecystitis

Cholecystitis is an inflammatory condition of the gallbladder, occurring because bile builds up in the organ, leading to inflammation, swelling, and infection. The bile normally passes from the gallbladder to the small intestine to aid in digestion, but there is a disruption in this flow with cholecystitis. Usually this disruption is due to gallstones. Cholecystitis is more likely to occur in females than males, and patients are frequently overweight. Patients will develop severe abdominal pain that is often present after eating a fatty meal. This pain is often aggravated with taking a deep breath. There may be bloating, nausea, and vomiting present. Oftentimes patients will complain of referred right shoulder pain. Abdominal ultrasound will often reveal gallstones, though a CT scan may be necessary. Treatment is with a cholecystectomy, usually done laparoscopically when possible. Some patients may have occasional flare-ups of cholecystitis that resolve spontaneously.

Pyloric stenosis

Pyloric stenosis occurs in infants when the pylorus, or opening between the stomach and duodenum, becomes enlarged. This prevents the transport of food from the stomach to the small intestine. Though there is no definite known cause, it is thought it may be genetic in nature. It is also thought that this condition develops after birth and not *in utero*.
The infant will have gradually worsening vomiting after meals. Projectile vomiting is not uncommon, and the child will act fussy and hungry even after eating. Constipation is common, and dehydration will eventually develop. The infant will also show a slower degree of weight gain and may begin losing weight. On exam, an olive-shaped mass can be palpated in the abdomen due to the enlarged pylorus. Treatment is by surgical correction of the pyloric sphincter. This is usually a very successful surgery that results in full recovery from the condition.

Hepatitis A, B, and C

Hepatitis A is a viral infection of the liver that is transmitted through the fecal-oral route by infected individuals and can be contracted through contaminated food and water, especially raw shellfish. It causes abdominal pain, nausea and vomiting, and jaundice. Arthritis may also develop. Symptoms generally resolve spontaneously within 2 months. Hepatitis B is a blood-borne viral infection and is contracted through contact with blood and body fluids of infected individuals. It causes abdominal pain, nausea and vomiting, jaundice, and may lead to liver failure. Treatment is usually limited to symptomatic control and the condition usually resolves on its own. Chronic conditions are treated with interferon or lamivudine. Hepatitis C is also contracted through blood and body fluids. It is the most serious form of viral hepatitis and is the leading cause of liver transplants. The symptoms are the same as the other forms of viral hepatitis, though liver failure or liver cancer can develop. Treatment is generally with pegylated interferon and ribavirin.

Cholelithiasis

Cholelithiasis is the development of gallstones from cholesterol and other fatty byproducts within the gallbladder. These can block the ducts leading from the gallbladder, causing cholecystitis. Symptoms can vary depending on which duct is blocked by the stone. Ducts leading to the pancreas can cause acute pancreatitis with severe abdominal pain and vomiting. Blockage of ducts leading to the liver can result in jaundice. Generally, patients will experience nausea and vomiting, abdominal pain that may refer to the right shoulder, and bloating. Patients may have several flare-ups of pain from the gallstones and may hold off on having surgery. Some patients can have gallstones and be asymptomatic. Patients who do not undergo surgery for correction of this condition should be advised to avoid fatty foods that can aggravate the problem and contribute to enlargement of the gallstones or development of new stones. Cholecystectomy to remove the gallbladder and stones and removal of a stone from a duct may be necessary.

Pancreatitis

The most common cause of pancreatitis is excessive alcohol consumption, in both binge drinkers and chronic alcoholics. Pancreatitis can also occur from cholelithiasis and associated duct blockage. Some autoimmune disorders, such as cystic fibrosis, can also leave patients susceptible to pancreatitis. High triglyceride levels can cause a patient to be more susceptible to developing pancreatitis. Symptoms include severe abdominal pain that radiates into the back. Patients may have intractable vomiting. Electrolyte imbalances can develop due to the lack of digestive enzymes in the stomach. Treatment of pancreatitis is mostly symptomatic. Patients should be NPO, and tube feedings though a nasogastric tube may be necessary. This allows the pancreas to rest and heal. IV fluids and correction of electrolyte imbalances are necessary. Sometimes the damage to the pancreas is severe enough to warrant surgical resection of a portion of the organ. Patients may go on to develop a chronic form of the disease.

Diverticulitis

Diverticula are outpouchings in the large intestine that commonly develop during the aging process. This is due to weakening of the intestinal walls with decreased smooth muscle integrity. Diverticulitis occurs when digestive matter becomes trapped within these outpouchings, leading to swelling, inflammation, and infection. Diverticula can rupture if the condition becomes severe. Patients will generally complain of left lower abdominal pain. Patients may complain of bloating and gas with diarrhea. Nausea and vomiting may be present, along with fever. Diverticulitis is generally treated with IV fluids and antibiotics. Patients should be kept NPO and receive feedings through a nasogastric tube. Patients will need to make some dietary changes and avoid small particulate matter in the diet, such as foods with seeds (sesame seeds, berry seeds, etc.) and popcorn. Diverticulitis usually resolves without surgery, but resection of the affected portion of the intestine may be necessary in severe cases.

Appendicitis

Appendicitis occurs due to blockage and inflammation of the appendix from feces or a foreign body. Certain forms of cancer can also cause inflammation of the organ. Blockage of the appendix will lead to swelling, inflammation, infection, and abscess formation. Appendicitis should be surgically treated immediately to prevent eventual rupture of the organ and subsequent peritonitis. Patients will complain of periumbilical pain that gradually worsens and eventually migrates to the right lower abdomen. Nausea and vomiting are usually present early on. Fever may also be present. A CT scan or ultrasound may show an enlarged appendix. The WBC will be elevated, possibly up to 15,000. If the diagnosis is not confirmed with CT or ultrasound, but other possible diseases that could cause patients' symptoms have been ruled out, the organ is still usually removed to prevent the potential rupture of the appendix. The appendectomy can usually be performed laparoscopically.

Irritable bowel syndrome

Irritable bowel syndrome (IBS) is very common and may affect up to 20% of Americans. It usually occurs in response to stressors, either psychological or physical, and can be severe enough to be debilitating. Patients will complain of intermittent periods of bloating, painful gas, and alternating diarrhea and constipation. Some patients may have predominantly diarrhea or constipation while others alternate between the two. A pattern of symptoms may be discernible after people eat certain foods or during periods of stress. Chronic illness may also cause IBS and lead to flare-ups of the condition. Fiber supplements to bulk the stool can help with the constipation while antidiarrheals may help with the diarrhea. Avoiding the triggering factors that lead to flare-ups can also help control symptoms. If chronic illness is the cause, managing the illness to prevent episodes of IBS can be helpful. There is research being conducted on medications specifically formulated to treat the symptoms of IBS.

Intussusception

Intussusception is a telescoping of the small intestine or colon that causes blood flow to be blocked and prevents the movement of food and feces through the bowel. It usually occurs in children, rarely in adults, and there is usually no known cause. Children will have nausea, vomiting, and fever. They may have diarrhea with "currant jelly" stools because of the frank blood that is present. There will be abdominal pain that may be severe, but it can be intermittent. On exam, there may be a palpable mass in the abdomen and abdominal tenderness. Treatment of intussusception is usually successful with a barium or air enema. This forces the bowel to straighten and slides the telescoped portion of the bowel back to normal. If there is damaged or dead tissue, surgery may be necessary to resect the ischemic portion of bowel. Most children recover well after treatment without recurrence of the condition.

Crohn's disease

Crohn's disease is an inflammatory condition that can affect any portion of the digestive tract, from the mouth to the anus. It causes breaks in the mucosal lining of the tract, and patients may experience periods of remission during which the symptoms are not present. The cause of Crohn's disease is not known, but it is thought to be due to a bacterial infection, an autoimmune response, or possibly genetic factors. Patients with Crohn's disease will complain of abdominal pain with or without fever and poor appetite. There may be evident weight loss with the disease. Patients frequently have diarrhea, possibly with blood present. Because Crohn's disease can occur at any point in the digestive tract, symptoms may be more focused on a particular area, such as the mouth or anus. There is no cure for Crohn's disease. Treatment is symptomatic with the goal being to reduce inflammation within the digestive tract. This can be accomplished with anti-inflammatory drugs, possibly steroids, and antibiotics.

Ulcerative colitis

Ulcerative colitis is an inflammatory disease that affects the mucous membranes lining the rectum and large intestine. The cause of ulcerative colitis is not clearly understood, but it is thought that to be immune-mediated due to infection with a virus or bacteria. There is a genetic-tendency for the disease, also. Ulcerative colitis is not caused by stress though this can aggravate the symptoms of ulcerative colitis. Patients will complain of abdominal pain with diarrhea. There may be obvious blood in the stool. Many people experience a spasm of the rectum, causing an urge to defecate but inability to do so. Treatment is with anti-inflammatory drugs and sometimes short-term steroids to help control the inflammation within the colon. There are immunosuppressant medications available that will help suppress flare-ups of the condition. Antidiarrheals and pain relievers may also be helpful. If mucosal damage is severe, surgery may be necessary to resect the damaged portion of the large intestine.

Toxic megacolon

Toxic megacolon usually occurs in those patients who suffer from inflammatory bowel disease. It results in a distended colon and can be a life-threatening condition. Patients may complain of abdominal distention and pain, with or without fever. Toxic megacolon can progress to the development of shock symptoms. Patients may appear dehydrated and have a rapid heart rate. Abdominal x-rays will show the dilated colon. WBC may be elevated and potassium may be decreased if patients are dehydrated. The colon is rested for 24 hours to try and reduce the distention. If this is not affective, surgery is usually done to resect that section of the colon. This condition can lead to shock and death, so prompt treatment is necessary. Patients should be hydrated with IV fluids and any electrolyte imbalances should be corrected. Steroids may be given to reduce inflammation within the organ and antibiotics will be useful if patients become septic.

Bowel obstruction

A bowel obstruction can be caused by improper function of the organ or by mechanical obstruction. An ileus is not caused by mechanical obstruction. It can be due to medications, infection, ischemia, injury, or manipulation during surgery. Mechanical obstruction of the bowel can occur from tumors, adhesions, hernias, or impacted stool. Patients will complain of abdominal pain and cramping in the absence of regular bowel movements or gas. They may have vomiting and a full, bloated feeling. On exam, bowel sounds may be high-pitched or tingling in nature early on, but eventually there will be absent bowel sounds. Treatment involves resting the bowel. A nasogastric tube will be inserted and set to low suction to decompress the gut. This often improves patients' sensations of bloating and stops the vomiting. If the condition is severe, a portion of bowel may need to be resected, especially if blood flow is compromised or if a severe infection develops.

Anorectal abscess

An anorectal abscess, or infection in the anal or rectal areas, can have several causes. An anal fissure can become infected, or an anal gland can become blocked, leading to abscess formation. Anal sexual intercourse can also place a patient at risk for developing an anorectal abscess. An anorectal abscess will cause patients significant pain with the development of an indurated, inflamed area near the anus. This may feel like a hard, hot lump at the edge of the anus. Patients may have very painful bowel movements or may develop constipation because of the fear of having a bowel movement. If the abscess ruptures, pus may be discharged through the rectum. Diagnosis is made per clinical assessment. The abscess will need to be drained and if it is deep or very extensive, surgery may be necessary. Sitz baths can help with some of the inflammation, and antibiotics will be necessary to help cure the infection.

Anal fissure

An anal fissure is a small tear in the tissue surrounding the anal sphincter. It is caused by excessive stretching of the anal sphincter, as with a large bowel movement. Patients will complain of pain at the anus, especially with bowel movements. They may have noticed bright red blood in their stool or on toilet paper following a bowel movement. There may also be a history of constipation present. A rectal exam will be extremely painful for these patients. The anal sphincter should be visually assessed to identify the anal fissure. Anal fissures usually resolve without treatment. If the fissures are very painful, Sitz baths may be soothing. A topical anesthetic can be used if the pain is preventing patients from having a bowel movement. To prevent recurrence, stool softeners and a diet high in fiber and fluids should be recommended to keep bowel movements regular and prevent constipation.

Pilonidal cyst

A pilonidal cyst is a cyst that forms at the base of the coccyx and becomes infected. It occurs at the superior end of the cleft between the buttocks. Pilonidal cysts occur in equal numbers of men and women. Some believe that a pilonidal cyst occurs due to ingrown hair in the region. Another theory is that it may be due to repeated trauma in the sacral and coccyx area. The cyst will form like a typical abscess with a red, indurated area at the base of the spine. Patients may or may not have a fever, but the cyst will be painful. If it opens, pus will drain from the cyst. Diagnosis is made per clinical assessment. As initial treatment, warm Sitz baths may help to prevent abscess formation. If an abscess does continue to develop, antibiotics may be given to resolve the infection. If this is not effective, surgical incision and drainage will be necessary, followed by oral antibiotics.

Hemorrhoids

Hemorrhoids occur when the veins surrounding the anus and rectum become engorged and swollen. Hemorrhoids commonly occur with excessive straining with a bowel movement, such as when constipated, and during pregnancy because of the increased pressure applied to the pelvic floor. Hemorrhoids can also occur as a result of anal sexual intercourse and as part of the aging process. Hemorrhoids can be internal or external. Internal hemorrhoids can bleed and will cause patients to have bright red blood on the toilet paper after a bowel movement. If hemorrhoids protrude through the anus, they will be painful. Diagnosis is made per clinical exam-external hemorrhoids are visibly noticeable and occur on the outside of the anus. They are painful and may itch or bleed. Most hemorrhoids will resolve without treatment, but topical ointments are available to help relieve the swelling and pain. Sitz baths can also help to relieve the inflammation. If severe or recurrent, surgery may be necessary to remove the hemorrhoids.

Niacin and niacin deficiency

A niacin, or vitamin B_3, deficiency can lead to a condition called pellagra. This can occur due to malnutrition with a lack of niacin in the diet, or because of a malabsorption syndrome that prevents the body from absorbing niacin. The "3 D's" can occur with advanced pellagra:
- Dementia.
- Diarrhea.
- Dermatitis.

Patients may experience weakness and have obvious signs of malnutrition, such as weight loss. Excoriations and signs of inflammation can be present on the skin. Patients may be irritable or short-tempered before the dementia becomes evident. Treatment of a niacin deficiency involves replacing the niacin so patients have normal serum levels of the vitamin. If malabsorption is the cause of the deficiency, measures should be taken to correct this condition if possible. Carcinoid or other gastric tumors may cause obstruction that prevents absorption of the niacin, and these should be surgically removed, if possible, to allow absorption.

Hernias

Hiatal hernias occur when the upper segment of the stomach protrudes through the diaphragm, causing a telescoping affect around the distal esophagus. Incisional hernias occur at the site of an abdominal surgical incision and result in a portion of bowel protruding through the abdominal wall. Inguinal hernias occur in the groin through a weakened portion of the inguinal canal. Umbilical hernias occur at the umbilicus due to a weakened area of the abdominal fascia, causing the bowel to protrude through the umbilical opening. Ventral hernias can occur anywhere there is a weakened area in the abdominal wall; they cause a section of bowel to protrude through the opening. Hernias are treated surgically. Hiatal hernias may require a Nissan fundoplication procedure in which the lower esophagus is reinforced with mesh to strengthen the area surrounding it, preventing the stomach from extending up around the esophagus. All other hernias are repaired by weaving a mesh material at the site of the weakened area to strengthen the wall.

Riboflavin and riboflavin deficiency

Riboflavin, or vitamin B_2, is a water-soluble vitamin. It is necessary for normal cell growth, development, and energy production. Riboflavin also helps in red blood cell production. A deficiency in riboflavin may be due to malnutrition, though this is rare in industrialized countries. It can also be caused by a malabsorption syndrome that prevents riboflavin from being absorbed. Symptoms of riboflavin deficiency include swelling of the mucous membranes, sore throat, and canker sores on the lips or in the mouth. Dermatitis may develop without adequate levels of riboflavin, as can certain types of anemia. If due to malnutrition, obvious muscle wasting and weight loss will be evident. Treatment is by replacement with riboflavin. If there is an underlying malabsorption disorder causing the deficiency, then this should be treated if possible. Riboflavin is excreted from the body through urine. There are no known cases of poisoning by riboflavin from taking excess supplements or by consuming too many foods high in riboflavin.

Vitamin A and vitamin A deficiency

Vitamin A is a fat-soluble vitamin and is helpful in boosting the immune system as well as help with maintaining bone and teeth integrity. Vitamin A helps to keep the eyes healthy and makes night vision possible. It is thought that vitamin A may help to prevent some forms of cancer. A primary vitamin A deficiency can be due to malnutrition and is rare in developed countries. Malabsorption systems that prevent absorption of fats may prevent absorption of vitamin A. Deficiency in vitamin A can lead to diarrhea, infection, respiratory disorders, night blindness and eventual complete blindness. Skin disorders can also occur with a lack of vitamin A. Vitamin A deficiency is treated by giving supplemental vitamin A. If a malabsorption syndrome is the cause of the deficiency, this should be corrected if possible. Disorders that disrupt the absorption of fat, necessary for vitamin A absorption, should be treated if possible.

Vitamin D and vitamin D deficiency

Vitamin D is a fat-soluble vitamin that plays a vital role in calcium absorption into the bones to provide healthy, strong teeth and bones. Vitamin D is readily found in dairy products and fish. A deficiency of vitamin D leads to a condition called rickets in children and osteoporosis in adults. Rickets will produce a bowing of the legs of children because of bone softening. Bone growth will also be stifled without vitamin D. Osteoporosis in adults places these individuals at higher risk of developing a compression fracture or large bone fracture because of brittle bones. Vitamin D supplements are available, often combined with calcium, for those who require extra doses of the vitamin. Increasing dairy products and fortified foods in the diet will also increase vitamin D intake. Vitamin D is known as the "sunshine vitamin" and is produced within the skin after exposure to sunlight. Daily sun exposure (15-20 minutes) can help increase a person's vitamin D level.

Vitamin C and vitamin C deficiency

Vitamin C is a vital substance that all humans need to prevent illness. It is responsible for the proper formation of blood vessels and is useful in wound healing. It is also necessary for cartilage formation. A deficiency in vitamin C causes an illness known as scurvy. Historically, this was seen in those who were at sea for extended periods of time and did not have access to foods rich in vitamin C. Scurvy causes discoloration of the skin, similar to liver spots. It also causes breakdown of collagen and some connective tissues, leading to tooth loss and immobility. The skin can easily break down and form ulcerative wounds if a person does not have adequate vitamin C intake, and this can eventually lead to death.

Treatment of a vitamin C deficiency requires dietary changes that increase a person's consumption of foods rich in vitamin C, such as citrus fruit. Supplements are also available to help with replacement of the vitamin.

Lactose intolerance

Lactose intolerance develops in those individuals who are lacking in the enzyme lactase, which breaks down the sugar in milk. There are no known specific causes for lactose intolerance. Patients will complain of bloating or abdominal pain shortly after eating dairy foods. There can also be cramping diarrhea, which is very common, along with nausea. Patients may have painful gas. Diagnosis of true lactose intolerance can be done in a few different ways. Patients can be tested after fasting overnight and given a dairy-rich drink. The blood is then measured over two hours to assess glucose levels. If the glucose levels remain low, there is a deficiency in lactase. Another test is by giving a lactose-rich drink to patients and the measure hydrogen levels in the breath. These should remain low, but will be elevated with lactose intolerance. Treatment is with dietary changes to avoid lactose-rich foods and beverages. Calcium supplementation may be necessary to ensure patients are receiving adequate amounts.

Vitamin K and vitamin K deficiency

Vitamin K is a fat-soluble vitamin that is found in abundant supply in green, leafy vegetables. It plays a vital role in the clotting cascade to prevent excessive bleeding. A deficiency in vitamin K is very rare, but it can be seen in those individuals with a form of malabsorption syndrome that prevents that absorption of fats from the GI tract. This will lead to a decrease in the amount of vitamin K that is absorbed from foods. The blood thinning drug warfarin (Coumadin®) blocks the function of vitamin K in the clotting cascade, which promotes bleeding and a decreased clotting time. Treatment of a vitamin K deficiency can be reversed with injectable vitamin K. This is also given to infants shortly after birth to help prevent excessive bleeding. A malabsorption syndrome that prevents absorption of fats from the digestive tract should be treated, if possible, to prevent the malabsorption of vitamin K.

Phenylketonuria

Phenylketonuria, or PKU, is a disorder in which an infant is not able to digest phenylalanine, a protein found in most foods. This causes phenylalanine to accumulate in the bloodstream and leads to severe brain damage and mental retardation. Screening is done nationwide at birth to identify infants suffering from this condition. Patients who do have PKU may have lighter skin and hair because phenylalanine helps to produce melanin in the body. These children will be developmentally delayed and show signs of mental retardation. They are more likely to suffer from a seizure disorder, jerky movements, and hyperactivity. PKU is diagnosed by an elevated serum phenylalanine, or by identifying PAH mutations by molecular analysis for prenatal diagnosis. PKU can be treated, but early identification is necessary. All children should be tested at birth for the presence of PKU. If PKU is diagnosed, a diet very low in phenylalanine should be strictly followed. If this is adhered to, mental retardation can be mild and there may be minimal impairment in function. If this diet is not closely followed, mental retardation will result.

Genitourinary System

Benign prostatic hyperplasia

Benign prostatic hyperplasia, or BPH, is a benign enlargement of the prostate gland. There is no definite known cause though it may be familial. Whenever there is a change in the size of the prostate gland, a complete assessment should be done to ensure it is not cause by a malignancy. Patients will complain of urinary frequency or urgency. Oftentimes they may have to urinate frequently, but only in small amounts. There may also be dribbling present at the end of the urinary stream and a decrease in the force of the urinary stream. Patients may have recurrent urinary tract infections. The prostate gland will feel smooth and enlarged on rectal exam, and the PSA is mildly elevated. It is important that other diagnosis be ruled out, especially carcinomas, stricture, infections, and contractures. A combination of history, physical and labs are used to make diagnosis. All men with BPH should be advised on the following behavioral modifications: reduce alcohol and caffeine, avoid fluid before bedtime or certain activities, and practice double voiding to more fully empty the bladder. Medications that help slow the growth of the prostate include Flomax® or Hytrin®. If symptoms of upper urinary tract injury develop, surgery may be necessary to remove a portion of the prostate.

Hydrocele

A hydrocele is a collection of fluid in the scrotum, surrounding the testicles. This is most common in infant boys and usually absorbs within the first year of life. Occasionally, the fluid does not absorb because the fluid is not able to flow back into the abdomen. A hydrocele can also occur in adult males, usually over 40, due to an injury or infection. Patients do not usually have any pain in the scrotum when a hydrocele is present. Pain will be present if an infection is the cause, or if there has been an injury to the scrotum. The main concern patients will have is of the enlargement of the scrotum. To help differentiate hydrocele from hernia, a mass, or a hematocele, the hydrocele will make the scrotal sac transilluminate due to the fluid. Ultrasound can be used if needed as well. Most of the time, a hydrocele will resolve spontaneously. Rarely, surgery may be necessary to remove the hydrocele from the scrotum. A fine needle aspiration can also be done to drain the fluid from the scrotum.

Cryptorchidism

Cryptorchidism occurs when one or both of the testicles fail to descend into the scrotum. This can be due to prematurity, low birth weight, or hormone balance abnormalities. In most boys, the testes will descend within the first 3 months of life. Cryptorchidism resolves in most infants by the first birthday, but about 1% of infants will not have resolution. The absence of one or more testes from the scrotum is a sign of cryptorchidism. The initial newborn exam includes palpating the scrotum to feel that both testes are there. They may be palpable a little further up the inguinal canal on one or both sides. Repeated checks should be done at follow-up visits to ensure the testicles descend. Some will descend spontaneously in the first three to four months, but if they are not descended by 6 months of age, surgical intervention will be needed as it is very unlikely for them to spontaneously descend after that time. Surgery may be performed to force the testes to descend into the scrotum. Hormonal treatments with HCG may be helpful to naturally cause them to descend. Complications include testicular torsion, infertility, testicular cancer, and inguinal hernia.

Paraphimosis

Paraphimosis is a condition that occurs in the uncircumcised male. It occurs when the foreskin of the penis becomes trapped behind the glans. The foreskin can normally be retracted manually and will slide back over the glans on its own or with little effort. The foreskin will become edematous and patients will complain of pain from the constriction. Paraphimosis can cause compromise of the blood flow and may lead to gangrene if untreated. A lubricant can be used to assist in sliding the foreskin over the glans to its normal position. The Dundee technique, in which a small gauge needle is used to create punctures in the foreskin, can also be used. The edematous fluid is then compressed from the tissue so the foreskin can be slid down. If these procedures fail, surgery may be necessary to create a slit in the foreskin to enable it to slide back to its normal position. A circumcision should be performed in these patients to prevent reoccurrence.

Varicocele

A varicocele is an engorgement of the veins of the pampiniform plexus. This plexus is part of the spermatic cord that travels through the inguinal canal, terminating in the testes. A varicocele is more likely to occur in the left testis because the veins from there run vertically into the renal vein. The veins from the right testis empty into the inferior vena cava. A varicocele is usually idiopathic in nature but can be caused by compression preventing the veins from draining. This condition usually occurs in males ages 15-25, but a malignant tumor should be considered in patients who develop a varicocele after the age of 40. Patients will complain of a heavy, aching, fullness in the affected testicle. On exam, the testicle may appear visibly enlarged with engorged veins. When palpated, the testicle may feel like a "bag of worms." A scrotal support may be used to try and resolve the condition on its own. If this is not effective, surgery may be necessary.

Cystitis

Cystitis, or a urinary tract infection (UTI), is an infection of the bladder. It is more common in women because of an anatomically shorter urethra, but can also occur in men. It is most common in women aged 30-50 and in men over 50 because of enlargement of the prostate obstructing urine flow. A UTI is caused by bacteria that travel up the urethra to the bladder to multiply. Women are more susceptible to developing a UTI after frequent sexual intercourse because of exposure to bacteria. It often occurs in conjunction with pyelonephritis. Signs and symptoms include burning on urination and frequent urination of small amounts of urine. Patients may have lower abdominal pain with or without a fever. Urinalysis will show WBCs and RBCs, positive nitrates, and bacteria. Culture and sensitivity should be done to isolate the causative organism, which is frequently *Escherichia coli*. For uncomplicated cystitis- nitrofurantoin, TMP-SMX, or pivmecillinam are the drugs of choice, but local susceptibility patterns should be taken into account. Urethral anesthetizing medications can be given to reduce the pain. Patients should have another urinalysis if there are recurrent symptoms or symptoms persist 48-72 hours after antimicrobial therapy has been started. Complications include pyelonephritis and hematuria.

Testicular torsion

The testicle is usually held in place by the tunica vaginalis, which allows little movement. Some males are born with a congenital anomaly that allows the testicles to move easily and rotate horizontally on the spermatic cord. This leaves them susceptible to developing testicular torsion in which a testicle can twist on the spermatic cord. This causes obstruction of blood flow to the testicle. Patients will complain of a sudden, severe testicular pain. This may occur after activity or while sleeping. Trauma may also contribute to a testicular torsion. The testicle may appear swollen or discolored, and the affected testicle may appear elevated when compared to the other. Patients may have nausea and vomiting. Treatment should be emergent because of the risk of tissue death from decreased blood flow. The torsion may be resolved by manually manipulating the testicle back into a normal position, but surgery may be necessary. With tissue death, an orchiectomy may be performed. Complications include infertility and tissue death of the testicle.

Prostatitis

Inflammation or infection of the prostate gland may be acute or chronic. Acute prostatitis is usually caused by a bacterial infection. Chronic prostatitis can be due to inflammation from a variety of causes, including urine backing up into the gland causing inflammation, interstitial cystitis, or spasms of the urinary sphincters. Patients with either form of prostatitis will complain of lower abdominal pain and pain on ejaculation, but a fever will be much more pronounced in patients with the acute form of the condition. Urinary frequency, decreased stream, and urgency will be present with both. On exam, the prostate gland will feel boggy and enlarged. Patients with acute prostatitis will have severe pain with palpation of the gland. Urine culture and gram stain can help guide therapy. On CBC, leukocytosis will be evident if acute. For acute prostatitis, TMP/SMX or a fluoroquinolone are the usualy drugs of choice, but check local susceptibility patterns. Chronic prostatitis may benefit from muscle relaxants and anti-inflammatory agents. Surgery may be necessary to remove all or a portion of the prostate if the symptoms of chronic prostatitis cannot be controlled.
Complications include acute urinary retention (will need bladder drained by suprapubic cath), prostatis abscess, sepsis, infertility, and epididymitis.

Epididymitis

The epididymis is located on the posterior surface of each testicle and functions to store sperm. It can become inflamed and infected, resulting in epididymitis. Epididymitis is most common in males under age 35 and is frequently due to a bacterial infection from a sexually transmitted disease, such as chlamydia or gonorrhea. Patients will complain of pain in the affected testicle, exacerbated with straining, such as with a bowel movement. They may also have pain with urinating and lower abdominal pain. There may be visible blood in the semen with pain on ejaculation. High fever and chills are common, along with enlarged inguinal lymph nodes. By clinical assessment, the testicle will feel warm and swollen with a palpable enlarged epididymis. To make differential diagnosis, rule out STDs with NAA testing, rule out urinary infection with a UA and urine culture. If the patient complains of testicular pain, perform an ultrasound to rule out testicular torsion. Treatment depends of severity. For antibiotic treatment, ceftriaxone plus doxycycline is the treatment of choice. Ice, NSAIDS, and elevating the scrotum are helpful. For those who appear septic, with extreme pain, consult urologist for possible surgical exploration. Patients positive for C. trachomatis or N. gonorrhoeae should be counseled on condom use to prevent future STDs, and partners should be evaluated. Complications include abscess of the scrotum, epididymo-orchitis, and infertility.

Wilms tumor

A Wilms tumor, or nephroblastoma, is a renal carcinoma that affects children usually ages 3-8. It is thought that a Wilms tumor begins to form while *in utero*. Some of the cells that would normally develop into renal cells fail to develop, and this mutation goes on to form a tumor. The condition is usually diagnosed by age 1, though sometimes it may be as late as age 5. Often a mass can be palpated in the abdomen and in the back over the affected kidney. A Wilms tumor can grow large before causing any pain in the child, so it may go undiagnosed until it becomes large enough to be palpable. There will frequently be visible blood in the urine. The child may become constipated and have nausea and vomiting. This may be accompanied by weight loss. Treatment comprises surgery, chemotherapy, and radiation, or a combination of all three treatments.

Pyelonephritis

Pyelonephritis is a severe infection of the kidneys. Pyelonephritis can be life-threatening if not treated promptly. Chronic renal damage, which may impair renal function, can occur without treatment. Commonly, pyelonephritis is caused by a urinary tract infection (UTI) that spreads from the bladder, through the ureters, and to the kidneys. The symptoms of pyelonephritis are similar to a UTI, only more severe. Urinary frequency, urgency, decreased stream, painful burning on urination, lower abdominal pain, and foul-smelling urine are present. Patients may have a high fever with chills. On exam, there will be pain to percussion over the costovertebral angle over the kidneys. Urinalysis will show elevated WBCs and RBCs with many bacteria. Treatment is with appropriate antibiotic therapy. For moderate cases cephalosporins and fluoroquinolones are used. If severe, patients may require hospitalization with IV antibiotics; most commonly beta lactam/betalactamase inhibitors or carbapenems are used. There is a risk of urosepsis with pyelonephritis, so treatment should begin immediately after diagnosis.

Nephrotic syndrome

Nephrotic syndrome is a condition that occurs due to damage to the microvascular system within the kidneys. It leads to excess excretion of protein in the urine and leaking of serum proteins out of the vessels, causing edema. There is also an increased risk of blood clot development. Nephrotic syndrome can be caused by chronic renal failure that occurs due to a primary renal disease or diabetic nephropathy. Other chronic conditions that can cause nephrotic syndrome include lupus erythematosus and amyloidosis. Nephrotic syndrome can cause a good deal of edema, especially in the extremities and face. There may be noticeable weight gain due to the retained fluid. Patients will have a feeling of general malaise and may or may not have a fever. Urinalysis will show very high levels of protein. Diagnosis is made in the presence of hypoalbuminemia and proteinuria > 50 mg/kg/day.
Treatment focuses on treating the underlying cause and controlling the symptoms of nephrotic syndrome. ACE inhibitors can be given to control hypertension and diuretics to reduce the edema. Anticoagulants may be necessary to prevent blood clot formation.
Complications include chronic kidney disease, infections, thombus, emboli, hypercholesterolemia, and hypertension.

Acute glomerulonephritis

Acute glomerulonephritis is an infection of the kidneys that affects the glomerular filters within the organs. It is usually sudden in onset and can lead to permanent kidney damage of not treated promptly. The cause of acute glomerulonephritis can be *streptococcal* infection, virus, or occur bacterial endocarditis. Patients will be acutely ill with glomerulonephritis. They will have a decrease in urinary output with a dark tea-stain color to their urine due to hematuria. The urine may appear foamy because of a high protein level. Edema can be quite profound, affecting the extremities and face. Blood pressure will be elevated due to the increased fluid load. Urinalysis, GFR, and the patient's age help disclose most likely cause of the glomerulonephritis. Serum creatinine, serum albumin, and urine for protein are ordered along with a renal biopsy to confirm the diagnosis. Interpreting these together can help discover etiology. Treatment focuses on treating the underlying cause. If due to a recent *streptococcal* infection or bacterial endocarditis, appropriate antibiotic therapy should be prescribed. The condition will usually resolve on its own with management of the symptoms, such as ACE inhibitors to control hypertension and diuretics to reduce the edema. Some patients may need dialysis during the acute episode.

Hyponatremia

Hyponatremia can be due to syndrome of inappropriate antidiuretic hormone secretion (SIADH) and suddenly stopping steroid treatment without tapering the medication. Hypomagnesemia can also cause a decrease in sodium levels. Mild hyponatremia will result in nausea and vomiting and other vague flu-like symptoms. Moderate hyponatremia causes muscular effects of weakness and muscle pain. Severe hyponatremia causes changes in mental status with lethargy and psychosis. If severe, seizures can occur that may lead to coma and possibly even death. Decreases in the sodium level may be the result of dilutional effects from over-hydration. Fluid restrictions can be implemented to return the sodium levels to normal. If hyponatremia is severe, IV fluids with high sodium content can be administered along with a diuretic to increase fluid output. If an abnormality in the amount of ADH is present, as with SIADH, an antibiotic can be given to correct this. If the SIADH is due to malignancy, treatment of the cancer can help to correct the condition. Significant diuresis may be necessary if fluid overload is causing a dilutional hyponatremia.

Polycystic kidney disease

Polycystic kidney disease is a condition in which groups of cysts form within the kidneys. It can potentially lead to high blood pressure and even renal failure. Polycystic disease is not limited to the kidneys and can affect other organs as well, but the kidneys are usually the most severely affected. This is a genetic condition that can be autosomal dominant or autosomal recessive. Patients may complain of abdominal pain and an increasing abdominal girth due to enlarging kidneys. They may have frequent urination or gross blood visible in the urine. High blood pressure is usually present and early signs of renal failure may be evident with elevated serum BUN and creatinine levels. Diagnosis is suspected with a family history of polycystic kidney disease and confirmed with bilateral and multiple cysts on ultrasound or CT scan. Treatment of polycystic kidney disease is focused on treating the symptoms and preventing renal failure. Close monitoring and control of blood pressure is necessary. If the cysts become large, they may need to be surgically drained to prevent compression on surrounding organs.

Hypokalemia

Hypokalemia is defined as a potassium level <3.5. Increased excretion of potassium, such as with diuretics or with dehydration through diarrhea and vomiting, can cause decreased levels of potassium. Various antibiotics can also cause hypokalemia. Because potassium and sodium have an inverse relationship, an increase in sodium levels can cause hypokalemia. Hypokalemia can cause cardiac dysrhythmias and an increased heart rate. Decreased blood pressure may be present along with mental status changes, such as somnolence or even seizures. If potassium levels drop severely low, fatal cardiac dysrhythmias can occur with cardiac arrest. EKG changes include flattened T waves and ST depression, similar to cardiac ischemia. Treatment consists of oral potassium or IV solutions with added potassium chloride. Potassium-rich foods can be given to increase intake of potassium. Patients must be closely monitored for signs and symptoms of hyperkalemia as potassium supplements are given, especially cardiac effects. Other electrolyte levels, especially sodium, should be closely monitored for abnormalities.

Hypernatremia

Hypernatremia can be caused by a decrease in fluid intake or dehydration. Diabetes insipidus can result in changes in antidiuretic hormone levels, which can alter sodium regulation. Renal dysfunction can alter the excretion of sodium and result in higher levels within the blood stream. Hypermagnesemia can also cause an increase in sodium levels.

S/S: If renal dysfunction is contributing to increased water wasting, increased urinary output will be present. If dehydration is the cause, excessive sweating and dryness of the oral mucosa can be present. Patients may have had some nausea and vomiting with a decrease in oral fluid intake if that is the cause of the dehydration. Nervous system effects include changes in mental status with irritability, somnolence, or seizures. Deep tendon reflexes may be depressed. Patients should be treated for dehydration if this is the cause and IV fluids provided to correct the imbalance if the renal system will allow this. If caused by increases in magnesium levels, then the hypermagnesemia should be treated.

Hypocalcemia

Hypocalcemia can be caused by under secretion of parathyroid hormone, resulting in more calcium remaining in the bones and less being circulated into the bloodstream. Calcium requires vitamin D to be absorbed in the GI tract, so a vitamin D deficiency can lead to hypocalcemia. This can also result from an alteration in renal function. With hypocalcemia there is excitability of the nervous system. Patients may exhibit spasm of the facial muscles (a positive Chvostek's sign). Mental status will be altered, and patients may even experience hallucinations. The heart rate may become irregular, and changes may be present on EKG. Muscle spasms can occur in the smooth muscle, such as the bronchial passages, leading to respiratory arrest. Treatment can be with calcium replacement if calcium levels have dropped dangerously low. Serum calcium values should be monitored regularly to assess for resolution of the condition and to detect if the calcium levels are decreasing further. Seizures precautions may be necessary if patients develop alterations in motor activity.

Hyperkalemia

Hyperkalemia is defined as a potassium level >5.5. Potassium is excreted through urine so any dysfunction that results in a decreased urinary output can cause increased serum potassium levels. Any process that causes blood cell destruction, such as hemolytic anemia, can cause a rise in potassium levels. Various medications can also lead to hyperkalemia.

S/S: Neuromuscular symptoms of weakness, lethargy, diminished reflexes, and tingling of the extremities may occur. Hyperkalemia causes a decreased heart rate and cardiac dysrhythmias. EKG changes include a wide QRS complex and elevated T waves. GI symptoms of nausea, vomiting, and diarrhea may be present. Normal potassium levels are achieved by increasing the excretion of potassium. This can be done with diuretics that increase potassium excretion through urine. Kayexalate binds with potassium to increase secretion and can be given rectally by enema. This will cause increased excretion of potassium through the GI tract. IV fluids high in glucose concentration can cause potassium to move from the extracellular to the intracellular space.

Hypomagnesemia

Hypomagnesemia is defined as a serum magnesium level <1.8. Magnesium is stored in the liver, and liver failure can cause the magnesium stores to be depleted. Some antibiotics and diuretics can cause a decrease in magnesium levels. Magnesium is responsible for maintaining normal electrolyte levels within the cells, so changes in sodium and potassium levels may affect magnesium levels. Magnesium has an adverse relationship with calcium levels, so if there is an increase in calcium, there will be a concomitant decrease in magnesium. Signs and symptoms include changes in mental status and somnolence, decreased reflexes, and/or seizures. Vasodilation may cause erythema and hypotension. There may be a decrease in respiratory rate. To treat hypomagnesemia, magnesium sulfate can be given. There are also medications that help to decrease the amount of magnesium that is excreted through the renal and urinary systems. Potassium and sodium levels should also be closely monitored to ensure these remain within normal limits.

Hypercalcemia

Hypercalcemia is an increased level of calcium in the serum, >10.5. Calcium levels within the bloodstream are controlled by many factors, one of which is parathyroid hormone. This causes calcium to be reabsorbed by the bones if the level is too high or causes it to escape the bones and enter the circulating bloodstream if levels are too low. Any tumors affecting this process can alter calcium levels and cause an elevated calcium level. Calcium is excreted by the renal system, and any alteration in kidney function could result in hypercalcemia. An increase in heart rate can occur. Patients will have changes in mental status with lethargy and somnolence being present. There may be a decrease in the peripheral reflexes because of malfunction in nerve transmissions. Decreased urinary output due to kidney dysfunction may occur. Treatment consists of IV steroids, and Gallium nitrate may be used with cancer-induced hypercalcemia. Patients should be encouraged to increase activity levels and perform light exercise as tolerated to build bone density.

Metabolic acidosis

Metabolic acidosis is a condition in which there are excess hydrogen ions within the system, resulting in a decrease in serum pH levels. This can be due to excessive intake of acidic substances, such as aspirin products, methanol, or antifreeze. Diabetes can also be a cause of metabolic acidosis. Metabolic dysfunction can also cause decreased secretion of hydrogen, leading to retention of more acid than the body needs. The body will try to compensate for this condition by increasing the respiratory rate and increasing the depth of respirations in an effort to "blow off" some of the excess hydrogen through carbon dioxide. Patients may become stuporous, and death may result without treatment. Lab studies will reveal a decrease in serum pH levels and possibly elevated chloride levels. If diabetes is the cause, glucose levels will often be very high. Treatment can be accomplished through IV fluids, but if severe, bicarbonate infusions may be necessary. Treating the underlying cause should be the focus of treatment.

Metabolic alkalosis

Metabolic alkalosis occurs when the pH of the blood becomes too elevated. This can occur due to a decrease in hydrogen ions or a direct increase in bicarbonate ions. The means by which these two actions occur is usually through the GI tract or through the renal tubule system. With the loss of hydrochloric acid in the stomach, such as with vomiting or NG tube suctioning, an alkalotic state can develop. Renal dysfunction or diuretic use can cause decreased secretion of bicarbonate ions, and this raises the bicarbonate levels. Signs and symptoms include signs of hypocalcemia (Chvostek's sign, changes in mental status), hypervolemia, and hypertension. Signs of bulimia, such as dental caries and electrolyte abnormalities may be present. Lab studies show an elevated serum pH, elevated bicarbonate levels, and possibly elevated aldosterone levels. Treatment consists of correction of the underlying cause. IV sodium chloride can help to restore the acid-base balance. If edema is present, potassium chloride should be used to balance electrolytes and reduce the edema.

Respiratory acidosis

Respiratory acidosis is due to a depressed respiratory system that prevents carbon dioxide from being "blown off," leading to elevated acid levels. This can be an acute or chronic condition that may or may not require treatment. Some common causes are primary respiratory illness that causes a depressed respiratory system, CNS dysfunction that affects the respiratory center in the hypothalamus, or unknown cause. Patients may exhibit a decreased respiratory rate with mental status changes, somnolence, or stupor. If chronic in nature, patients may appear largely asymptomatic. Pulse oximetry will show a decrease in O_2 saturation. If severe, patients may appear cyanotic, especially in the nail beds and circum-orally. Treatment may not be necessary if this is a chronic condition and patients are not especially symptomatic. Otherwise, the underlying cause should be treated. Medications can be given to make respirations more productive. Mechanical ventilation with intubation may be necessary.

Respiratory alkalosis

Respiratory alkalosis usually occurs due to an excessive loss of carbon dioxide through respirations. This can occur with chronic respiratory illnesses or may be acute in nature. When chronic, the body will compensate and adjust to the excess loss of chloride by decreasing excretion of bicarbonate ions through the urine. Chronic respiratory alkalosis will not cause patients to experience any symptoms. When acute, patients may experience light-headedness, dizziness, paresthesias, and syncope. This can be seen with hyperventilation. On exam, patients may be visibly hyperventilating or short of breath and carpopedal spasms may be present. Fever can raise the respiratory rate and lead to hyperventilation, which can cause respiratory alkalosis. Treatment is by treating the underlying cause. Frequently, the chronic form of the condition is not treated. With symptomatic respiratory alkalosis, effort should be made to correct the acid-base imbalance by slowing down the respiratory rate and administering oxygen. If fever is the cause, antipyretics should be given and the underlying cause of the fever should be treated.

Leiomyoma

Leiomyomas, or uterine fibroids, are very common benign uterine tumors. They usually form during the childbearing years, and most women are not aware they have them because they are frequently asymptomatic. Leiomyomas may be caused by genetic factors or hormones, especially estrogen and progesterone. Most women are asymptomatic from leiomyomas. When they do produce symptoms, patients will complain of heavy bleeding that may or may not be associated with menstrual periods. Leiomyomas may be large enough to cause abdominal or pelvic pain and pressure. If compressing on the colon, they can cause constipation. If applying pressure to the bladder, they can cause urinary frequency or incontinence. A hysterectomy can be performed to remove the uterus if the symptoms are severe and the woman is not planning to have any more children. Laser ablation can also be attempted to shrink the tumors. Medications may be tried, such as gonadotropin-releasing hormone agonists or androgen hormones to reduce symptoms.

Hematologic System

Sickle cell anemia

Sickle cell anemia is a genetic form of anemia that affects the red blood cells. Patients will be anemic and will have episodes of pain, particularly in the extremities. Swollen hands and feet are common and extreme pain can develop during a sickle cell crisis. Sequestration syndrome can occur in which the organs are affected, especially the spleen. Diagnosis is confirmed per electrophoresis, PCR, or direct DNA testing. Treatment includes prophylactic penicillin for children from 2 months to 5 years to prevent pneumonia, IV fluids to prevent dehydration, Analgesics (morphine) during painful crises, folic acid for anemia, oxygen for congestive heart failure or pulmonary disease, blood transfusions with chelation therapy to remove excess iron OR erythropheresis, in which red cells are removed and replaced with healthy cells, either autologous or from a donor. Hematopoietic stem cells transplantation is the only curative treatment, but immunosuppressive drugs must be used and success rates are only about 85%, so the procedure is only used on those at high risk. Partial chimerism uses a mixture of the donor and the recipient's bone marrow stem cells and does not require ablation of bone marrow. There are many serious complications including organ damage, stroke, MI, priapism, blindness, and pulmonary hypertension.

Vitamin B12 deficiency

A deficiency in vitamin B12, or pernicious anemia, can occur in those who do not consume enough foods high in B12, such as dairy products and meat. It is most often due to a lack of intrinsic factor in the stomach. This factor is necessary for the absorption of B12. Past surgeries to remove portions of the GI tract can also decrease the absorption of B12. A deficiency of vitamin B12 can cause chronic fatigue and a loss of appetite. Patients may appear pale and short of breath. Paresthesias may develop in the extremities, and the condition can progress to the point of mental changes, such as confusion. Treatment consists of vitamin B12 replacement. This can be administered by intramuscular injection or nasal spray. Treatment begins with daily doses of the vitamin supplement, but then decreases to once monthly. Vitamin B12 levels should be monitored to measure the effectiveness of treatment.

Clotting disorders

Factor VII disorder is due to a lack of extrinsic factor, which is necessary to complete the clotting cascade. A prolonged PT and normal PTT will be present. Treatment is with infusions of plasma, factor VII concentrates, or recombinant factor VII. Factor IX disorder is also called hemophilia B. It is a genetic disorder found on the X chromosome so it affects males more than females. A prolonged PTT, normal PT, normal bleeding time, and normal fibrinogen levels will be present. Treatment is with infusions of factor IX. Factor XI disorder is also called Rosenthal syndrome or hemophilia C. It occurs in both males and females and is more common in the Jewish population. It is also more common in children with Noonan syndrome. A prolonged PTT and normal PT will be present. Infusions of fresh frozen plasma (FFP) are the primary treatment. Factor XI concentrates are also available for treatment.

Infectious Diseases

Epstein-Barr infection

Most people are carriers of the Epstein-Barr virus, but may not have developed an active infection from the virus. It is a form of herpes virus (human herpesvirus 4), and is responsible for causing infectious mononucleosis. It is transmitted through saliva.

Symptoms of an Epstein-Barr infection include swollen painful lymph nodes, extreme fatigue, and sore throat. Fever may also be present. This is most common in teenagers or college-age young adults. The white blood cell count will be elevated with increased lymphocytes in the differential. A Mono Spot test will be positive for infection.

Treatment is supportive, and antibiotics are not helpful in treating this viral infection. Analgesics, increased fluid intake, and rest will help to relieve some of the symptoms. Warm salt water gargles can help with the sore throat. The symptoms of the infection may last for several weeks. A patient will not contract mononucleosis again after the initial exposure to the Epstein-Barr virus.

Pinworm infection

The pinworm is a type of roundworm. The worms will lay eggs within the digestive tract and then they travel to the anal area where they are usually found. Pinworms can be effectively treated, but serious complications can develop if the infestation is severe. Pinworms are more prevalent in warmer areas of the country and infestations occur more frequently in children. Pinworms are highly contagious. As a patient itches the anal area where the eggs are located, the eggs cling to the fingers and can easily be transmitted to other people either directly or through food or surfaces. The eggs can thrive for 2-3 weeks on an inanimate object. Patients will have anal itching that can be intense. Itching is usually worse at night and can cause insomnia. Abdominal pain, nausea, and vomiting can also occur. Anti-parasitic medications are given to kill the pinworms and their larvae. The most effective drugs used are Pin-X® and Albenza®. The entire family should be treated because pinworms are so contagious.

Syphilis

Syphilis is caused by the spirochete *Treponema pallidum* and has increased in incidence over the last 10 years; it is associated with risk-taking behavior such as drug use. The disease has 3 phases, with an incubation period of about 3 weeks:

- Primary: chancre (painless) in areas of sexual contact, persisting 3 to 6 weeks.
- Secondary: General flu-like symptoms (sore throat, fever, headaches) and red papular rash on trunk, flexor surfaces, palms, and soles, and lymphadenopathy occur about 3 to 6 weeks after end of primary phase and eventually resolves.
- Tertiary (latent): Affects about 30% and includes CNS and cardiovascular symptoms 3 to 20 years after initial infection. Gummas (granulomatous lesions) may be widespread.

Diagnosis is made by dark-field microscopy (primary or secondary) or serologic testing. The CDC provides treatment protocol for different populations. Treatment for primary, secondary, and early tertiary is benzathine penicillin G 104 million units IM in 1 dose. For tertiary treatment consists of benzathine penicillin G 2.4 million units IM weekly for 3 weeks. Complications include dementia, meningitis, neuropathy, thoracic aneurysm, aortic aneurysm, and cardiac valve disease.

Lyme disease

Lyme disease can occur from a bite from an infected deer tick. It is more prevalent in heavily wooded areas. Those who spend time outdoors, especially in wooded areas or tall grass, are more at risk for being bitten from an infected deer tick. Having exposed skin when walking in these types of areas will also increase the risk of developing Lyme disease.

The bite from an infected deer tick will leave an erythematous area on the skin and the tick may still be attached. A few days later, a bull's eye rash can develop that may be small or large. Lyme disease can progress to cause severe joint pain, paresthesias, Bell's palsy, confusion, fatigue, and heart palpitations. Antibiotic treatment with doxycycline or amoxicillin is started immediately after diagnosis. It may be necessary to treat with IV infusions of antibiotics, depending on the severity of the disease. Supportive therapy with pain relievers may help with the pain associated with Lyme disease.

Musculoskeletal System

Boxer's, Colles', and scaphoid fractures

Boxer's fracture occurs at the distal end of the fifth metacarpal bone. It earned its name because it is usually caused by force of a fist hitting a hard surface, as with boxing. It usually resolves within 4-6 weeks with rest, compression, and elevation. Casting may or may not be necessary depending on the severity of the fracture. Colles fracture occurs at the distal end of the radius. It is usually caused by breaking a fall with an outstretched hand, causing extreme force to be applied to the arm. Depending on severity, a cast is applied for 6 weeks until the fracture has healed. Surgery may be necessary with a displaced fracture. Scaphoid fracture occurs from a fall on an outstretched hand. This will cause tenderness in the anatomic snuffbox at the base of the thumb in the wrist. There is risk of interrupted blood supply to the small bone with this fracture. Treatment is with casting, sometimes up to 10-12 weeks, and surgery may be necessary.

Nursemaid's elbow

Nursemaid's elbow is a subluxation of the radial head. It occurs in children under 6-years-old. A pulling mechanism on the arm, such as when swinging a child, causes the radial head to pull out of the capsule in which it sits. This results in partial dislocation, or subluxation, of the arm. The child will initially experience pain with this condition. The child may continue to act normally but will refuse to use the affected arm. There is no actual deformity of the arm visible, but the child will guard the arm and prevent any movement of it to prevent pain. A nursemaid's elbow is easily reduced. The child's arm should be extended, the hand supinated, and then the elbow flexed so the hand touches the shoulder. If this does not reduce the subluxation, the arm may be placed in a sling and orthopedic evaluation obtained to determine whether surgery is warranted. The parents should be advised to avoid swinging or pulling the child to prevent this from happening again.

Gamekeeper's thumb

Gamekeeper's thumb, or skier's thumb, is injury to the ulnar collateral ligament of the thumb. It is caused by a force that hyperextends the thumb away from the hand toward the body, as when falling on a ski pole. It earned its name from gamekeepers in Europe injuring the ligament while breaking rabbits' necks. Patients will have significant pain with this injury and, depending upon severity, it can be disabling. The pain is greatly exacerbated when trying to grasp or pinch anything, like when holding car keys. The area may be edematous, erythematous, or ecchymotic. Exam may reveal ligament instability. Treatment consists of immobilization of the ligament, possibly with casting depending on severity, and pain relievers. Surgery may be necessary if the ligament injury is not healing or if there is a complete non-healing tear. Stretching of the ligament may be necessary following immobilization to regain normal range of motion.

De Quervain's tenosynovitis

De Quervain's tenosynovitis is a condition in which there is inflammation in the abductor pollicis longus and extensor pollicis brevis tendons in the thumb. They are held together in the thumb by the extensor retinaculum. If the tendons become inflamed and swollen, the retinaculum cannot expand to accommodate the inflammation, leading to tenosynovitis. This can be caused by overuse of the thumbs. The pain is reproducible with moving the thumb away from the palm and backwards. Arthritis and trauma can also cause edema in the tendons, leading to this condition. Pregnancy can cause water retention, which may lead to constriction and pain of the tendons. Treatment consists of resting the thumbs. Ice can be applied to relieve the pain. Anti-inflammatory drugs may help with pain relief, also. Splints can be applied that restrict the thumb movements and reduce pain. If conservative treatments do not help, steroid injections into the tendons may reduce the inflammation. As a last resort, surgery can be done to release the extensor retinaculum.

Carpal tunnel syndrome

Carpal tunnel syndrome occurs when there is irritation and pressure applied to the median nerve within the carpal tunnel of the wrist. It can have no known cause, but most patients have experienced some type of repetitive movement of the hands that caused irritation within the carpal tunnel. Signs and symptoms are gradually progressive and include numbness or tingling of the thumb, index, and middle fingers. Symptoms can be elicited by tapping on the inner wrist over the carpal tunnel (Tinel's sign). Symptoms may be worse at night and may wake patients. Patients may describe grip strength weakness and frequent dropping of objects at home. EMG and nerve conduction testing will reveal a diagnosis of carpal tunnel syndrome. Cock-up wrist splints should be tried to help relieve pressure on the nerve and reduce the symptoms. Anti-inflammatory drugs and resting the hands and wrists may help. Surgery to release the ligament over the carpal tunnel usually resolves the condition.

Lateral epicondylitis

Lateral epicondylitis, or tennis elbow, occurs due to overuse of the extensor muscles in the forearm. These muscles attach to a tendon that attaches to the lateral epicondyle of the elbow. With overuse, such as with playing tennis, inflammation in the tendon can occur. Patients will complain of pain and tenderness over the lateral epicondyle, aggravated with extending the fingers and wrist. Hand or wrist weakness may develop. All symptoms will become worse while picking up an object. Testing involves having patients extend the wrist or fingers against resistance. This will reproduce the pain. Treatment includes rest of the elbow and forearm. A splint can be worn at the elbow to relieve pain and ice can be applied. Anti-inflammatory drugs may also help. Steroid injections can be performed in the tendon at the lateral epicondyle. Exercises can be done, also, to help strengthen the extensor muscles of the forearm.

Medial epicondylitis

Medial epicondylitis, or golfer's elbow, occurs due to overuse of the flexor muscles in the forearm. These muscles attach to a tendon that attaches to the medial epicondyle of the elbow. With overuse, such as with golfing, inflammation in the tendon can occur. Patients will complain of pain and tenderness over the medial epicondyle, aggravated by flexing the fingers and wrist. Hand or wrist weakness may develop. All symptoms will become worse while grasping an object. Testing involves having patients extend the palm outward and attempt to flex the wrist toward the arm against pressure. This will reproduce the pain. Treatment includes rest of the elbow and forearm. A splint can be worn at the elbow to relieve pain and ice can be applied. Anti-inflammatory drugs may also help. Steroid injections can be performed in the tendon at the medial epicondyle. Exercises can be done, also, to help strengthen the flexor muscles of the forearm.

Cauda equina syndrome

Cauda equina syndrome is a condition in which there is severe compression of the nerve roots exiting the spinal canal from the cauda equina below the termination of the spinal cord at L1. It is usually caused by an acute herniated nucleus pulposus (herniated disc) or can occur due to progressive degenerative changes causing severe spinal stenosis in the lower lumbar spine. Patients will usually have low back pain with pain radiating into one or both of the lower extremities. There will be saddle anesthesia present along with bowel and bladder incontinence. The lower extremities will be numb and/or weak. There will also be depressed or absent reflexes in the lower extremities. Steroids can be started to reduce the inflammation, but this is usually only until surgery is performed. Treatment of cauda equina syndrome is urgent surgical intervention. If treated promptly, there is a chance that patients' symptoms will be reversed. The longer the symptoms are present, however, the less likely patients will reach a full recovery.

Ankylosing spondylitis

Ankylosing spondylitis is an inflammatory form of arthritis that can affect any of the joints in the body. It most commonly affects the joints in the vertebral column and the sacroiliac joints. The inflammation that occurs causes bony overgrowth, especially in the spine, and leads to fusion of the vertebral bodies. When it occurs at the joints of the ribs and spine, rib cage mobility can be affected, restricting respirations. Patients will complain of pain and stiffness in the affected joints. This will lead to a stooped posture and possibly depressed respirations. Iritis and inflammatory bowel disease is also common with ankylosing spondylitis. X-rays will show the bony fusion that occurs, especially in the vertebral column. Blood testing includes CRP, ESR, and CBC to check for inflammation. Genetic testing for the HLA-B27 gene indicates a person's predilection for developing this condition. Treatment includes pain relievers and anti-inflammatory drugs. Steroids may be necessary to decrease inflammation. Infusions of Embral® or Remicade® may also help to decrease symptoms.

Spinal stenosis

Spinal stenosis occurs when there is disc or bony material, causing narrowing of the spinal canal. In the upper spine, this can cause compression of the spinal cord, and in the lower lumbar spine it will cause compression on the nerves of the cauda equina. Spinal stenosis is most often degenerative in nature. It can also occur with traumatic disc herniation or spondylolisthesis. Patients will complain of pain in the affected portion of the spine with pain, numbness, and/or weakness extending into the upper or lower extremities, depending on location. With spinal cord stenosis, there will be profound weakness and hyperactive reflexes/spasticity. Symptoms of neurogenic claudication are due to lumbar spinal stenosis and include pain that is aggravated with walking and standing. These are usually somewhat relieved with sitting and leaning forward. Symptoms may be slightly relieved with anti-inflammatory drugs and pain relievers. Surgical correction can be performed with a laminectomy or X-Stop procedure that relieves the pressure being applied to the spinal canal.

Herniated nucleus pulposus

A herniated nucleus pulposus, or herniated disc, can occur anywhere in the spinal column. The disc can bulge in one direction of may be central. If this occurs above the level of L1, there is a risk of spinal cord compression. Patients will complain of pain at the level of the spine where the herniation occurs, along with radicular pain following the dermatome of the affected nerve. For example, if the herniation occurs at L5-S1, patients may complain of sciatic-type pain. Patients may develop numbness or tingling in the affected dermatome, along with weakness of the affected limb. Patients should be started on anti-inflammatory drugs and pain relievers. Often, the symptoms will resolve with conservative treatment. Physical therapy to help with pain relief and stretching and strengthening can help. Steroids, either orally or per epidural injection, can help to reduce the inflammation. Surgery can also be done with a microdiscectomy to remove the portion of the disc that has herniated.

Slipped capital femoral epiphysis

A slipped capital femoral epiphysis is a condition in which the proximal femoral growth plate becomes unstable. This can occur because of trauma causing a Salter-Harris fracture, obesity, or abnormal growth of the bone and cartilage in the growth plate itself. It is most commonly detected in children from 10-16 years of age. It usually occurs unilaterally, but may occur bilaterally, especially in children under the age of 10. Patients will develop a limp that becomes progressively worse. They will complain of pain in the hip, groin, thigh, or even in the knee. X-rays will show displacement of the femoral head, from mild to severe. Surgical repair is necessary to correct this condition. An open reduction and internal fixation of the femoral head is performed to stabilize the joint. With severe disease, the child may end up with a discrepancy in the leg lengths, which can lead to chronic limp.

Avascular necrosis

Avascular necrosis usually affects the upper femur at the hip but can occur in other bones as well. It occurs when there is a loss of blood supply to the bone. Chronic steroid use can cause this condition, as can radiation treatments to the area or chemotherapy. Alcoholism can lead to occlusion of the vessels providing blood to the bones and may lead to avascular necrosis. Chronic medical conditions, such as sickle cell anemia and lupus, may also cause this condition. Pain is the most common symptom of avascular necrosis. Patients may have noticed a gradual progression of the pain or may develop a pathologic fracture. X-rays will show the dead bone tissue once the condition is advanced. MRI is more sensitive in detecting early disease. Treatment should focus on treating the underlying cause and restoring blood supply to the bone. Joint replacement or bone grafting may be necessary. A core decompression procedure can remove the inner layer of bone to help regenerate the blood vessels, restoring blood supply.

Septic arthritis

Septic arthritis is an infection in a joint, most commonly the knee though other joints may be affected. This is usually due to a bacterial infection that has spread to the joint, but it can be caused by fungus also. The most common bacterial causes are *Staphylococcus aureus* or *Neisseria gonorrhea*. Patients will complain of significant pain in the affected joint with fever and chills. They may have some nausea and vomiting. They may or may not be aware of a recent bacterial infection elsewhere in their body. The joint will appear red, swollen, hot, and very tender to the touch. Aspiration of the infectious material in the knee will show purulent discharge, possibly with some blood present. Culture and sensitivity testing of the infectious material should be performed. Treatment is with IV antibiotics started at the time of diagnosis. This will be followed by a course of oral antibiotics. If the condition is severe, surgery may be necessary to flush the joint to remove the infectious material.

Osgood-Schlatter disease

Osgood-Schlatter disease is a condition in which inflammation develops around the tibial tuberosity at the knee. It occurs with repeated stress on the patellar tendon, such as with running and kicking, and can cause the tendon to slightly pull away at its attachment to the tibial tuberosity. In severe cases, the tendon can completely tear at its attachment point. This is most common in active children, usually in their early teens, involved in sports. Patients will complain of pain in the knee at the tibial tuberosity. There may be swelling, redness, and decreased motion of the knee present. The pain is aggravated with running, kicking, and squatting. Rest will usually resolve the condition. Mild analgesics, NSAIDs, and ice can also help to relieve the pain. This condition can last for weeks to months, so it can be frustrating to the child to limit sports activities. Rarely, surgery is necessary if the tendon has torn and is not healing on its own.

Osteosarcoma

Osteosarcoma is a type of bone cancer that occurs in bones as they are growing. It commonly affects children and young adults from 10-20 years of age. Some hereditary diseases, such as hereditary retinoblastoma, may make children more susceptible to developing bone cancer. Exposure of the bone to high doses of radiation can also increase the risk of this disease. Oftentimes, osteosarcoma will occur without any known cause. Patients will complain of bone pain and may not be diagnosed until they suffer a pathologic fracture. There may be swelling at the site of the cancer. Patients will be fatigued and may or may not have a fever. The most common treatment for osteosarcoma is surgery to remove the affected portion of the bone. Chemotherapy may be necessary before surgery to shrink the tumor, and it may be used again after surgery. Radiation therapy may also be used to help destroy the cancer cells. In some cases, the cancer can spread to other organs of the body.

Osteoporosis

Osteoporosis is a condition in which there is a decrease in the bone mineral density. It is more common in women than men and is usually post-menopausal. Estrogen is thought to be bone-protective and, with the decrease in estrogen levels after menopause, the bones may begin to weaken. Medications, such as chronic steroid use, can also contribute to the loss of bone density. Smokers and those with a hormonal imbalance, such as hyperparathyroidism, are also more susceptible to developing osteoporosis. Patients may suffer an osteoporotic fracture, such as a compression fracture, as a result of little or no trauma. A DEXA bone density scan will show a bone density of at least 2.5 standard deviations below the value for peak bone mass. Treatment includes weight-bearing exercise, calcium and vitamin D supplementation, or bisphosphonates or other newer medications that promote absorption of calcium by the bones. If possible, glucocorticoids should be weaned if they are the cause of osteoporosis.

Osteoarthritis

Osteoarthritis is a very common condition that occurs due to overuse of the joints. It is characterized by a wearing down of the cartilage within the joints and is a gradually progressive condition. The cause of the condition is use of the joints, especially overuse, and it commonly occurs in the large joints, such as the hips and knees. It can affect any joint in the body. Patients will complain of pain in the affected joint, especially with activity. There may be swelling in the joint. On exam, crepitus can be felt with flexion and extension of the joint. X-rays will show joint space narrowing because of the worn down cartilage. Treatment includes anti-inflammatory drugs and rest of the affected joint when it is painful. Exercise should still be performed but not to the point that pain occurs. Physical therapy may help with muscle strengthening, and exercises that decrease the stress on joints can be helpful. When osteoarthritis is severe, surgery may be necessary to replace the joint.

Gout

Gout occurs when there is an accumulation of uric acid in the blood, leading to urate crystals settling in a joint. Gout can be due to excess consumption of foods that are high in uric acid, or can be due to decreased excretion of uric acid by the kidneys. It usually affects the big toe joint but can occur in other joints. It is more common in men than women. Patients will complain of a sudden onset of severe pain in the affected joint. Even light pressure on the joint causes significant pain. The joint will appear red and swollen and will be very tender when examined. Treatment includes rest of the affected joint and NSAIDs to decrease the inflammation. Colchicine may be given during an acute attack if it is tolerated. Allopurinol can be taken on a regular basis for prevention of acute episodes for those with chronic gout. Allopurinol increases excretion of uric acid. Patients should also be counseled on dietary changes to decrease their intake of foods high in uric acid.

Fibromyalgia

Fibromyalgia is a condition in which patients feels fatigued and has pain "all over." This condition affects the muscles and joints and is diagnosed when no other cause of the symptoms can be found. There is no known cause of fibromyalgia, but it is believed to be a condition in which the body's nervous system becomes hypersensitive to painful stimuli, leading to over activity of the pain receptors in the body. Patients will complain of chronic fatigue accompanied with pain that affects almost the whole body. Signs of depression may also be present. Many patients with fibromyalgia will also suffer from irritable bowel syndrome and chronic headaches. Treatment consists of anti-inflammatory drugs. Narcotic analgesics have not proven to be effective in treating this condition. Current treatment guidelines recommend an SSRI antidepressant to help relieve patients' symptoms. Lyrica® (pregabalin) is an anti-seizure medication that is the first drug indicated for the treatment of fibromyalgia, and it may help relieve the symptoms.

Polyarteritis nodosa

Polyarteritis nodosa is an autoimmune condition in which inflammation occurs within the arteries. It can occur anywhere within the body, but it most often affects the kidneys, intestines, muscles, and joints. It has no known definite cause, but it is often seen in patients who have been diagnosed with hepatitis B. Patients will complain of pain in the area of the body that is affected by the arterial inflammation. Abdominal pain with bowel involvement, weight loss, and fever are common symptoms. If the inflammation is severe, there can be ischemia of the bowel, kidney, or other affected organs. Treatment includes high doses of anti-inflammatory drugs, oral and/or IV, such as prednisone or Cytoxan®. Immunosuppressant drugs, such as Imuran®, can be helpful. If patients have hepatitis B, appropriate therapy should be started to treat this condition. If polyarteritis nodosa is severe and tissue death has occurred, surgery may be necessary to remove the ischemic tissue.

Pseudogout

Pseudogout is very similar to gout, except the causative agent is different. With pseudogout, the pain and inflammation is due to deposition of calcium pyrophosphate dihydrate crystals within a joint. The most common joints affected by pseudogout are the knees, but it can also occur in the other large joints of the body. Patients will complain of a sudden onset of severe pain in the affected joint. Even light pressure on the joint causes significant pain. The joint will appear red and swollen and will be very tender when examined. Treatment includes NSAIDs to reduce the inflammation in the affected joint. Colchicine may be effective in helping to reduce the symptoms, though it can cause several gastrointestinal side effects and may not be well tolerated. Maintenance therapy with colchicine can also be prescribed to help reduce the number of acute attacks of pseudogout. Aspiration of the joint fluid can be performed to relieve pressure on the joint and help to decrease pain.

Polymyalgia rheumatica

Polymyalgia rheumatica is a condition in which patients experience muscle stiffness and aching throughout their bodies. Polymyalgia rheumatica can be insidious in onset or occur very quickly. It is more common in adults over the age of 50, and it may resolve after 1 or 2 years. Polymyalgia rheumatica is an autoimmune disorder, and it is not known exactly what triggers this disease to occur. Patients will complain of muscle pain and stiffness in various locations of the body. As the disease progresses, it will affect both sides equally but may begin in a unilateral distribution. Patients may have a generalized feeling of weakness or malaise, fever, weight loss, and fatigue. Anemia of chronic disease can also develop in time. Treatment of the muscle pain is attempted with NSAIDs. Treatment with corticosteroids may be necessary as symptoms become debilitating. Patients should be counseled on the risks of long-term steroid use and should be closely monitored.

Polymyositis

Polymyositis is a connective tissue disease in which inflammation occurs in the muscles. It most commonly affects the muscles in the proximal large joints, such as shoulders and hips, and is gradually progressive in onset. A definite cause is not known, but it may be due to an autoimmune reaction. Patients will complain of a slow progression of muscle weakness and pain. This will commonly be present in the shoulders and arms, and patients will experience a sensation of fatigue after even light activity. They may have some dysphagia that has been progressive, also. The most common treatments for polymyositis are high dose anti-inflammatory drugs, including steroids, along with physical therapy. There are some experimental medications available that work by suppressing the immune system, but most of them are only available through clinical trials. Complications of polymyositis include possible pneumonia due to decreased chest wall muscle expansion or aspiration pneumonia due to dysphagia.

Rheumatoid arthritis

Rheumatoid arthritis is a progressive disease that affects the synovial linings of the joints. The body's white blood cells attack this synovial lining and destroy it, leading to deformity and destruction of the joint. It is usually diagnosed in middle age and is more likely to occur in females than males. Patients will have a gradual progression of joint pain that generally starts in the small joints of the hands, wrists, ankles, and feet first. It will eventually spread to include the larger joints of the body. They will notice swelling and possibly redness of the joints, along with decreased movement as the disease progresses. There is no cure for rheumatoid arthritis, but symptoms can be controlled. NSAIDs and pain medications can help with pain relief. Immunosuppressants, such as Imuran®, and TNF-alpha suppressants, such as Enbrel®, can help to prevent flare-ups of the condition and control symptoms. In severe cases, joint replacement surgery may be necessary.

Reiter's syndrome

Reiter's syndrome is a collection of three syndromes: arthritis, redness of the eyes, and urinary tract symptoms. This condition is also called reactive arthritis because it can occur in response to an infection somewhere in the body. The most common predisposing infection is *Chlamydia*. And symptoms of Reiter's usually appear 1-3 weeks following infection. Other less common bacteria that may cause Reiter's syndrome include *Salmonella* and *Shigella*. It is more common in young adult males. The arthritis primarily affects the joints in the lower extremities and spine. Sacroiliitis and spondylitis of the spine are common. Conjunctivitis and uveitis also usually occur, and these symptoms may wax and wane during the course of the illness. Patients will have complaints of dysuria, urinary frequency, discharge, and prostatitis in men. Symptomatic treatment is indicated for Reiter's syndrome. If there is an active infection, appropriate antibiotics should be given. NSAIDs and corticosteroids can be helpful.

Sjögren's syndrome

Sjögren's syndrome is an autoimmune disorder that is often seen with other types of connective tissue disorders. It is not known what causes Sjögren's syndrome though it is suspected that hereditary factors may play a part. There may also be a link with a bacterial or viral infection. Sjögren's syndrome is more common in women than men. The primary symptoms seen with Sjögren's are dry eyes and a dry mouth. Rarely, it can cause lung, kidney, or liver damage. Since it is commonly seen in conjunction with other connective tissue disorders, symptoms of those accompanying diseases may also be present. There are medications that can help specifically with the dry eyes and dry mouth associated with Sjögren's syndrome. Systemic medications to treat the symptoms include corticosteroids and immunosuppressants, especially if another connective tissue disorder is present. If dry eyes are severe, surgery can be performed to block small openings in the eyelids that drain tears from the eyes, thereby retaining moisture within the eyes.

Systemic lupus erythematous

Lupus is a condition in which the body's immune system turns against itself and begins attacking organs, tissues, and blood cells. There is no definite known cause of lupus, but it is thought that genetic factors may play a part in developing the disease. There may be some influence from environmental factors as well. The malar rash (butterfly) across the nose and cheeks is common with lupus, and patients may complain of other skin lesions that come and go. Joint pain and stiffness is common, as is Raynaud's phenomenon. Patients may have chronic fatigue and weakness, along with depression. There is no known cure for lupus, but the symptoms can usually be controlled. NSAIDs and corticosteroids can help to decrease inflammation during an acute flare-up. Some of the symptoms of lupus respond to anti-malarial drugs though it is not known why. Immunosuppressant medications may also be helpful in decreasing the symptoms of lupus.

Scleroderma

Scleroderma is a condition in which hardening of the skin and connective tissues occurs. This can become progressively worse and lead to involvement of the organs. There is no definite known cause of scleroderma, but it is an autoimmune connective tissue disorder. It is more common in women than men. Patients will complain of some areas of thickened or hardened skin that will not go away. As the condition progresses, the skin becomes stiffer and range of motion of the limbs is decreased. Scleroderma can even affect the organs, such as the stomach, and lead to decreased gastric motility. It can also affect the kidneys, and when severe, result in renal failure. Topical medications can be used to help decrease inflammation over the thickened areas of skin. NSAIDs and corticosteroids can help with pain as stiffness occurs. Medications to improve circulation can help, as can immunosuppressants to decrease the symptoms and progression of scleroderma.

Neurologic System

Cerebral palsy

Cerebral palsy is a condition that develops due to brain damage during development. It affects a child's motor development and may or may not be accompanied by mental retardation. Cerebral palsy affects motor function by causing the muscles to be flaccid and weak or rigid and spastic. It can be caused by infections in the mother during pregnancy or improper brain development after birth. Parents will notice their children are not reaching developmental milestones, like sitting up, crawling, or walking, as they should. The limbs will appear under-developed and flaccid or, more commonly, stiff and rigid. The child will be uncoordinated and hyper-reflexic. There is no cure for cerebral palsy. Physical therapy and kinesiotherapy can help with stretching the muscles and preventing contractions due to rigidity. Muscle relaxants can also be given to help decrease rigidity in the limbs. If there are learning impairments, special education should be utilized to maximize the child's learning potential.

Guillain-Barré syndrome

Guillain-Barré is a condition in which inflammation occurs in the nerves throughout the body, resulting in muscle weakness and occasionally respiratory depression. There is no definite known cause of this disease, but over one-half of the people who suffer from Guillain-Barré have a history of a respiratory or gastrointestinal illness before they develop symptoms. It may be due to an autoimmune disorder. Patients will develop weakness and numbness in the extremities that gradually spreads up the limbs. Depending on the severity of the illness, patients may have paralysis of the diaphragm that requires mechanical ventilation. This can be accompanied with hypotension and bladder/bowel incontinence. Plasmapheresis can help to remove antibodies that may contribute to the symptoms of Guillain-Barré. Alternately, immunoglobulin intravenously can help decrease symptoms. The disorder generally begins to resolve after approximately 1 month. Most people make a full recovery from Guillain-Barré with a small portion of patients having some degree of residual weakness.

Bell's palsy

Bell's palsy is a condition in which the seventh cranial nerve, the facial nerve, is weakened or paralyzed. It can be caused by a viral infection, pregnancy, or an autoimmune condition. Patients will notice a rather rapid onset of weakness on one side of the face. This can occur quite suddenly or may come on gradually over the course of a couple of days. There will be difficulty closing the eye on the affected side, smiling, or clenching teeth, and a headache may be present. Some patients may experience pain in front of the ear on the affected side, usually a couple of days before the palsy sets in. Bell's palsy is almost always a self-limiting condition that last from a week to a few months. Giving corticosteroids early on may help reduce the symptoms and reduce inflammation surrounding the facial nerve. Antiviral medications may be helpful in reducing symptoms. Lubricating eye drops may be helpful with dry eye on the affected side.

Cluster headaches

Cluster headaches are characterized by periods when headaches will happen frequently, perhaps for a few days or months, and then go into remission without headaches for a period of time. There is no definite known cause of cluster headaches though it has been found that they are more common in males who are heavy drinkers and smokers. Dysfunction of the hypothalamus gland may also play a role. Cluster headaches are very severe and are more likely to occur at night. Patients will not usually have an aura or triggering event for the headache. They will describe a nasal congestion at the time of the headache, possibly with swelling around the eyes. Administering oxygen during a cluster headache can help decrease the severity and length of the headache. Imitrex® injections can also help at the beginning of the headache. Some patients respond well to dihydroergotamine or local anesthetics administered nasally.

Myasthenia gravis

Myasthenia gravis is a neurologic disorder that causes muscle fatigue with activity. It is an autoimmune disorder in which the body blocks the acetylcholine receptor sites at the neuromuscular junction. This leads to fewer nerve signals being sent to the muscle cells, resulting in weakness. It most commonly affects middle-aged men and women. There is no definite known cause of myasthenia gravis, but the thymus gland may play a role in producing the antibodies for the disease. Patients will complain of weakness with any activity, relieved with rest. They may have trouble with their eyelids drooping and difficulty chewing or swallowing. When severe, myasthenia gravis can even affect normal respirations. Diagnosis is by injecting Tensilon and monitoring for an improvement in symptoms. There is no cure for myasthenia gravis, but symptoms can be controlled with immunosuppressant medications. Plasmapheresis and immunoglobulin infusions may also help in reducing the symptoms. A small percentage of patients will improve after removal of the thymus gland.

Tension headaches

Tension headaches are the most common type of headache, and just about everyone has had one at some point in his/her life. It is thought headaches may be due to many factors. Changes in the balance of neurotransmitters within the brain may contribute as may fluctuating hormone levels. Increased alcohol, caffeine, or tobacco use may also cause tension headaches. Daily stress, lack of sleep, or missing a meal can also contribute to tension headaches. Patients will describe headache pain that usually feels like a band around the skull. It may affect the whole head or only one side. The headache can radiate down to the neck and cause neck and upper back pain. Rarely will people have nausea or vomiting with tension headaches. Decreasing stress and other lifestyle changes can help control chronic tension headaches. Avoiding alcohol and caffeine and quitting smoking can also help. NSAIDs and other pain relievers may help, but with excessive use, NSAIDs can contribute to rebound headaches.

Migraine headaches

Migraine headaches are fairly common and occur more in women than men. It is thought that there are several factors that may trigger a migraine. Changes in hormone levels during the menstrual cycle may trigger these, as can certain foods such as alcohol, chocolate, fermented or pickled foods, and caffeine. Stress and changes in the environment may trigger a migraine. Patients may or may not describe an aura before the headache begins. This can include a tingling sensation, change in smell or taste, or visual changes. The headache is severe and usually affects one side of the head. It may be accompanied by photophobia, phonophobia, or nausea and vomiting. Triptan medications at the first sign of a migraine can help to abort it or decrease the intensity of the pain. Pain relievers, ergot medications, and anti-emetics can also help. Prophylactic medication, such as beta-blockers, can also help to decrease the incidence of migraines.

Meningitis

Meningitis is an infection of the meninges that surround the brain and spinal cord. It is most often due to a virus and is self-limiting, but it can be fatal if a bacterium is the cause. The most common cause of bacterial meningitis is *Streptococcus pneumoniae*, with *Neisseria meningitides* as the second leading cause. *H. influenzae* and *Listeria monocytogenes* may also cause meningitis. Rarely, fungus can cause the disease. Patients will have a severe headache followed by lethargy and possibly seizures. They may describe neck pain and have neck rigidity on exam. A high fever is usually present along with photophobia. Diagnosis is by lumbar puncture and evaluation of CSF with gram stain and culture and sensitivity. While waiting for lab results to return, IV antibiotics should be started immediately. If the infection is thought to be viral in nature, supportive treatment is all that is necessary, and the illness will usually resolve within 10 days. Bacterial meningitis can be fatal and lead to multi-system organ failure.

Encephalitis

Encephalitis is a viral infection of the brain that can be primary or can occur due to a viral infection elsewhere in the body. The most common viruses to cause this are the herpes virus, especially herpes simplex, Epstein-Barr, and varicella-zoster. Arboviruses can cause encephalitis, such as Eastern and Western equine encephalitis or West Nile encephalitis. Patients may have few symptoms, or the disease may be severe. They may complain of a severe headache accompanied by nausea and vomiting. Visual changes may occur and seizures may be present. If encephalitis is severe, mental confusion and lethargy may be present. Treatment is mainly supportive. NSAIDs can help reduce the inflammation around the brain and narcotics can help with the pain. Anticonvulsants may be necessary if patients are having seizures. If a herpes virus is the causative organism, acyclovir may help to reduce symptoms and shorten the length of the illness. Research is being done on interferon as an immunosuppressant therapy to treat encephalitis.

Huntington's disease

Huntington's disease is a hereditary disorder of the neurological system. It causes destruction of brain cells and is progressive. It is an autosomal dominant disorder, which means only one parent needs to carry the gene for a child to develop the disease. Early symptoms include personality changes, impaired cognition, and depression. Physical signs include imbalance, uncontrollable facial expressions, lack of coordination, and sudden spasm-like movements. These symptoms gradually progress to the point where patients are incapacitated and cannot care for themselves. There is no cure for Huntington's disease and patients have a 10-30 year life expectancy after the onset of symptoms. Anticonvulsants, antipsychotics, and antidepressants can help with some of the symptoms. Physical therapy, occupational therapy, and kinesiotherapy can all help with maintaining range of motion and controlled movements of the limbs but will not be able to completely stop the progression of the disease.

Essential tremors

Essential tremors occur in older adults and usually affect the hands though occasionally they can be evident in the legs or even voice. They are not accompanied by any other symptoms, as seen with the tremor of Parkinson's disease, but can be debilitating if severe. Some patients have a genetic predisposition to developing essential tremors, but it is not known what causes the tremors in those who do not have a family history. Patients will complain of gradually progressive tremors in the hands or other areas. Tremors are most pronounced when performing simple activities, such as eating and drinking, and writing. The tremors usually stop when patients are resting and not moving but restart when they perform activities. Medications, such as beta-blockers and anticonvulsants, can help control the tremor in most patients. When the tremor is severe and not responding to medical management, a deep brain stimulator can be surgically implanted to try to control the tremor.

Generalized convulsive disorder

A generalized convulsive disorder occurs due to an abnormality in the electrical signals in the brain. Researchers believe a genetic abnormality causes a defect in these brain cells. Brain trauma, disease, or a stroke may also increase the chances of developing a convulsive disorder. Seizures associated with a generalized convulsive disorder may vary. The mildest of these would be a petit mal, or absence seizure, in which patients stare blankly or have very subtle movements. The other end of the spectrum is a grand mal, or tonic-clonic seizure, in which there is a loss of consciousness with generalized jerking and possibly loss of bowel or bladder control. Treatment is with anticonvulsants, but it may take several trials of drugs to find the most effective treatment for patients. Sometimes multiple medications are necessary. Rarely, surgery can be done if the seizure activity is arising from the frontal lobe of the brain. This procedure involves removing the small portion of the brain in which the seizures are originating.

Parkinson's disease

Parkinson's disease involves damage or destruction of the neurons that produce the neurotransmitter dopamine in the brain. Dopamine is responsible for allowing the body to move smoothly, without rigidity or jerkiness. The exact cause of Parkinson's is not clearly understood, though it is known that there are genetic tendencies with the disease as well as an increased incidence in people with chronic exposure to herbicides and pesticides. Symptoms usually occur after the age of 60 but may begin earlier. Patients will develop a shuffling gait, a tremor that may become severe, slowed movements, a flat affect, and sometimes dementia. It can affect speech and swallowing, and some patients may describe a loss of balance. Treatment is started with levodopa, which is converted to dopamine within the brain. It is frequently given with carbidopa, which increases its concentration within the brain. Other dopamine-agonist medications are also available to increase the dopamine levels within the brain. Surgically, a deep brain stimulator may help with movement disorders associated with Parkinson's.

Status epilepticus

Status epilepticus is a condition in which tonic-clonic or grand mal seizures occur and do not stop. It is considered a medical emergency because of the risk of asphyxiation or respiratory arrest during the seizure. Status epilepticus is most often due to patients not taking the seizure medications correctly but can also occur in acute illnesses such as meningitis, encephalitis, decreased glucose levels, or very high fever. Patients will exhibit signs of a grand mal seizure persisting after 3 minutes. There may be a known diagnosis of epilepsy or other illness. The airway of patients should be protected and intubation may be necessary. Anticonvulsants are given IV, and Valium is often the treatment of choice to stop the seizure. If the cause of the seizure is not immediately known, an EEG and other testing should be done. If an acute illness is suspected, a lumbar puncture should be done for CSF analysis. Blood cultures should also be drawn to assess for sepsis.

Generalized nonconvulsive disorder

A generalized nonconvulsive disorder occurs due to an abnormality in the electrical signals in the brain. Researchers believe a genetic abnormality causes a defect in these brain cells. Brain trauma, disease, or a stroke may also increase the chances of developing a nonconvulsive disorder. This disorder causes partial seizures. Simple partial seizures do not cause a loss of awareness, but rather a change in how things appear, taste, or smell. Patients do not have a change in motor activity with partial seizures. Complex partial seizures will cause a change in consciousness or loss of awareness with some motor changes, such as arm movements, lip smacking, repeated swallowing, or yelling out. Treatment is with anticonvulsants, but it may take several trials of drugs to find the most effective treatment for patients. Rarely, surgery can be done if the nonconvulsive seizure activity is arising from the frontal lobe of the brain. This involves removing the small portion of the brain in which the seizures are originating.

Transient ischemic attack

A transient ischemic attack (TIA), or "mini-stroke," occurs because of atherosclerosis in the brain's arteries. This buildup of cholesterol, or plaque, causes a temporary decrease in oxygen to a certain portion of the brain. About one-third of patients who have a TIA will eventually have a stroke, with most of those occurring within the next year. Patients will have symptoms similar to a stroke with possible hemiparesis, garbled speech, dizziness, and possible loss of vision in one eye. The difference between a stroke and a TIA is that, with a TIA, the symptoms will resolve spontaneously within 24 hours. There are no residual effects from a TIA. Patients who have had a TIA should be started on anticoagulant or antiplatelet medications. Low-dose aspirin should be given daily. Medications such as Plavix® or Aggrenox® help to prevent platelet aggregation but do not require routine lab work for monitoring like Coumadin®. Lifestyle changes should be implemented, including eating foods lower in fat and cholesterol, quitting smoking, and losing weight if necessary.

Psychiatry/Behavioral Science

Panic disorder

Panic disorder is a condition in which people experience extreme anxiety that may become severe enough to affect their lives and level of functioning. Panic disorder is characterized by panic attacks that may vary in intensity and frequency and usually occur in young adults. It is twice as likely to affect females. There have been links to panic disorder and exposure to trauma, substance abuse, family history, stress, and defects within the limbic system of the brain. Panic attacks experienced with panic disorder give patients a sense of extreme anxiety with rapid heartbeat, sweating, dyspnea, shaking, and dizziness. Patients may have a fear of leaving their homes or encountering crowds of people (agoraphobia), or panic disorder may be limited to feelings of anxiety during stressful situations. Treatment is with behavioral therapies to "talk themselves down" from developing a panic attack. Antidepressant therapy with SSRIs and anti-anxiety medications, such as benzodiazepines, can be helpful. Sensitization therapy with small doses of exposure to the anxiety-provoking stimulus can also be helpful.

Posttraumatic stress disorder

Posttraumatic stress disorder (PTSD) occurs following involvement in or witness to an extremely traumatic event. This can occur after abuse, from violence to patients or others, or from experiencing a natural disaster. The exact reason some people suffer from PTSD and others do not is not clearly understood. Symptoms of PTSD usually begin within 3 months of the triggering event but may occur up to years later. Patients will have flashbacks of the trauma, nightmares, irritability, anger, guilt, and possibly substance abuse. They may have difficulty in interpersonal relationships and anhedonia (inability to experience pleasure). Small reminders of the trauma can send them into an episode of anger or fear. Psychotherapy can be helpful in working through the guilt that may be experienced with PTSD. Developing coping skills to reduce anger that is triggered by reminders of the trauma can also be helpful. Medical treatment varies, depending on the predominant symptoms patients are experiencing. SSRIs and anti-anxiety medications are usually the mainstays of treatment.

Generalized anxiety disorder

Generalized anxiety disorder, or GAD, is a condition in which a person worries all the time about situations or conditions. This worry or stress is out of proportion with the general reaction of most people. It is thought that an imbalance in the neurotransmitters serotonin and norepinephrine may play a role in the development of GAD. GAD causes a generalized state of unrest with muscle tension, irritability, impatience, difficulty concentrating, and insomnia. People may appear very restless with shortness of breath, and they may complain of somatic symptoms such as nausea, diarrhea, or headache. Psychotherapy can be helpful for the treatment of GAD by having patients develop better coping skills and relaxation methods. Medical treatment is with benzodiazepines for anti-anxiety, such as Xanax® or Ativan®. SSRIs can also control symptoms. Prozac®, Effexor®, and Paxil® have been helpful in treating generalized anxiety disorder. Medical treatment may involve several trials of different medications to find the treatment that works best for patients.

Bulimia nervosa

Bulimia nervosa is an eating disorder characterized by episodes of bingeing and purging. Patients will eat excessive amounts and then feel disgusted with themselves and induce vomiting. The purging may also be accomplished with abuse of laxatives or diuretics. It is not entirely clear what causes bulimia, but a family history of eating disorders, along with a low self-esteem and striving for perfection, can contribute. Patients with bulimia may be thin or appear normal in size. Dental caries can occur because of damage from stomach acids during vomiting. Ulcers may develop in the throat and mouth. Electrolyte abnormalities can occur and may be life-threatening. Dehydration, hypotension, and cardiac dysrhythmias may also occur. Treatment includes psychotherapy to develop an improved self-esteem and healthy coping methods. The only medication that is indicated for treatment of bulimia is Prozac®, though anti-anxiety medications may also be helpful. Close medical monitoring is necessary to detect any life-threatening effects of bulimia.

Anorexia nervosa

Anorexia nervosa is an unhealthy obsession with body weight and shape. Patients avoid eating, or will only eat small amounts, to become as thin as possible. Anorexia is caused by an altered perception of body image along with underlying depression. There is often an obsession with perfection. The cause is not clearly understood, but it is known that a family history of eating disorders, along with low self-esteem and characteristics of obsessive-compulsive disorder, may contribute. Patients will appear extremely thin and may exercise excessively. Hair will be thin and nails will be brittle. The skin may be dry, and they may experience dizziness or syncope. Patients are often anemic and may have some electrolyte abnormalities. Menstruation may stop in females. Hypotension and cardiac dysrhythmias often develop. Treatment includes psychotherapy to help patients develop a better self-image and learn healthy coping methods. Antidepressants may help with some of the symptoms. Close medical monitoring is necessary to detect any possible life-threatening effects of anorexia.

Persistent depressive disorder

Depression is a common illness, and most patients experience more than one major depressive episode in a lifetime. Patients with persistent depressive disorder often have repeated episodes of depressive symptoms that are difficult to treat. The causes include a positive family history, imbalances in the neurotransmitters in the brain, and possibly environmental factors, such as tragedy in one's life. Signs and symptoms include anhedonia, sleep disturbances, unintentional weight loss or gain, crying for no reason, vague somatic complaints, and loss of concentration. Patients with major depression may develop irritability, restlessness, impatience, extreme fatigue, or low self-esteem. Treatment includes a combination of psychotherapy and antidepressant medications. In-patient treatment may be necessary in those contemplating suicide. Compliance with treatment is essential to prevent repeated episodes of the symptoms of major depression. It should be noted that suicide rates tend to be higher in patients as they are "coming out of" an episode of major depression, when their mood and outlook on life seem to be improving.

Adjustment mood disorder

An adjustment disorder is a stress and anxiety condition that occurs in response to some change in a person's life. Most people adapt to change with minimal stress-causing symptoms, but people with adjustment disorder develop excessive symptoms with minimal change in their lives. The cause of adjustment disorder is not known. Adjustment disorder will cause patients to exhibit signs of anxiety and depression in response to change. Patients may complain of sleep disturbances, extreme sadness, anhedonia, irritability, or even thoughts of suicide. They may exhibit behavior changes that are erratic, such as abusing drugs or alcohol, avoiding family, getting into legal or financial trouble, or destroying property. Children with adjustment disorder may have failing grades or may skip school. Treatment consists of psychotherapy to help work through the stress caused by the change in their lives and to develop healthy coping skills. If symptoms are severe, antidepressants may be helpful in relieving the symptoms of depression.

Bipolar disorder

Bipolar disorder is characterized by mood swings that range from major depression to mania. The severity of the disorder varies among patients, but it usually greatly affects a person's life. The exact cause of bipolar disorder is unknown, but it is thought that a positive family history, imbalances in the neurotransmitters in the brain, and some environmental factors may play a role in its development. The "low" points of bipolar disorder cause the classic symptoms of major depression with anhedonia, sleep disturbances, feelings of hopelessness, and possibly suicide. The "high" points occur during the manic phase. The characteristics of mania include restlessness, lack of sleep, aggressive behavior, pressured speech, inflated self-esteem, erratic behavior, and possibly legal or financial trouble. Patients can swing back and forth from these two states very quickly and frequently. Medical treatment of bipolar disorder is with mood stabilizers and antidepressants. Anti-anxiety medications may also be helpful. Some patients have responded well to anticonvulsants and antipsychotics.

Avoidant personality disorder

Avoidant personality disorder is a condition in which a person is very anxious or fearful of any social situations. They may be obsessive or exhibit odd behaviors that prevent them from functioning appropriately in social situations. There is no definite known cause, but social and biological factors may play a role in the development of avoidant personality disorder. These patients are often very uncomfortable in social situations and may appear to be extremely shy. They are very concerned about what others think about them and do not respond well to criticism or rejection. Interpersonal relationships are often very short-lived or do not occur at all because of their inability to overcome these feelings. Treatment of avoidant personality disorder is with a combination of psychotherapy and antidepressants or anti-anxiety medications. Antipsychotics may be necessary if patients are exhibiting any psychotic features with their disease. Therapy can be difficult, though, because of their difficulty with forming trusting relationships with therapists.

Antisocial personality disorder

People with antisocial personality disorder often repeatedly break the law, lie, cheat, steal, or harm others. They are often poor parents and are frequently imprisoned for their actions. The condition is most often noticed during the teenage years and symptoms tend to decrease as a person ages. It is more common in men and often develops in those who suffer abuse or neglect as a child. Symptoms include impulsiveness, repeated lying, stealing, aggression, and violence. Patients may be irritable, easily bored, or depressed. Oftentimes, these people appear to be very charming and fun to be around, but they will unexpectedly lash out at others or have very violent temper tantrums. Antisocial personality disorder is very hard to treat. A combination of psychotherapy with antidepressants or antipsychotics may help to control the symptoms. If patients are at risk of harming themselves or others, hospitalization with in-patient treatment may be necessary. The symptoms will often begin to decrease as patients enter middle age.

Histrionic personality disorder

Histrionic personality disorder is a condition in which a person is extremely emotional or dramatic. The condition is more common in women than men, and the cause is not completely understood though it is probably due to a combination of genetic and environmental factors. Symptoms of histrionic personality disorder include an obsession with the approval of others. These patients often are very dramatic and attention seeking. They may wear very revealing clothing and act out in a sexually promiscuous way. They may have multiple sexual partners and not become emotionally attached to any one person. They can have frequent mood changes and be impulsive. Treatment of histrionic personality disorder is often with a combination of psychotherapy and medications. Psychotherapy can be difficult because of patients' inability to form trusting relationships with the therapists. Antidepressants and anti-anxiety medications may help with the symptoms. Hospitalization may be necessary if patients are in danger of harming themselves.

Borderline personality disorder

Borderline personality development is a condition in which a person struggles with maintaining an even personality. They are constantly in a conflicting state in which they cannot regulate their emotions. This condition is more prevalent in women and is thought to occur due to a combination of child abuse or neglect, a positive family history, or a serotonin imbalance in the brain. Symptoms of borderline personality disorder include a rollercoaster of mood swings. They may be happy with their life situation one day and hate it the next day. This makes relationships very difficult. They frequently change jobs or move. They often have a low self-esteem and may even have tendencies to hurt themselves.
Treatment of borderline personality disorder is with a combination of psychotherapy and medications. Antidepressants and anti-anxiety medications can help control some of the symptoms. Hospitalization may be necessary if patients are at risk of harming themselves.

Obsessive-compulsive disorder

Obsessive-compulsive disorder (OCD) is a condition in which a person performs repeated activities or has obsessive thoughts that interfere with their daily lives. The condition frequently begins during adolescence and may be due to several factors. Environmental or genetic factors can increase the tendency to develop OCD. Low serotonin levels may also play a role. Excessive stress and disruption in one's life can lead to OCD. There is some preliminary research that shows there may be a link between *streptococcal* throat infection and the development of OCD.

Symptoms comprise obsessions and compulsions:
- Obsessions are thoughts that are constant, anxiety-provoking, and interfere with a person's ability to concentrate.
- Compulsions are the actions that come about because of the obsessive thoughts. These can be excessive washing and cleaning because of obsession with germs, or any other repetitive actions.

Treatment is psychotherapy and antidepressants. Both Paxil® and Zoloft ®have been approved for the treatment of OCD. These medications help to elevate serotonin levels in the brain.

Narcissistic personality disorder

Narcissistic personality disorder is a condition in which people have no regard for others and feel that they are superior to others. It occurs more frequently in males than females, and symptoms often become evident in early adulthood. Narcissistic personality disorder may be caused by abuse or neglect as a child or possibly from excessive pampering and spoiling as a child. It may also be related to an imbalance of neurotransmitters within the brain. Symptoms of narcissistic personality disorder are a combination of extreme boastfulness and conceit but with a very volatile self-esteem. Criticism from others can be devastating, but these patients will often put down those who do not praise them. They belittle others and have difficulty maintaining healthy relationships. These patients often praise their own achievements and take advantage of others to get what they want. The primary treatment for narcissistic personality disorder is psychotherapy. If there is underlying depression or anxiety, medications to treat these conditions may be helpful.

Schizoid personality disorder

Schizoid personality disorder is a condition in which people withdraw from society and avoid interaction with others. They often find relationships too distressing and feel more comfortable when they are isolated. The cause is thought to be extreme child neglect or abuse. They may have had parents who were uninvolved in their lives and did not exhibit any love toward them. Symptoms of schizoid personality disorder include self-imposed social isolation, a lack of social skills, indifference to criticism, and inability to maintain healthy relationships with others. They often have a flat affect and show very little emotion. These patients may have a low work ethic and be poor students. Psychotherapy is the mainstay of treatment with schizoid personality disorder. This is focused on developing social skills and helping patients find pleasure from interacting with others. Medications may be used to help treat some of the concomitant symptoms of depression or anxiety.

Paranoid personality disorder

Paranoid personality disorder is characterized by odd or eccentric behaviors that interfere with daily living. Risk factors include a positive family history of the disorder. Environmental factors, such as a history of child abuse or neglect, may also play a role in developing paranoid personality disorder. Symptoms of paranoid personality disorder include distrust of others, extreme sensitivity to criticism, and irritability. These patients often feel that others are "out to get them" and may find criticism in even the most innocent remark. They have difficulty maintaining healthy relationships and do not work well with others. They often isolate themselves emotionally from others because of the perception that others are out to hurt them. Treatment of paranoid personality disorder is with a combination of psychotherapy and medications. Antidepressants, anti-anxiety medications, and antipsychotics may be helpful in controlling some of the symptoms. Therapy can be difficult because of patients' inability to form trusting relationships with therapists.

Delusional disorder

Delusional disorder is a condition in which a person develops very strong beliefs in a specific situation that is not true, to the point that they alter their behaviors and life around this idea. This disorder may be caused by a combination of environmental or genetic factors though no specific cause is understood. Delusional disorder can take different forms. Patients may have delusions of grandeur, believing that they are above everyone else and in a much higher standing than they really are. They may have paranoid delusions that others are out to hurt them or others. They may have a belief that someone is in love with them. They may also have delusions that they are physically ill when there is nothing medically wrong. Treatment is with a combination of psychotherapy and medications. Antidepressants and antipsychotics may help to control the symptoms. Treatment can be difficult because patients firmly believe in their delusions.

Schizotypal personality disorder

Schizotypal personality disorder is a condition in which people isolates themselves from social situations because of extreme anxiety when interacting with others. They find their isolation very distressing, though, unlike the schizoid personalities who crave isolation. Risk factors include a combination of a family history of schizophrenia or environmental factors, such as abuse or neglect during childhood. Symptoms of schizotypal personality disorder include social isolation, anxiety and distress with isolation or social interaction, and a lack of relationships with others. These patients often develop a belief that they have magical powers, such as mental telepathy, and may exhibit odd behaviors. Their emotions may be unstable with occasional temper tantrums or rages. Treatment is with a combination of psychotherapy and medications. Antidepressants and antipsychotics may help to relieve some of the symptoms of this condition. Therapy can be difficult because of patients' inability to develop trusting relationships with therapists.

Schizoaffective disorder

Schizoaffective disorder is a combination of schizophrenic symptoms with a mood disorder. These patients may have hallucinations and delusions with depression, anxiety, or mania. The condition is thought to be caused by a combination of genetic, environmental, and biologic factors. Schizoaffective disorder will cause patients to have delusions and/or hallucinations consistent with schizophrenia. Along with these behaviors will be major depression, extreme anxiety, or episodes of mania. Patients may cycle between depression and mania, consistent with a bipolar component to the condition. Symptoms may become severe enough that patients can be at risk for harming themselves or others. Treatment consists of a combination of psychotherapy and medications to control the symptoms. Antidepressants, anti-anxiety medications, or antipsychotics may be used depending on patients' symptoms. Medications to stabilize mood may also be useful in decreasing the mood disorder component of the disease. Hospitalization may be necessary for in-patient treatment, especially if patients are at risk of hurting themselves or others.

Pulmonary System

Acute bronchitis

Acute bronchitis is an infection of the bronchial tree. This infection and inflammation causes the bronchial structures to secrete more mucus, which causes wheezing and a productive cough. This infection is usually caused by a virus. Patients with acute bronchitis will complain of a chronic cough, usually productive, and may describe some wheezing. They may have developed the common cold and feel that this has now started with symptoms in their lungs. They may say that the cough is worse at night and may or may not have a fever with this. Because acute bronchitis is usually caused by a virus, antibiotics rarely help to relieve the symptoms. Using a humidifier at night to moisten the air, drinking plenty of fluids to thin the mucus secretions, and resting should help to relieve the symptoms within a week. The cough of bronchitis may linger for several weeks as the bronchial tubes heal.

Acute epiglottitis

Acute epiglottitis is a medical emergency that can result in the epiglottis blocking the trachea if it is not treated immediately. It can be caused by the *H. influenzae* bacterium, but this is not often seen because of the immunization now available. *Streptococcus* and *Staphylococcus* are the most common bacteria to cause epiglottitis now. Trauma to the throat can also cause inflammation of the epiglottis. Patients with epiglottitis will have a muffled voice. There will be throat pain and usually a fever. Difficulty swallowing and breathing will also be present. Patients lean forward to breathe and may even be drooling if swallowing is too difficult. If epiglottitis is suspected, one should NOT attempt to visualize the epiglottis because this may cause more inflammation and could close the airway. Lateral neck x-rays will show an enlarged epiglottis (thumb sign). Treatment consists of second and third-generation cephalosporins. Patients should be kept calm, should avoid swallowing or talking, and intubation equipment should be kept on hand in case of airway obstruction.

Acute bronchiolitis

Acute bronchiolitis is a viral infection that causes inflammation of the upper and lower respiratory tract. This most often affects infants and young children because older children and adults have larger bronchial tubes that can accommodate this inflammation and the edema associated with it. Respiratory syncytial virus (RSV) is one of the viruses that can cause acute bronchiolitis in children. The parents of patients with acute bronchiolitis may describe hearing their child wheeze and cough frequently. The child may even appear short of breath. A low-grade fever is usually present. Rarely, the severe respiratory symptoms can lead to respiratory arrest. The cause of acute bronchiolitis is usually viral, so treatment is supportive with nebulizer treatments to decrease the inflammation and open the airways. Humidifier use to moisten the air can be helpful also. Antipyretics should be given to decrease fever, if present. Plenty of fluids should be given to prevent dehydration.

Influenza

Influenza is a viral infection that affects the entire respiratory system from the nose to the lungs. There are 3 strains of influenza virus: A, B, and C. Types A and B is the ones seen most often and the ones that the annual flu shot is most effective against. Type C is not as common. Though the symptoms can be very similar, the flu and the common cold differ in that the flu is very sudden in onset while a cold tends to come on slowly. A patient with the flu will have a high fever with chills and sweats, body aches, nasal congestion, dry cough, headache, and loss of appetite. Children may also have vomiting and diarrhea. Antibiotic treatment is not effective. Supportive treatment with rest, fluids, analgesics, decongestants, and cough suppressants can be tried. Usually the flu just needs to run its course, but it can linger up to several weeks. It can be life-threatening to the very young, the elderly, and the immunocompromised.

Croup

Croup occurs because of inflammation around the larynx and trachea. It occurs in children and causes a cough that sounds like a bark and is very distinguishable. It is most often caused by the parainfluenza virus, though sometimes by RSV, measles, or bacterial infections. The barking cough associated with croup is usually worse at night and can wake a child up from sleep. A fever and hoarseness are usually present. If children are old enough, they will complain of sore throat. Humidified air and cool drinks will help to ease the inflammation in the throat. Keeping children calm and decreasing the amount they talk will also help relieve the irritation. Sometimes, nebulizer treatments with corticosteroids or epinephrine can help to dilate the airways. Rarely, hospitalization is necessary with oxygen tent treatments or even intubation if very severe. In the rare case that bacteria is the cause of croup, appropriate antibiotics can be given to eradicate the causative organism.

Bacterial, viral, fungal, and HIV-related pneumonias

Bacterial pneumonia, or community-acquired pneumonia, is most commonly caused by *Streptococcus pneumoniae*. The balance of the cases of pneumonia is divided amongst *H. Influenzae*, *Moraxella catarrhalis*, atypical pathogens such as *Legionella* and *Mycoplasma* species, *Staphylococcus aureus*, and gram-negative organisms. Viral pneumonia is commonly caused by influenza A or B viruses. RSV can also cause viral pneumonia, as can the herpes virus, parainfluenza, adenovirus, and varicella viruses. Herpes and varicella virus pneumonias are rare. Fungal pneumonia is usually caused by *Histoplasma capsulatum*, *Coccidioides immitis*, or *Blastomyces dermatitidis*. This usually only occurs in those patients who are severely immunocompromised. Patients with this type of pneumonia often do not know they are infected until they become very ill. HIV-related pneumonia is most often caused by *Pneumocystis jiroveci*, though the immunocompromised patient is susceptible to contracting any type of pneumonia. Fungal pneumonias are also prevalent among patients with HIV.

Pertussis

Pertussis, or whooping cough, is a highly contagious respiratory infection caused by the bacterium *Bordetella pertussis*. Pertussis is becoming more common now because immunization from the DPT injection tends to wear off by adulthood. The symptoms come in 3 stages:
- The first stage, the catarrhal stage, is when there are symptoms of a cold such as runny nose, fever, sneezing, and mild cough.
- After one to two weeks, the second stage, or paroxysmal stage, begins. This is characterized by coughing spells that often leave the person breathless. These spells are followed by a loud inspiratory breath that makes a loud "whoop" sound.
- The third stage, or convalescent stage, lasts two to three weeks as the symptoms gradually fade.

It is questionable whether antibiotics help to shorten the duration of symptoms of pertussis. Erythromycin can be given for 7 days to help eradicate the bacteria. There are no proven effective treatments to treat the cough.

Tuberculosis

Tuberculosis (TB) is more prevalent in those who are homeless or who live in crowded conditions. TB is seen more often in those who are frequently exposed to the disease. Underdeveloped countries also have a higher prevalence of TB. The symptoms of active TB include night sweats, chronic cough with hemoptysis, fever, fatigue, and dyspnea. Loss of appetite, weight loss, and pleurisy are often common. A person can be exposed to TB and not contract the disease but will test positive on a PPD skin test. Prophylactic antibiotics can be given at that time to prevent the development of symptoms. Treatment includes multiple antibiotics. INH and rifampin are mainstays of treatment and should be continued for at least 6 months of treatment. Pyrazinamide and ethambutol are also usually given. Once diagnosed, patients with TB should be kept in isolation, and the local health department should be notified of an active case of TB in the community.

Pneumonia

Patients will present with symptoms of fatigue, productive cough with purulent sputum, fevers with chills, and dyspnea. Patients may have wheezes and crackles, fever, and a lung consolidation present on chest x-ray. Treatment of bacterial pneumonia is with antibiotics. There is growing resistance to many antibiotics, but first line treatment is with cephalosporins, macrolides, fluoroquinolones, or tetracyclines. Viral pneumonia causes a low-grade fever with a cough that is mildly productive. Muscle aches are common. Patients may be sick for several days before seeing a doctor. Treatment of viral pneumonia can be done with an anti-viral such as amantadine or rimantadine if started within 36 hours of the onset of symptoms. Otherwise, treatment is symptomatic. Fungal pneumonias have similar symptoms, but can also spread to become systemic. Treatment is with anti-fungals, depending on the infective organism. HIV-related pneumonias have symptoms according to the type of pneumonia that is present. Treatment depends upon the infective organism.

Carcinoid tumors

Carcinoid tumors occur in the neuroendocrine system and are most frequently found in the appendix or small intestine, though they may also be seen in the lung or pancreas. They are slow growing tumors and are frequently not diagnosed for several years. Patients with carcinoid tumors may be asymptomatic. If the tumor is outside the appendix, it will likely secrete serotonin, and symptoms of carcinoid syndrome can be seen (flushing, diarrhea, weight loss, loss of appetite, wheezing). Treatment of carcinoid tumors consists of surgical removal of the tumor. This may involve an appendectomy or small bowel resection. Chemotherapy may be given if the tumor has spread to other locations in the body. Radiation can also be given but is usually reserved for those carcinoid tumors that have spread to the bones to help relieve pain. Interferon injections may be given to help decrease the growth of the tumor, especially if it is affecting the liver.

Bronchogenic carcinoma

Bronchogenic carcinoma is the most deadly cancer in the United States and accounts for approximately 25% of all cancer deaths in this country. Bronchogenic cancer is primarily seen as lung cancer. Smoking is the most common risk factor, with almost all cases of this type of cancer occurring in smokers. Small cell carcinoma has the worst prognosis and has usually metastasized by the time it is diagnosed. A symptom of bronchogenic carcinoma is a progressively worsening cough with or without hemoptysis and dyspnea. Weight loss and fatigue may be present as the disease progresses. If metastasis is present, patients may experience bone pain, abdominal pain, or confusion, depending on the location of the metastasis. Some small cell tumors may serve as an ectopic source of hormone production, so symptoms that mimic an endocrine disorder maybe evident. Often, once diagnosed, prognosis is very poor with this disease. Treatment may involve surgery to debulk a large tumor or a lobectomy. This may be followed with radiation and/or chemotherapy depending on the location of the cancer.

Bronchiectasis

Bronchiectasis is a condition in which the bronchial tubes are dilated which prevents people from being able to clear mucus from their lungs. Bronchiectasis can occur in just one location of the lungs or may occur in several areas. It is most often due to inflammation or infection, such as with pneumonia. Chronic disease, such as cystic fibrosis, can cause bronchiectasis. Patients will have a productive cough of yellowish green sputum or even hemoptysis, and they may be short of breath. With chronic disease, recurrent pneumonia in the same location of the lungs may occur. If the bronchiectasis is due to chronic disease, regular postural drainage should be done to encourage drainage of mucus from the lungs. However, aspiration of a foreign body can damage the bronchial tubes. Inhaled corticosteroids can help to dilate the airways, and avoiding allergens can help to prevent further constriction of the airways. If due to pneumonia, appropriate antibiotic therapy should be given. In severe cases, a lobectomy can remove the damaged section of the lung.

Asthma

Asthma occurs when the airways are inflamed. These airways will constrict and produce more mucus, which causes difficulty breathing and the classic "asthma attacks." Asthma is frequently seen in multiple family members. It can be aggravated by allergen exposure, cold air, exercise, and stress. The symptoms of asthma include wheezing, difficulty breathing, and chest tightness. Symptoms may be worse during the night. Coughing spasms can also occur as the airways constrict and the lungs attempt to expel the extra mucus that is produced. Treatment can be divided amongst long-acting medicines and quick-acting "rescue" medications. The long-acting drugs used include inhaled corticosteroids, beta-2 agonists, leukotriene modifiers, and Cromolyn®. The short-acting medications are used when patients are having an acute exacerbation of the disease and include short-acting beta-2 agonists, ipratropium (Atrovent®), and corticosteroids. The best treatment is prevention by minimizing exposure to known allergens or triggers, using medications regularly, and not smoking.

Cystic fibrosis

Cystic fibrosis is an autosomal recessive genetic disorder. It causes excessive mucus production that leads to lung obstruction, deficient enzyme production that causes pancreatic dysfunction, and a less-than-competent immune system. Cystic fibrosis is diagnosed in childhood, usually after a child has had multiple lung infections or is exhibiting weight loss and failure to thrive. Symptoms include recurrent lung infection with excessive congestion, bowel obstruction due to thickened feces, and poor nutrition because of decreased vitamin absorption. There is no cure for cystic fibrosis. Life expectancy is usually into the 20s, but advances in treatment have extended this somewhat. Postural drainage can be performed regularly to promote drainage of lung secretions. Enzymes are taken orally to aid in digestion. Bronchodilators and chronic steroids are given to decrease irritation in the lungs and promote bronchodilation. In severe cases, lung transplantation can be performed though this still does not cure the disease.

Chronic bronchitis

Chronic bronchitis occurs when the bronchial tubes are irritated and inflamed, causing them to secrete excess mucus. This, in turn, causes the airways to become plugged and prevents adequate flow of oxygen. Smoking is the most common cause of chronic bronchitis. Occasionally chronic exposure to dust and other irritants can cause chronic bronchitis. Diagnosis is made by symptoms of a productive cough for at least 3 months during a 2-year period, most often in a smoker. This is not accompanied by an acute illness or cold symptoms, and patients are afebrile. Patients may complain of shortness of breath and occasional chest pain with wheezing. They may be chronically fatigued and have a feeling of general malaise. Treatment is symptomatic and may include bronchodilators to widen the airways. Patients may require supplemental oxygen at home if hypoxia is severe. Patients should quit smoking to help decrease irritation to the lungs.

Pleural effusion

A pleural effusion is an accumulation of fluid in the pleural space. This can result in excessive pressure applied to the lungs. It is frequently caused by infections, such as pneumonia, or chronic disease, as seen with CHF or lung cancer. Patients will complain of a cough and shortness of breath. They may have pleuritic chest pain. Decreased breath sounds may be heard, and there will be dullness to percussion over the lung fields. The effusion is evident on chest x-ray and may be better-examined by CT imaging. Diuretics may be used to decrease the effusion if is it due to CHF. A thoracentesis may be done to draw the fluid off the lungs and to diagnose whether it is infective in nature or if it contains malignant cells. If the fluid is infective in nature, it could result in the formation of an abscess around the lungs. If the fluid collection increases, a pneumothorax can occur due to the pressure applied to the outside of the lung.

Emphysema

Emphysema occurs when the alveoli lose their elasticity and do not completely empty of air with expiration. This causes hyperinflation of the lungs with difficulty drawing in the oxygen needed to take another breath. The most common cause of emphysema is smoking. A deficiency in alpha-1-antitrypsin protein can also lead to emphysema. Patients will feel short of breath and easily fatigued. They will have a chronic, mild, usually non-productive cough. Over time, patients will develop the appearance of a barrel chest and clubbing in their fingernails. Treatment consists of inhaled bronchodilators to decrease the cough, though they are not as effective as they are with asthma. Steroids can help to decrease inflammation in the lungs, though they are not extremely effective. Quitting smoking is the best treatment to help prevent progression of the disease. Patients may require supplemental oxygen at home. Rarely, surgery can be done to remove the damaged tissue.

Pulmonary embolism

A pulmonary embolism (PE) occurs when a thrombus travels to the lungs and causes obstruction of the airway. PE can be caused by a deep vein thrombosis that travels to the lungs, by any conditions that cause the blood to be hypercoagulable, or by cardiac dysrhythmia. Patients with a PE will become suddenly short of breath and may complain of chest pain, shoulder pain, sweating, or cough. On exam, the blood pressure may be low and there may be decreased breath sounds throughout the lungs. Patients may become unconscious. Oxygen is given first to help patients. Blood thinners will also be started, usually heparin first. Injectable Lovenox® or oral Coumadin® may be given later. Patients will need to stay on Coumadin® because of the risk of recurrent PE. Once a PE is confirmed, "clot buster" thrombolytic drugs may be given to break up the clot. Throughout all treatment, medications may need to be given that will help keep patients' blood pressure at a normal level.

Primary, secondary, traumatic, and tension pneumothorax

A primary pneumothorax usually occurs in young, tall males. This happens when a bleb ruptures on the lung, causing collapse of a portion of the lung. This does not occur because of chronic lung disease. If small, it can be monitored with chest x-rays. If large, hospitalization with a chest tube may be necessary. A secondary pneumothorax occurs with chronic lung disease, such as COPD or cystic fibrosis. It can be life-threatening and may require a chest tube for treatment. A traumatic pneumothorax occurs when there is trauma to the chest wall that results in air entering the chest cavity. This can result in a small pneumothorax that can be monitored or it may be large enough to require a chest tube. A tension pneumothorax occurs when air becomes trapped in the pleural space and cannot escape. This will result in a worsening pneumothorax that will eventually cause the structures in the pleural cavity to shift. It can be life-threatening and should be treated urgently with a chest tube.

Cor pulmonale

Cor pulmonale is right-sided heart failure. This can occur because of prolonged pulmonary hypertension or an increase in pressure within the right ventricle. Chronic lung disease, such as COPD or cystic fibrosis, can lead to cor pulmonale. Patients may complain of increasing shortness of breath and fatigue. They may have chest pain that is exacerbated with activity and that is not entirely relieved with rest as the disease progresses. On exam, patients may have an increase in jugular venous distention, ascites, hepatomegaly, or lower extremity edema. The focus of treatment with cor pulmonale is to treat the underlying cause. Calcium channel blockers are generally given, and patients may require anticoagulant therapy to prevent complications of the condition. Vasodilators can also be given as can medications that will help to optimize cardiac function. Oxygen may be given for patients to use at home in order to supply their bodies with extra oxygen in order to improve oxygenation of the blood.

Pulmonary hypertension

Pulmonary hypertension is a rise in pressure within the pulmonary artery carrying blood to the lungs. It can be caused by left-sided heart failure, especially as the ejection fraction decreases and the left ventricular function decreases. There are many medical conditions that can also cause pulmonary hypertension, such as cirrhosis, sickle cell disease, scleroderma, and congenital heart disease. The symptoms of pulmonary hypertension include shortness of breath, which becomes progressively worse, and fatigue. Patients may also complain of a cough, sometimes with hemoptysis, and may even have syncopal episodes. Chest pain may also occur as the condition becomes advanced. The treatment of pulmonary hypertension focuses on treating the underlying cause. Treatment includes diuretics, beta-blockers, and ACE inhibitors for heart failure. Digoxin or other medications to improve cardiac function may also be helpful. Calcium channel blockers, vasodilators, and anticoagulants may also be useful in treating pulmonary hypertension and in preventing complications from this condition.

Pneumoconiosis

Pneumoconiosis is an occupational lung disease that is due to inhaling particulate matter. It can be due to inhaling the dust from coal, asbestos, silica, beryllium, iron, and other materials. The specific type of pneumoconiosis will vary depending upon the material inhaled. For example, asbestos workers can develop asbestosis while those who work with silica develop silicosis. Patients will complain of progressively worsening shortness of breath that is more pronounced during activities. They will also have a chronic cough that may be productive or nonproductive. On exam, there may be decreased breath sounds present. Chest x-ray may show consolidated areas where the inhaled dust has damaged the lung tissue. There is no known treatment for the pneumoconiosis diseases. Supportive treatment with supplemental oxygen may be necessary. Patients should avoid any future contact with causative substances and if they smoke, they should quit in order preventing any further damage to the lung tissue or any additional exacerbation of the illness. In very severe cases, lung transplantation can be performed.

Pulmonary fibrosis

Pulmonary fibrosis is a condition in which the alveoli become damaged and are replaced by fibrotic scar tissue. This results in a thickening of the alveolar tissue, preventing the transfer of oxygen. The cause of pulmonary fibrosis is uncertain, but it is thought there may be a genetic tendency for people to develop this disease. It is also thought that inhaled environmental agents, including cigarette smoke, may increase the likelihood of developing pulmonary fibrosis. Patients may complain of shortness of breath, especially during activity. They may have a dry, hacking cough and fatigue. Patients may have a loss of appetite with significant weight loss. On exam, there may be decreased breath sounds and a decrease in oxygen saturation with pulse oximetry. There is no curable treatment for pulmonary fibrosis. Supplemental oxygen can be given to help with shortness of breath. In severe cases, a single lung transplant may be performed.

Acute respiratory distress syndrome

Acute respiratory distress syndrome (ARDS) occurs when there is inflammation and fluid accumulation within the lungs. ARDS can be caused by pneumonia, trauma, shock, aspiration, or chemical burns. The onset of this condition is usually 1-3 days following the triggering event. ARDS can be life-threatening, and patients are treated in the ICU. Patients will have rapid respiratory decline to the point of respiratory arrest. Patients may become unconscious and multisystem organ failure can occur. Patients may also be hypotensive, and cardiogenic shock can set in. On exam, crackles may be heard in the lungs because of fluid accumulation. Cyanosis is frequently present. Maintaining proper oxygenation is the mainstay of treatment. Patients are usually placed on ventilators until they can be weaned off and are able to breathe on their own. If a lung infection is present, appropriate antibiotics should be given. Diuretics may be given to decrease the fluid accumulation within the lungs.

Sarcoidosis

Sarcoidosis is an inflammatory disease that starts in the lungs but may go on to affect every organ system in the body. It is usually self-limiting and will resolve within a few years, but in rare cases it may be fatal. The cause of sarcoidosis is not known, but it is thought it may be due to an immune response after exposure to a certain bacteria, virus, or toxin. Signs and symptoms vary depending on the organ system affected. With lung disease, patients may complain of shortness of breath with a chronic cough. A skin rash, aching joints, weight loss, fatigue, and red or watery eyes may also be present. Lab tests may reveal an elevation in ACE and calcium, but this is not definitive for diagnosis. Bronchoscopy can be performed for granuloma samples and confirmation of the diagnosis. There is no cure for the disease but treatment may help to control some of the symptoms. High-dose anti-inflammatory drugs are given and steroid therapy is necessary for treatment of severe symptoms.

Aspiration of foreign body

Aspiration of a foreign body is commonly seen in children. It can occur in patients with swallowing difficulties as they aspirate food, liquids, or medications because of dysphagia. Frequently patients will have a persistent cough and the feeling the something is "stuck" in their throats. Wheezing or stridor may be heard, depending on the location of the blockage within the airway. If severe, the airway may be completely blocked, and this could cause patients to collapse and go into respiratory arrest. On exam, decreased breath sounds may be present on one side due to blockage of the main bronchus. Wheezing may also be heard in any portion of the lungs. Treatment is focused on removing the object. In severe cases, the Heimlich maneuver should be given to forcefully expel the object from the airway. In emergency cases, an emergency tracheostomy may be performed to create a new airway below the level of the obstruction. In patients who are stable, bronchoscopy can be performed to physically remove the object.

Hyaline membrane disease

Hyaline membrane disease affects premature infants. It occurs when infants are born before the lungs are producing adequate amounts of surfactant. Surfactant helps to prevent the lungs from collapsing. As the airways collapse, infants will struggle more and more to breath until they become acidotic and multisystem organ failure begins. The most common symptom of this condition is respiratory distress in the premature infant. Surfactant is usually present after week 35 of gestation, and amniotic fluid can be tested for adequate production of the substance. The baby can become cyanotic and become more dyspneic. Respiratory arrest can occur after the baby becomes exhausted. Treatment includes mechanical ventilation with positive pressure. Artificial surfactant can be given through the endotracheal tube. Babies may suffer permanent respiratory illness because of hyaline membrane disease, but others make a full recovery and suffer no consequences. The best treatment is maintaining a healthy pregnant to prevent premature birth.

Reproductive System

Endometriosis

Endometriosis occurs when the tissue that makes up the uterine lining is also present outside the uterus. This can occur on the fallopian tubes, the ovaries, or outside of the uterus. It will thicken with hormonal changes that occur during the menstrual cycle and will shed, causing irritation to the surrounding structures. When severe, endometriosis can cause adhesions and severe pain. The cause of endometriosis is unknown. The most common symptom is cramping pain, especially during menstruation. Bleeding can be excessively heavy. Infertility may occur as scar tissue and adhesions form. These may interfere with normal release of the mature egg from the ovary. Oral contraceptives can help maintain hormone levels to prevent excessive symptoms from this condition. Medications to prevent the secretion of hormones by the ovaries can also help to decrease the symptoms. Laparoscopic surgery can be done to remove the tissue from the ovaries and fallopian tubes and decrease the symptoms and increase chances of pregnancy. As a last resort, hysterectomy may be performed.

Ovarian cysts

Ovarian cysts are relatively common and occur on the surface of the ovaries. Most do not produce symptoms, but some women can have significant symptoms from these cysts. Cysts can occur in the follicle when the egg does not release from the maturing follicle and continues to grow, leading to a cyst. These generally resolve without treatment. A corpus luteum cyst occurs after the egg ruptures, and the follicle becomes the corpus luteum. It seals itself off and begins to expand as fluid accumulates in it to form a cyst. The follicular cysts generally do not cause symptoms. The corpus luteum cysts, however, can grow to be 4 cm wide and may cause significant abdominal pain. These can also rupture, which will cause sudden, severe abdominal pain and syncope. Oral contraceptives may prevent cyst formation with the menstrual cycle by regulating hormone secretion. If symptoms are persistent, surgery may be necessary to remove the cysts from the ovary. If a cyst ruptures, removal of the ovary may be necessary.

Metritis

Metritis is an infection of the uterine lining that occurs following childbirth, usually due to retained fragments from childbirth. It can be life-threatening if not promptly treated and should be considered as a diagnosis in any woman who develops a fever after childbirth. The first symptom will be a fever with chills and patients may complain of lower abdominal or pelvic pain. The uterus will be tender on palpation and the vaginal discharge present will have a foul odor. This can develop rapidly into peritonitis, pelvic abscess, and septic shock. This can cause coagulopathies with possible deep vein thrombosis or pulmonary embolism. Treatment consists of prompt administration of multiple IV antibiotics. Blood transfusion may be necessary if septic shock develops. The antibiotics should be continued for at least 48 hours after the fever resolves. Manual exam should be performed to attempt to remove any retained placental fragments, and surgery may be necessary to irrigate the uterus or to do a hysterectomy if symptoms do not resolve.

Incompetent cervix

An incompetent cervix refers to a cervix that will not remain completely closed during pregnancy, placing the baby at risk for premature birth. This can be due to past trauma to the cervix, such as from surgery or D&C. Previous deliveries that were traumatic to the cervix may lead to an incompetent cervix, as can genetic anomalies that cause a malformed cervix. Unfortunately, an incompetent cervix is usually diagnosed after a second or third-trimester miscarriage occurs. The incompetent cervix can usually be detected on prenatal ultrasound or pelvic exam. Patients may or may not have some bleeding in the second or third trimester. The cervix can be reinforced with a cerclage procedure, which involves placing purse string sutures in the cervix to draw it closed. This affectively sutures the cervix closed to prevent premature dilation. These sutures are usually removed in the last few weeks of pregnancy to prevent tearing of the cervix as it tries to dilate.

Cervicitis

Cervicitis is inflammation or infection of the cervix. This usually occurs due to sexually-transmitted diseases, such as chlamydia or gonorrhea. Chemical irritation from lubricants, spermicides, or douching may also cause cervicitis. Bacterial vaginitis may also cause a bacterial infection of the cervix. Patients will complain of lower pelvic pain that is aggravated during sexual intercourse. They may have noticed an increase in vaginal discharge that is yellow or grayish in color with a foul odor. Frequent, burning urination may be present. The inflammation of the cervix may cause bleeding between menses. Fever may or may not be present depending on the severity of infection. A Pap smear with *Gonorrhea* and *Chlamydia* cultures should be done for definitive diagnosis. Appropriate antibiotics should be started to prevent spreading of the infection, which could lead to pelvic inflammatory disease or a pelvic abscess. If the irritation is chemical in nature, patients should stop using the causative agent.

Rectocele

A rectocele occurs when the supportive connective tissue separating the rectum and vagina weaken, leading to a prolapse of the rectal wall into the vagina. This is usually due to any type of trauma that weakens the supportive tissue in this area, such as childbirth or repeated heavy lifting.

In some women, the decrease in estrogen that occurs after menopause may cause laxity of these connective tissues, leading to a rectocele. Patients may or may not experience symptoms from a rectocele, depending on its severity. There may be a sensation of a mass present in the vagina. Patients may have chronic constipation or have the sensation that the rectum is not completely emptied following a bowel movement. Occasionally, patients may experience episodes of fecal incontinence. A pessary can be inserted to support the vaginal wall and prevent the rectum from bulging into the vagina. If symptoms are very bothersome, surgery may be necessary to strengthen the connective tissue.

Cystocele

A cystocele occurs when the supportive connective tissues separating the bladder and vagina weaken, leading to a prolapse of the bladder into the superior end of the vagina. This can occur after childbirth or after lifting heavy objects for a period of time. A chronic cough can repeatedly strain these connective tissues, leading to a cystocele. Obese women are more likely to develop a cystocele. Patients may be able to feel a mass in the vagina, and there may be a feeling of pressure in the lower abdomen or pelvis. Stress incontinence may be present, especially when patients are laughing or coughing. If urine is being retained in the bladder, patients may develop recurrent urinary tract infections. A pessary can be inserted to provide extra support to these connective tissues and prevent the bladder from prolapsing into the vagina. If symptoms are very bothersome and not relieved with more conservative measures, surgery may be necessary to strengthen the support underneath the bladder.

Fibrocystic breast disease

Fibrocystic breast disease is a condition in which women develop lumps in the breasts that come and go. There is no increased risk of breast cancer in patients who have this condition. It is thought that the fibrocystic masses felt in the breasts may be due to changing hormone levels during the menstrual cycle. Patients will complain of a breast mass that may change in size, especially during their menstrual cycles. These masses are usually painful and may radiate into the axillae. The breasts may feel full and heavy. Occasionally there will be a small amount of greenish-brown nipple discharge. Ultrasound exam will show cystic masses within the breasts. There is no definitive cure for fibrocystic breast disease. Wearing a bra with extra support may help to provide some pain relief. It is thought that caffeine may worsen the condition, so limiting caffeine in the diet may help. Women should be encouraged to perform monthly self-breast exams one week after a period when cysts are at their smallest.

Vaginitis

Vaginitis is an inflammation of the vagina that is not necessarily due to an infection. Though infection from bacteria, viruses, or yeast can cause this inflammation, it can also be due to decreased estrogen levels following menopause, causing the vaginal walls to be drier and easily irritated. The symptoms will depend upon the cause of the inflammation, but all types will usually cause vaginal itching or burning and pain with sexual intercourse. Bacterial infections cause a foul-smelling vaginal discharge that may be grayish in color. Fungal infections cause a white curd-like discharge. Vaginal trichomoniasis infection can cause a green-yellow vaginal discharge. Menopause-induced vaginitis will cause itching and irritation of the vagina and painful intercourse. There may be pain present during urination, as well. Treatment varies, depending on the cause of the inflammation. Appropriate antibiotics or antifungals may be necessary for infections. Estrogen cream can help with the vaginal dryness that occurs after menopause.

Abruptio placenta

Abruptio placenta occurs when the placenta prematurely begins separating from the uterine wall. It is a medical emergency that can place the unborn child and mother at risk. Frequently, the cause of the placental abruption is unknown. However, it can occur following some type of trauma that occurs, such as a bad fall or car accident in which there is some degree of trauma to the mother. Patients will have a sudden onset of abdominal or back pain with uterine contractions that are very close together, usually one after another. Vaginal bleeding will occur, and there may be pelvic tenderness to palpation on exam. If ultrasound determines that the placental abruption is very minor and the child is stable, the mother may be closely monitored on bed rest. If the symptoms should worsen, however, treatment is to deliver the baby as quickly as possible, usually via emergency C-section. If the baby is at term developmentally, a vaginal delivery may be attempted if the child's heart rate is stable.

Mastitis

Mastitis is a condition in which bacteria enter the breast tissue through a milk duct or a fissure in the skin, caused by breastfeeding. Mastitis usually occurs within the first few weeks of breastfeeding, but may occur later on, also. Rarely, this condition occurs in women who are not breastfeeding. Patients will complain of a painful area of the breast that is reddened and warm. They may feel very fatigued with a fever generally >101°F. A burning pain may be present constantly or only while breastfeeding. On exam, patients will appear generally ill. The area of the breast infected will be edematous and erythematous. The location of the infection may appear indurated. Appropriate antibiotic therapy should be given to treat the infection, with attention to the safety of the antibiotic while breastfeeding. Patients should be encouraged to continue breastfeeding and apply warm compresses to the infected area.

Placenta previa

Placenta previa occurs when the placenta forms very close to the cervix, or even overlies the cervix. A female who has scarring of the inner uterus may develop this condition because of scar tissue preventing attachment of the placenta higher in the uterus. A malformed uterus can also cause placenta previa to develop. Females carrying multiple embryos at once can also develop this condition. Bleeding is the most common symptom present in pregnant women with placenta previa. The amount and duration of bleeding late in pregnancy will depend upon how much of the cervix is covered by the placenta. There is a risk of massive bleeding and danger to the unborn child if the cervix begins to dilate, causing the placenta to tear prematurely. Treatment depends upon the severity of symptoms. Patients should be on bed rest, possibly hospitalized if the condition is severe. If bleeding is persistent, the baby should be delivered via C-section as soon as possible, even if premature, to prevent further fetal distress.

Ectopic pregnancy

An ectopic pregnancy occurs when a fertilized egg fails to implant in the uterine lining. It most often will implant within the fallopian tube but can implant within the ovary, abdomen, or down low in the neck of the cervix. An ectopic pregnancy often occurs without any known cause, but scar tissue or a malformation of the tube can cause this to occur. Patients may or may not know they are pregnant. They will complain of gradually worsening abdominal pain, usually one-sided, with vaginal bleeding. Rupture of the fallopian tube can occur as the ovum enlarges, and this will cause severe stabbing pain on the affected side. Syncope may occur if the tube ruptures. Treatment is removal of the ovum. An injection of methotrexate can reduce the size of the ovum and cause dissolution of the cells, but this may require more than one injection. If rupture of the fallopian tube occurs, emergency surgery will be necessary to attempt to repair the tube or remove it.

Premature rupture of the membranes

Premature rupture of the membranes is a condition in which the amniotic sac ruptures before labor begins. This refers to situations in which the female is at least at 37 weeks gestation. This can occur early and is called preterm premature rupture of the membranes. Premature rupture of the membranes can occur because of infection of the amniotic membrane. Patients with poor diet and lack of prenatal care are also more at risk. Smokers and women who abuse alcohol or drugs during pregnancy may also be at increased risk. Patients will experience a trickle or a sudden gush of amniotic fluid from the vagina. This may be accompanied by vaginal bleeding. Contractions are not present. Treatment consists of bed rest and imminent delivery of the baby. Vaginal delivery can be performed if the baby and mother are stable. Pitocin may be needed to start contractions if they have not started within 24 hours after rupture.

Practice Test

Practice Questions

1. A 45-year-old male comes to the emergency room after being involved in a head-on motor vehicle accident earlier in the day. The patient notes that he struck his head, but he did not experience any loss of consciousness. His blood pressure is 190/110, his respirations are irregular, and his electrocardiogram (EKG) shows sinus bradycardia with a heart rate of 42 beats per minute. The patient's symptoms are part of which clinical triad?
    a. Beck's triad
    b. Charcot's triad
    c. Cushing's triad
    d. Bergman's triad

2. All of the following are minor manifestations of acute rheumatic fever as described by the modified Jones criteria EXCEPT
    a. Erythema marginatum
    b. Leukocytosis
    c. Elevated erythrocyte sedimentation rate (ESR)
    d. Arthralgia

3. A 19-year-old woman comes to the office complaining of a painful rash on her elbows and knees. The rash appears as raised erythematous areas topped with silvery, scaling skin. She reports, "The rash is very itchy." She had similar symptoms several weeks before, but they spontaneously resolved without treatment. Which of the following is most likely to be the diagnosis?
    a. Impetigo
    b. Tinea corporis
    c. Rosacea
    d. Psoriasis

4. During a colonoscopy, the gastroenterologist notices that the patient's colon wall has a "cobblestone" appearance. Which of the following is the most likely diagnosis?
    a. Celiac sprue
    b. Crohn's disease
    c. Ulcerative colitis
    d. Whipple's disease

5. You are evaluating an obese 37-year-old female in the ER. She has been complaining of right-sided abdominal pain and excessive flatulence. She normally has the pain after eating, but it usually resolves on its own. This episode has persisted for several hours. On physical examination, you palpate her right-upper quadrant while she takes a deep inspiration. Discomfort during this maneuver is referred to as a positive:
    a. Brudziński's sign
    b. Psoas sign
    c. Murphy's sign
    d. Levine's sign

6. You are acting as the first assist in the operating room, and the surgeon asks you to close an abdominal incision with an absorbable suture material. Based on the following choices, which suture would be your pick?
    a. Dermabond
    b. Vicryl
    c. Silk
    d. Nylon

7. All of the following are symptoms of esophageal achalasia EXCEPT
    a. Acid reflux
    b. Dysphagia
    c. Hematochezia
    d. Chest pain

8. Which of the following is NOT part of CREST syndrome?
    a. Calcinosis
    b. Sclerodactyly
    c. Solar urticaria
    d. Esophageal dysmotility

9. A 20-year-old female recently diagnosed with chlamydia comes to your office for swelling and pain in her knees bilaterally. The most likely diagnosis for this woman's complaints is
    a. Sjögren's syndrome
    b. Reiter's syndrome
    c. Turner syndrome
    d. Down syndrome

10. A 26-year-old female comes to the ER with complaints of white vaginal discharge and pelvic pain. She admits to having unprotected sex. On physical examination, she has an inflamed cervix and cervical motion tenderness. Which one of the following two-medication pairs should she receive prior to leaving the ER?
    a. Ceftriaxone 250 mg IM and clindamycin 300 mg po
    b. Clindamycin 300 mg po and azithromycin 1 gm po
    c. Mefoxitin 2 gm IV and azithromycin 1 gm po
    d. Ceftriaxone 250 mg IM and azithromycin 1 gm po

11. A 19-year-old male patient is brought to the ER by his mother for altered mental status. She notes that he "hasn't been acting normally" since the morning. He has a known history of depression and anxiety for which he does not take medication and chronic back pain for which he takes codeine. On physical examination, his pupils are 2 mm bilaterally and he is lethargic, but he is able to be aroused. His heart rate is 44, his blood pressure is 78/44, and his respiratory rate is eight breaths per minute. Which of the following medications may reverse his symptoms and confirm your suspected diagnosis?
    a. Oxycodone
    b. Naloxone
    c. Prednisolone
    d. Buspirone

12. You diagnose an adult patient in your clinic with streptococcal pharyngitis. The patient has a known anaphylactic reaction to penicillin. Which of the following medications would be an acceptable substitute?
    a. Cefepime
    b. Cephalexin
    c. Augmentin
    d. Clarithromycin

13. You are examining a five-year-old patient for a wellness examination. During the examination, you notice that the child has painful-looking, swollen joints and notching of the maxillary incisors. The child has a past medical history of being blind and deaf. Based on his past medical history and examination findings, the patient most likely has a history of
    a. Congenital syphilis
    b. Down syndrome
    c. Osgood–Schlatter disease
    d. Turner syndrome

14. A 45-year-old male presents to your clinic with a painful, erythematous bump on his right eyelid of three days' duration. The eyeball itself is unaffected. His vision is unaffected. He has no crusting on the eyelids or lashes. The most likely diagnosis is
    a. Xanthelasma
    b. Hordeolum
    c. Mongolian spots
    d. Felon

15. A 66-year-old male comes into the office complaining of painless, yellowish, raised patches on his eyelids bilaterally for the past several weeks. He has no other skin lesions and has had no history of these lesions before. He has a known history of hyperlipidemia for which he is noncompliant with medications. What is the most likely diagnosis?
    a. Dermoid cyst
    b. Impetigo
    c. Mongolian spots
    d. Xanthelasma

16. Parents of a five-year-old boy bring him to the ER, noting that he has had worsening ataxia, nausea, vomiting, and headaches. He has no significant medical history. His parents deny recent trauma or recent travel. A magnetic resonance imaging (MRI) scan of the brain shows a tumor in the middle of the cerebellum with mild hydrocephalus. The most likely diagnosis is
    a. Schistosomiasis
    b. Melanoma
    c. Medulloblastoma
    d. Hygroma

17. A patient in the ER is noted to have right-upper quadrant tenderness, a temperature of 102.1° F, and jaundice. This patient most likely has which one of the following conditions?
    a. Ascending cholangitis
    b. Acute appendicitis
    c. Choledocholithiasis
    d. Acute pyelonephritis

18. You have been evaluating a young woman in the office for amenorrhea of eight weeks' duration. Her urine pregnancy test is positive. During the pelvic examination, you notice a bluish discoloration on the vaginal mucosa. Based on her lab findings and physical examination, the name for this bluish discoloration is called
    a. Levine's sign
    b. Kerning's sign
    c. Chadwick's sign
    d. Obturator sign

19. A 58-year-old male comes to the ER with a painful, red, swollen big toe. He has a known history of gout. Based on his past medical history and your examination findings, your first-line treatment would be
    a. Colchicine
    b. Zyloprim
    c. Tetracycline
    d. Amantadine

20. You suspect a patient has benign positional vertigo. Which of the following maneuvers may help aid in your diagnosis?
    a. Dix–Hallpike test
    b. Electroencephalogram (EEG)
    c. Transcranial Doppler ultrasound (TCD)
    d. Phalen's maneuver

21. A 10-year-old child is brought to your office. On physical examination, she is short in stature, has a short wide neck, broad forehead and tongue, and small ears. She has a medical history of mild cognitive and cardiac defects. Which of the following chromosomal defects is most likely the cause for her condition?
    a. 13
    b. 21
    c. 23
    d. 24

22. A patient comes to the ER complaining of pain with inspiration, fever, and palpitations. He recently underwent a coronary artery bypass graft two weeks prior. A cardiology consult is called. The cardiologist tells you he noted "electrical alternans" on your patient's electrocardiogram (EKG). Based on the medical history and EKG findings, you diagnose the patient with
    a. Pericardial tamponade
    b Myocardial infarction
    c. Pneumothorax
    d. Heart murmur

23. A patient comes into the ER complaining of dull, constant, left-sided chest pain for the previous six hours. He is diagnosed with an inferior-wall myocardial infarction (MI). What do you expect the electrocardiogram (EKG) and troponin levels to show?
    a. ST depression in leads V1 through V6 and normal troponin
    b. ST elevation in leads I, aVL, V5, and V6 and elevated troponin
    c. ST elevation in leads II, II, and aVF and elevated troponin
    d. ST depression in leads V7, V8, and V9 and normal troponin

24. You are evaluating a 72-year-old man in the ER for dizziness and syncope. An electrocardiogram (EKG) shows an increasingly prolonged PR interval on consecutive beats followed by a dropped QRS complex. Based on the EKG findings, you are most likely to suspect what type of heart block?
   a. First-degree heart block
   b. Second-degree heart block
   c. Third-degree heart block
   d. Asystole

25. Treatment of asymptomatic sinus bradycardia includes
   a. Continuous telemetry monitoring
   b. Atropine
   c. Epinephrine
   d. Transcutaneous pacing

26. Which of the following is NOT a characteristic of Beck's triad?
   a. Distended jugular veins
   b. Hypotension
   c. Muffled heart sounds
   d. Hypertension

27. All of the following may trigger an asthma attack EXCEPT
   a. Sinusitis
   b. Allergies
   c. Warm air
   d. Smoke

28. Which of the following cells release insulin?
   a. Alpha cells
   b. Beta cells
   c. Gamma cells
   d. Delta cells

29. Which of the following is NOT a complication of diabetes mellitus?
   a. Atherosclerosis
   b. Renal insufficiency
   c. Neuropathy
   d. Hypotension

30. All of the following medications are used to treat *Helicobacter pylori (H. pylori)* infections EXCEPT
   a. Clarithromycin, metronidazole, esomeprazole
   b. Amoxicillin, tetracycline, omeprazole
   c. Omeprazole, metronidazole, amoxicillin
   d. Pantoprazole, esomeprazole, clarithromycin

31. All of the following are true about peptic ulcers EXCEPT
   a. Obesity is a major risk factor
   b. It is most commonly caused by *H. pylori*
   c. It can be diagnosed with a stool antigen test
   d. Symptoms are exacerbated by the use of nonsteroidal anti-inflammatory drugs (NSAIDs)

32. In Parkinson's disease, the deterioration of which neurotransmitter is primarily responsible for its symptoms?
    a. Norepinephrine
    b. Epinephrine
    c. Serotonin
    d. Dopamine

33. A person who is diagnosed with Parkinson's disease would have damaged neurons in what area of the brain?
    a. Hippocampus
    b. Pituitary
    c. Substantia nigra
    d. Medulla oblongata

34. Which of the following is most likely associated with left bundle branch block?
    a. Pulmonary embolus
    b. Mitral valve prolapse
    c. Severe aortic valve disease
    d. Pericardial tamponade

35. A 26-year-old female is hospitalized for sickle-cell crisis. Upon admission, she was also found to have a right-lower extremity deep venous thrombus. While examining the patient, you notice that her oxygen saturation on room air drops to 89%, her heart rate is 122, and her respirations are 35 breaths per minute. She is short of breath and complaining of chest pain. Her arterial blood gas (ABG) is normal, and her electrocardiogram (EKG) shows sinus tachycardia. After administering supplemental oxygen, what is your next course of action?
    a. Order a troponin level and wait for the results
    b. Order a computed tomography (CT) angiogram of the chest
    c. Order a CT of the chest without contrast
    d. Repeat the ABG in one hour

36. Which of the following is NOT part of the tetralogy of Fallot?
    a. Atrial septal defect
    b. Narrowing of the pulmonary outflow tract
    c. Right ventricular hypertrophy
    d. Overriding aorta

37. Which of the following is the most common congenital heart defect?
    a. Ventricular septal defect
    b. Tricuspid atresia
    c. Aortic stenosis
    d. Tetralogy of Fallot

38. What is the most common side effect seen with the use of angiotensin-converting enzyme (ACE) inhibitors?
    a. Liver failure
    b. Hypotension
    c. Erectile dysfunction
    d. Cough

- 146 -

39. Which of the following is a gram-positive cocci and is frequently the cause of common skin infections and abscesses?
    a. *Haemophilus influenzae*
    b. *Streptococcus pneumoniae*
    c. *Staphylococcus aureus*
    d. *Staphylococcus pseudintermedius*

40. Which of the following is a treatment for Addison's disease?
    a. Insulin
    b. Somatropin
    c. Synthroid
    d. Cortisol

41. Which of the following is NOT a complication in patients who have chronic obstructive pulmonary disease (COPD)?
    a. Cor pulmonale
    b. Myocardial infarction
    c. Hypotension
    d. Pneumonia

42. Parents bring their toddler into your office. They've noticed that their daughter has had delayed growth, poor weight gain, clay-colored stools, and frequent episodes of pneumonia. You order a sweat chloride test. If the result is positive, what is the most likely diagnosis?
    a. Pneumonia
    b. Cystic fibrosis
    c. Bronchitis
    d. Respiratory syncytial virus

43. Which of the following is TRUE regarding sickle-cell anemia?
    a. It is an autosomal-dominant disease
    b. Heterozygotes are usually asymptomatic
    c. It is due to a defective chromosome 18
    d. It increases your risk of diabetes

44. A 41-year-old female presents to the office with dysuria, frequency, urgency, and lower abdominal discomfort. She denies having fever, chills, back pain, vaginal discharge, nausea, or vomiting. She is in a monogamous relationship and has no history of sexually transmitted diseases. A urine pregnancy test is negative. The urinalysis is positive for leukocytes, bacteria, and nitrites. She has no drug allergies. What is the next step in your medical management?
    a. Prescribe ceftriaxone 250 mg IM x 1 dose
    b. Prescribe azithromycin 1 gm po x 1 dose
    c. Prescribe Augmentin 875 mg po BID x 7 days
    d. Prescribe ciprofloxacin 500 mg po BID x 7 days

45. A 27-year-old patient who is 17 weeks pregnant is diagnosed with a urinary tract infection. She has no drug allergies. What would be your first-choice antibiotic?
    a. Macrobid
    b. Bactrim
    c. Ciprofloxacin
    d. Moxifloxacin

46. A 26-year-old female is seen in your office and diagnosed with chlamydia. This is her fifth sexually transmitted disease in two years. Which of the following interventions in NOT appropriate?
    a. Advise her to not tell her partners; they may shun her if they know
    b. Counsel her on the use of condoms and other safe-sex measures
    c. Treat her with ceftriaxone and azithromycin
    d. Order a pregnancy test

47. An 18-year-old male comes to your clinic with a history of periods of "elation and energy" following periods of "sadness and anxiety." He denies suicidal ideation, phobias, new stress or recent trauma, and hallucinations. The physical examination is normal, and the patient is neurologically intact. He has no other significant past medical history. What would be the most likely diagnosis?
    a. Dysthymic disorder
    b. Bipolar disorder
    c. Posttraumatic stress disorder
    d. Adjustment disorder

48. A patient recently diagnosed and treated for a urinary tract infection by her primary care doctor now presents to the ER with bright-orange urine of two days' duration. Her urinary tract infection (UTI) symptoms are improved. She cannot recall the medications she was prescribed, but she notes that her symptoms started after taking the medications. She denies allergies to medications, recent travel, or eating new food. Which of the following is most likely the cause for her symptom?
    a. Pilocarpine
    b. Percodan
    c. Pepcid
    d. Pyridium

49. A woman comes to your clinic for advice on how to help prevent kidney stone infections. Which of the following is the best advice you would give her?
    a. Increase fluid intake, increase carbohydrate intake
    b. Decrease fluid intake, increase calcium intake
    c. Increase fluid intake, limit calcium intake
    d. Decrease fluid intake, decrease protein intake

50. A 32-year-old woman comes to your office complaining of a several-week history of unexplained sadness and anxiety. She no longer enjoys engaging in her extracurricular activities. She denies traumatic events, phobia, hallucinations, or suicidal ideation. She has no significant past medical history. She's never had these symptoms before. Which of the following medications may be beneficial for your patient?
    a. Levothyroxine
    b. Escitalopram
    c. Amiodarone
    d. Haloperidol

51. A 14-year-old female patient is brought to your office by her parents with complaints of heavy menses, easy bruising, and recurrent nosebleeds. Her mother notes that she has similar but milder symptoms. Her hemoglobin is 9.8. Her blood work shows that she has a factor VIII clotting deficiency. Which of the following is the most likely diagnosis?
    a. Von Willebrand disease
    b. Thalassemia
    c. Hemophilia
    d. Myeloma

52. A 52-year-old male is brought to the ER after falling 10 feet from a ladder and landing on his buttocks. He notes mild pain but has the feeling of "pins and needles" going down both of his lower extremities. He is also complaining of feeling like he has to urinate but is not able to do so. On physical examination, he has decreased lower extremity reflexes, decreased motor strength, and decreased rectal tone. What is the most likely diagnosis?
    a. Fibromyalgia
    b. Greenstick fracture
    c. Cauda equina syndrome
    d. Kyphosis

53. A 13-year-old child is brought to your office complaining of a several-week history of left hip and knee pain. His parent notices that he has been walking with a progressive limp. The child denies trauma or strenuous activity. He has no significant medical problems. On physical examination, you notice that his left leg is slightly shorter than his right. His joints are not swollen or painful. What is the most likely diagnosis?
    a. Developmental dysplasia of the hip
    b. Paget's disease
    c. Slipped capital femoral epiphysis
    d. Osteitis pubis

54. A 66-year-old patient presents to your clinic with progressive bowing of her left femur and tibia as well as pelvis for several months. She notes that she has had two spontaneous leg fractures in the past four months. Her only medical issues are diabetes and gout; she is compliant with her medication regimens. On physical examination, she has notable pelvic enlargement on the left side only. She has bowing of the left leg. Her joints are painful, but they are not red or swollen. Her blood work shows that her serum alkaline phosphatase is elevated. Her computed tomography (CT) scan shows multiple bony deformities on her pelvis and left leg. Based on her lab findings and medical history, which of the following medications would NOT be helpful in treating this patient?
    a. Nonsteroidal anti-inflammatory drugs (NSAIDs)
    b. Calcitonin
    c. Fosamax
    d. Colchicine

55. A 55-year-old female presents to the ER with painless vision loss from her right eye of 30 minutes' duration. She denies photophobia, headache, nausea, vomiting, visual disturbances prior to the vision loss, trauma, or periorbital pain. She has a known history of uncontrolled hypertension and transient ischemic attacks. What is the most likely diagnosis?
    a. Acute angle closure glaucoma
    b. Retinal artery occlusion
    c. Conjunctivitis
    d. Retinal detachment

56. A parent brings her five-year-old daughter into the ER for worsening sore throat, fever, and respiratory distress. The child's oral temperature is 102.5° F. She is drooling and unable to open her mouth. You suspect epiglottitis. Which of the following would NOT be your next course of action?
    a. Administer IV penicillin immediately
    b. Direct visualization of the oropharynx with a tongue depressor
    c. Call a stat ear, nose, and throat (ENT) consultation
    d. Order a lateral cervical spine x ray

57. The most common bacterial pathogen of otitis externa is
    a. *Haemophilus influenzae*
    b. *Pseudomonas aeruginosa*
    c. *Aspergillus*
    d. *Staphylococcus aureus*

58. A 12-year-old child comes to the office with right-sided ear pain, purulent otorrhea, and a fever of 100.5° F. Her father notes that she just returned from a beach vacation, where she spent the majority of her time in the ocean. On physical examination, palpation of her tragus produces pain. Based on her medical history and physical examination, what is your next step?
    a. Stat ear, nose, and throat (ENT) consult
    b. Ofloxacin eardrops
    c. Clindamycin po
    d. Computed tomography (CT) scan

59. A 58-year-old male comes to the office with intermittent vertigo, nausea, tinnitus, and hearing loss. His hearing loss only occurs with the acute vertigo attacks and then returns to baseline. His symptoms started after he had gotten better from a cold about four weeks ago. He notes that although these symptoms are persistent, they are starting to improve. This patient has no significant past medical history. His physical examination is normal. Based on his examination and his medical history, what is the most likely diagnosis?
    a. Labyrinthitis
    b. Ménière's disease
    c. Mastoiditis
    d. Otitis media

60. A 69-year-old male presents to your office with difficulty urinating. He complains of urinary frequency, but decreased urine output. His *prostate-specific antigen* (PSA) is slightly elevated. On digital rectal examination, he has an enlarged prostate, but no masses or nodules. His urinalysis is normal. What medication would you prescribe for this patient?
    a. Terbinafine
    b. Tegretol
    c. Tramadol
    d. Tamsulosin

61. A female patient has been diagnosed with gestational diabetes, but the diabetes is not controllable by dietary modifications. What is your first step in her medical management?
    a. Start Novolin
    b. Start glyburide
    c. Start pioglitazone
    d. Start glimepiride

62. A patient comes to your clinic, concerned because his brother has just been diagnosed with type 2 diabetes. His father and paternal grandmother were also diabetics. His fasting blood sugar is 98, and his hemoglobin A1C is 5.2. What is the next step in the management of this patient?
    a. Recheck his hemoglobin A1C in a week
    b. Recommend a low-sugar diet and exercise
    c. Start Lantus and metformin
    d. Start metformin only

63. A 35-year-old woman comes to your office for her annual wellness visit. Her examination and vital signs are normal. She has no significant past medical history. She states that her father was diagnosed with colon cancer when he was 48 years old. At what time should this patient get her first colonoscopy?
    a. This year
    b. At 38 years old
    c. At 48 years old
    d. At 50 years old

64. A mother brings her unvaccinated child to the ER with a deep whooping cough. The child is diagnosed with pertussis. Which medication can you prescribe to the mother to help prevent her child from spreading the illness to others?
   a. Augmentin
   b. Clindamycin
   c. Erythromycin
   d. *Guaifenesin*

65. A father brings in his three-year-old son to the ER with a "barking" cough, runny nose, and a fever of 100.5° F. The child attends day care. He has no other significant past medical history. On physical examination, he is noted to have the aforementioned cough, clear rhinorrhea, and mild wheezing bilaterally. He is not in any acute respiratory distress. Based on his physical examination and medical history, what is the most likely diagnosis?
   a. Pneumonia
   b. Cystic fibrosis
   c. Respiratory syncytial virus (RSV)
   d. Asthma

66. A 26-year-old man is rushed to the emergency room with chest pain and shortness of breath that developed suddenly. A family member notes that he has smoked a half a pack of cigarettes per day for five years, but he has no other known medical problems. On physical examination, there is no evidence of trauma. He has normal breath sounds on the left but decreased breath sounds on the right. A chest x-ray shows lung markings on the left, but not on the right. Based on his past medical history, presentation, and x-ray, what is the most likely diagnosis?
   a. Pneumonia
   b. Secondary pneumothorax
   c. Pulmonary carcinoma
   d. Spontaneous pneumothorax

67. A 30-year-old man comes to the ER with a two-week history of hemoptysis, fever, and chills. He has no significant past medical history. A chest x-ray shows multiple cavitary lesions. Based on his chest x-ray and his symptoms, what is your diagnosis?
   a. Bronchitis
   b. Tuberculosis
   c. Pneumothorax
   d. Lung cancer

68. A 19-year-old patient comes to your clinic complaining of recurrent nasal congestion. She states that her primary care doctor gave her a nasal spray. It helped her symptoms for the first three days. She continued to use it for another four days, and the nasal congestion reoccurred. Which of the following medications are most likely to blame for her symptoms?
   a. Oxymetazoline hydrochloride
   b. Benzonatate
   c. Ofloxacin
   d. Guaifenesin

69. A 58-year-old male patient comes to your office concerned because he has a family history of heart disease and would like to be worked up. His father and older brother died of heart attacks. This patient's LDL is 150. His weight, vital signs, stress test, two-dimensional echocardiogram, and electrocardiogram (EKG) are normal. He has no significant past medical history. What medications would you recommend for this patient?
   a. A baby aspirin and amlodipine
   b. Amlodipine and simvastatin
   c. A baby aspirin and metoprolol
   d. A baby aspirin and simvastatin

70. A mother brings her one-month-old son into your office for evaluation. He has had poor weight gain, even though he seems to be constantly hungry. She states that the child has an episode of projectile vomiting after almost every feeding. You notice that the child's abdomen is distended, and you palpate an olive-shaped mass in the epigastrium. Based on the medical history and physical examination, what is the most likely diagnosis?
   a. Gastroesophageal reflux disease (GERD)
   b. Gastritis
   c. Pyloric stenosis
   d. Mallory–Weiss tear

71. A 69-year-old male with a history of alcohol abuse comes to the ER after having an episode of hematemesis following binge drinking. Recently he's also been noticing black, tarry stools. He states that he's vomited blood on several occasions, but these episodes have been becoming more frequent. He denies unintentional weight loss or gain, abdominal pain, diarrhea, fever, recent illness, history of bleeding disorders, or lymphadenopathy. His stool guaiac is positive. His physical examination is normal. He currently feels fine. Based on his medical history and physical examination, what is the most likely diagnosis?
   a. Celiac sprue
   b. Whipple's disease
   c. Mallory–Weiss tear
   d. Pyloric stenosis

72. A mother brings her toddler into the office for an evaluation. The mother notes that the child's right eye deviates toward her nose. The child has had this condition since she was an infant. Her pupils are equal and reactive. Based on her medical history and physical examination, what is the most likely diagnosis?
   a. Exotropia
   b. Hypertropia
   c. Esotropia
   d. Hypotropia

73. A father brings his child to the ER noting a two-day history of red eyes, low-grade fever, and crusting of the eyelids and eyelashes. He states that many of her classmates have similar symptoms. On physical examination, the child has erythematous conjunctiva bilaterally with golden crusts on her eyelids and lashes. The child denies pain. The child's pupils are equal and reactive, and her vision is normal. She has no medical problems. Based on her medical history and physical examination findings, what is the most likely diagnosis?
  a. Allergic conjunctivitis
  b. Bacterial conjunctivitis
  c. Viral conjunctivitis
  d. Dacryoadenitis

74. A six-year-old patient comes to the ER and is diagnosed with bacterial conjunctivitis. She has no past medical history and is up to date on all of her vaccinations. What is the next step in your medical management?
  a. Erythromycin
  b. Trifluridine
  c. Ciprofloxacin
  d. Famciclovir

75. A 68-year-old female newly diagnosed with hyperlipidemia comes to the ER after she noticed her entire body turning a reddish color and associated mild itching. She was just started on a new medication for her high cholesterol last week, but she cannot remember the name. She denies recent travel, new soaps or detergents, new foods, chest pain, shortness of breath, or palpitations. Other than her generalized flushing and pruritus, her physical examination seems normal. What medication has most likely caused her symptoms?
  a. Atorvastatin
  b. Rosuvastatin
  c. Simvastatin
  d. Niacin

76. A 58-year-old man presents to the ER with a temperature of 101.5° F, productive cough with yellow sputum, shaking chills, and mild dyspnea for the past two days. His oxygen saturation is 98% on room air. A chest x-ray shows an infiltrate on the lower left lobe. He has no significant past medical history. What is the next step in your medical management?
  a. Start po antibiotics and discharge home
  b. Order a computed tomography (CT) scan of the chest
  c. Admit to the hospital and start intravenous (IV) antibiotics
  d. Obtain an arterial blood gas (ABG)

77. A patient with hyperlipidemia that you have recently placed on niacin develops mild generalized flushing and pruritus. What would NOT be the next step in your medical management?
  a. Discontinue the medication immediately
  b. Continue the medication and adjust the dosage
  c. Give Decadron and Benadryl for symptomatic relief
  d. Have the patient take nonsteroidal anti-inflammatory drugs (NSAIDs) prior to niacin dose

78. A father brings his two-year-old son to the ER for a three-day history of runny nose, a temperature of 100.5° F, and nasal congestion. Today, the child developed a barking cough. The child is not in any respiratory distress, and his appetite, fluid intake, and urinary output have all been normal. What is the next step in your medical management?
    a. Discharge home, recommend fluids and humidified air
    b. Discharge home with oral steroids only
    c. Discharge home with oral steroids and oral antibiotics
    d. Discharge home with oral antibiotics only

79. An HIV-positive patient is diagnosed with *Pneumocystis* pneumonia. What is the first-line treatment?
    a. Gentamicin
    b. Trimethoprim-sulfamethoxazole
    c. Augmentin
    d. Corticosteroids

80. A newborn is diagnosed with phenylketonuria (PKU). What can you do as a health-care provider to minimize the sequelae of this disease?
    a. Prescribe Ritalin
    b. Prescribe Dilantin
    c. Advise routine blood work
    d. Advise parents about dietary restrictions

81. What is the most effective way to prevent the spread of communicable diseases?
    a. Maintaining a sterile environment
    b. Wearing gloves
    c. Hand washing
    d. Wearing a face mask while working with sick patients

82. Which of the following is NOT a way to prevent listeriosis?
    a. Thoroughly rinse raw produce
    b. Refrain from ingesting unpasteurized milk
    c. Limit intake of processed meats during pregnancy
    d. Refrain from eating fish or seafood during pregnancy

83. What is the most effective way to prevent rabies infection?
    a. Immediately obtaining the rabies vaccine
    b. Immediately cleansing the wound
    c. Administering po Augmentin
    d. Administering IV clindamycin

84. Which of the following is NOT a way to treat scabies?
    a. Lotrimin cream
    b. Permethrin cream
    c. Washing linens and clothing in hot water
    d. Avoiding contact with infected people

85. A 24-year-old man presents to the ER with worsening left-sided abdominal pain radiating to the back, temperature of 100.5° F, shaking chills, nausea, and vomiting of three days' duration. On physical examination, he has mild left-epigastric pain with moderate left-sided costovertebral angle tenderness. His urinalysis is positive for red blood cells only. His white blood cell (WBC) count is 16,000. His basic metabolic panel, amylase, lipase, and liver function tests are normal. Based on his medical history, physical examination, and lab results, what is the most likely diagnosis?
    a. Hepatitis
    b. Cholecystitis
    c. Appendicitis
    d. Nephrolithiasis

86. Which of the following is the least likely to cause a cardiac arrest?
    a. Hyperkalemia
    b. Hypervolemia
    c. Hypokalemia
    d. Hypovolemia

87. An 11-year-old male is brought to the ER by his mother with a one-day history of sudden, right-sided abdominal pain, nausea, and vomiting. These symptoms are not related to food intake. There is no history of trauma, recent travel, ingesting raw or rare foods, or diarrhea. His only medical problem is asthma. During his physical examination, he cries out in pain while you gently shake the bed. He displays moderate discomfort when you flex his right leg at his hip and his knee. What is the most likely diagnosis based on his medical history and examination findings?
    a. Nephrolithiasis
    b. Appendicitis
    c. Cholecystitis
    d. Hepatitis

88. A mother brings her 16-year-old daughter to the ER for a two-day history of fever, nausea, vomiting, photophobia, and severe constant generalized headache. There is no history of trauma. The child has no significant past medical history. During her physical examination, she flexes her hip and knee when you flex her neck. Based on her presenting symptoms and her examination, what is the most likely diagnosis?
    a. Subarachnoid hemorrhage
    b. Migraines
    c. Vestibulocerebellar syndrome
    d. Meningitis

89. A 56-year-old man comes to the ER with dull, nonradiating left-sided chest pain, nausea, and vomiting for the past four hours. The chest pain is not related to activity. He denies a history of similar symptoms. You notice that his blood pressure is 80/45 and that his electrocardiogram (EKG) shows sinus tachycardia with a rate of 123. His oxygen saturation is 99% on room air. During his physical examination, you notice that his neck veins are bulging. Auscultation of his heart reveals quiet systolic and diastolic sounds. His breath sounds are coarse bilaterally. Based on his symptoms and physical examination, what is the most likely diagnosis?
    a. Pericardial tamponade
    b. Pneumothorax
    c. Aortic dissection
    d. Stable angina

90. A patient's electrocardiogram (EKG) shows a prolonged PR interval that regularly precedes a QRS complex. The PR interval remains unchanged. What is the most likely diagnosis based on the EKG findings?
   a. First-degree heart block
   b. Second-degree heart block (Mobitz type I)
   c. Second-degree heart block (Mobitz type II)
   d. Third-degree heart block

91. A 19-year-old female patient comes to your office with her parent, who is concerned about the deterioration of her daughter's health over the past several months. The daughter admits to being depressed. Her vital signs and weight are normal. On physical examination, you notice that she has multiple cavities and gingivitis. The patient admits that she sometimes forces herself to vomit after meals to help control her weight. Based on her medical history and physical, what is the most likely diagnosis?
   a. Anorexia nervosa
   b. Panic disorder
   c. Bulimia nervosa
   d. Dysthymic disorder

92. A 28-year-old male patient is brought to your clinic by his brother, who states that his brother's behavior is becoming increasingly erratic. He has intermittent episodes of agitation. The patient has been stating that he has been seeing and talking to his father, even though his father passed away five years ago. The patient also has been having trouble concentrating and often skips from different topics during a conversation in a few minutes. The patient confides in you that his brother is "part of a conspiracy to lock him away." The patient's labs are all normal and so are his vital signs. His physical examination is normal as well. A computed tomography (CT) scan of the brain shows no acute abnormalities. Based on his medical history, physical examination, and labs, what is the next step in your management?
   a. Start haloperidol and a psychiatry referral
   b. Start paroxetine and a psychiatry referral
   c. Start escitalopram and a psychiatry referral
   d. Start zolpidem and a psychiatry referral

93. Parents bring their one-month-old son to your clinic for failure to thrive, pallor, dark urine, and jaundice since birth. His vital signs are normal. His complete blood count (CBC) and iron panel show hemolytic anemia. His platelets, white blood cell (WBC) count, liver function tests, amylase, and lipase are normal. On physical examination, the child is mildly lethargic but easily aroused. You notice that he has jaundice. Based on his past medical history, physical examination, and labs, what is the most likely diagnosis?
   a. Leukocytosis
   b. Thrombocytopenia
   c. Glucose-6-phosphate dehydrogenase (G6PD) deficiency
   d. Von Willebrand disease

94. One of your pediatric patients has just been diagnosed with thalassemia major. The parents ask you what they can do to limit the severity of symptoms and improve their child's quality of life. What suggestions do you give them?
   a. Blood transfusions and iron supplements
   b. Limit folate and iron intake
   c. Folate supplements and regular blood transfusions
   d. Avoid nonsteroidal anti-inflammatory drugs (NSAIDs), legumes, and henna

95. A 24-year-old female who is twenty-six weeks pregnant comes to the ER for sudden onset of bright-red, painless vaginal bleeding. She has no medical problems; she does not smoke, drink, or use drugs, and hasn't had any prior complications during this pregnancy. Other than the vaginal bleeding, she does not have any symptoms. Her complete blood count (CBC) is normal. An ultrasound reveals that the placenta is touching the top of the cervix. What is the most likely diagnosis based on her symptoms, labs, and ultrasound findings?
   a. Placental abruption (abruptio placentae)
   b. Premature rupture of membranes
   c. Dystocia
   d. Placenta previa

96. A 35-year-old woman who is six weeks pregnant comes to the ER for mild vaginal bleeding and mild low-back pain. Her transvaginal ultrasound is negative for an intrauterine pregnancy. Her serum beta human chorionic gonadotropin (HCG) is normal. What is the next step in your medical management?
   a. Stat surgical consult for laparoscopy
   b. Repeat her beta HCG and ultrasound in two days
   c. Discharge home and recommend bed rest
   d. Administer methotrexate

97. A child has been recently diagnosed with impetigo. Which of the following recommendations would NOT prevent the spread of the infection?
   a. You may touch the skin lesions once antibiotics have been started
   b. Wash hands thoroughly after touching the patient
   c. Clean all clothes and bed linens in hot water
   d. Do not share personal care items with the patient

98. You diagnose a patient with tinea corporis. Which of the following medications would treat this condition?
   a. Erythromycin
   b. Ketoconazole
   c. Mupirocin
   d. Metronidazole

99. A father brings his 13-year-old son to the ER. He states that the foreskin of his son's penis is "stuck." The penis is mildly swollen and erythematous. The testes are normal. Upon physical examination, you note that the foreskin cannot be reduced. The most likely diagnosis is
   a. Phimosis
   b. Hydrocele
   c. Paraphimosis
   d. Cryptorchidism

100. A two-month-old male is brought to your clinic for a routine wellness examination. During his physical examination, you notice that you cannot palpate his left testicle. Your next step in his medical management is to
    a. Recommend a surgical consult for possible orchiopexy
    b. Recommend a computed tomography (CT) scan
    c. Recommend hormone injections
    d. Recommend to monitor the child for now

101. A 22-year-old male comes to your clinic with a painless mass on his right testicle of two weeks' duration. He denies trauma, lymphadenopathy, or prior infection. His complete blood count (CBC) and chemistry are normal. A physical examination reveals a soft, fluctuant, nontender mass. You shine a flashlight at the mass, which transmits light. Based on his medical history and physical examination, what is the most likely diagnosis?
    a. Hydrocele
    b. Testicular torsion
    c. Varicocele
    d. Cryptorchidism

102. A 21-year-old patient in the hospital for sickle-cell crisis is newly diagnosed with a pulmonary embolus. She has no past medical history other than sickle-cell disease. Which of the following would NOT be part of your medical management once the patient's oxygenation status is stabilized?
    a. Surgery consult for an inferior vena cava (IVC) filter
    b. Start heparin infusion
    c. Administer analgesics for the chest pain
    d. Repeat D-dimer in one week

103. A 30-year-old patient in your clinic tells you that he seems to get the flu every year. Other than smoking a half a pack of cigarettes per day for the past five years, he is healthy. He asks you how he can avoid contracting the flu this year. Which of the following is NOT part of your recommendations?
    a. Frequent hand washing while at work or at a public venue
    b. Obtaining the influenza vaccine in the fall
    c. Avoid the influenza vaccine because he is not in a high-risk group
    d. Decrease his tobacco use

104. All of the following medications will treat atrial fibrillation EXCEPT?
    a. Lanoxin
    b. Furosemide
    c. Metoprolol
    d. Warfarin

105. A patient visits your office for his annual wellness examination. He tells you he had recently become ill after visiting the southwest part of the United States. He had painful red lumps on his lower legs, blood-tinged sputum, loss of appetite, fever, night sweats, and headache. The symptoms spontaneously resolved on their own without treatment. A doctor who saw him in the ER while he was in the southwest said he had valley fever. The patient's vital signs and physical examination are normal. He has no past medical history. Based on his symptoms and medical history, what illness did your patient most likely have?
    a. *Pneumocystis* pneumonia
    b. Tuberculosis
    c. Respiratory syncytial virus (RSV)
    d. Coccidioidomycosis

106. Which of the following can make a definitive diagnosis of ventricular septal defect?
    a. Echocardiogram
    b. Chest x ray
    c. Electrocardiogram (EKG)
    d. Auscultation with a stethoscope

107. A mother brings in her six-year-old daughter to the ER for syncope, worsening chest pain, shortness of breath, and dizziness. The mother notes that her daughter always seems to have cold legs. The child has a past medical history of Turner syndrome. A chest x-ray shows cardiomegaly. A cardiologist is called, who notes the figure 3 sign on the chest x-ray. Based on the medical history, presentation, and imaging findings, what is the most likely diagnosis?
    a. Tetralogy of Fallot
    b. Coarctation of the aorta
    c. Hypoplastic left heart syndrome
    d. Tricuspid atresia

108. A 56-year-old female patient with a history of alcohol abuse presents to the ER with dizziness, chest pain, palpitations, and syncope. A cardiologist viewing her electrocardiogram (EKG) mentions that the QRS complex twists around the isoelectric baseline. What cardiac arrhythmia is the cardiologist most likely describing?
    a. Bundle branch block
    b. Sick sinus syndrome
    c. Torsades de pointes
    d. Atrial fibrillation

109. A 24-year-old woman presents to your clinic with persistent chest pain and shortness of breath, which commonly occur at rest. Exercise does not induce her symptoms. She has been to the ER several times with these symptoms. Her electrocardiogram (EKG), troponin level, chest x ray, and two-dimensional echocardiogram are all normal. She had a prior cardiac catheterization one year ago, which was negative. Her physical examination is normal; palpation of her chest wall does not reproduce symptoms. She has no medical problems. She admits to smoking a pack of cigarettes a day for five years. What is the most likely diagnosis?
    a. Prinzmetal's angina
    b. Unstable angina
    c. Stable angina
    d. Costochondritis

110. Which of the following can be the cause of syndrome of inappropriate antidiuretic hormone (SIADH)?
    a. Squamous-cell carcinoma
    b. Large-cell carcinoma
    c. Adenocarcinoma
    d. Small-cell carcinoma

111. A patient presents to the ER with suspected infective endocarditis. Which of the following tests would be the least helpful diagnostic aid?
    a. Computed tomography (CT) scan of the chest
    b. Echocardiogram
    c. Chest x-ray
    d. Blood cultures

112. A patient has come to your clinic for multiple visits over the past several weeks with a persistently borderline elevated blood pressure. Today it is 138/88. He has no family history of hypertension. He smokes less than a half a pack of cigarettes per day, but otherwise he has no medical problems. Which of the following would be recommendations to help him lower his blood pressure without medications?
    a. Limit tobacco use, increase sodium intake, increase physical activity
    b. Decrease stress, increase tobacco use, increase physical activity
    c. Decrease sodium intake, increase physical activity, limit tobacco use
    d. Limit tobacco use, decrease sodium intake, decrease physical activity

113. You are evaluating a 52-year-old female patient in your office for the first time. During auscultation of her heart, you hear a midsystolic click. The murmur gets louder when she stands up. The patient informs you that she has a known history of a heart murmur. She denies chest pain, dyspnea, dizziness, and palpitations. Her electrocardiogram (EKG) is normal. Her echocardiogram reveals a mitral valve that does not fully close. What is your next step in her medical management?
    a. Recommend cardiology referral for possible catheterization
    b. Order a computed tomography (CT) scan of the chest
    c. Monitor for now; no intervention is needed
    d. Order a repeat EKG in one month

114. A 61-year-old male presents to the ER with the sudden onset of dull, throbbing, left-sided chest pain radiating to his jaw and back, nausea, vomiting, and diaphoresis. An electrocardiogram (EKG) shows an inferior wall non-ST segment elevation myocardial infarction (NSTEMI). His vital signs are as follows: BP, 165/98; pulse, 92 beats per minute; pulse oximetry, 93% on room air; and respirations, 26 per minute. The patient is awake and alert, but in moderate pain. After administering oxygen, which of the following would be the next step in your medical management?
    a. Order metoprolol, morphine, and clopidogrel
    b. Order aspirin, metoprolol, and nitroglycerin
    c. Order an echocardiogram and troponin level
    d. Order metoprolol, aspirin, and clopidogrel

115. A 68-year-old male comes to the ER after having an episode of left-sided chest pain radiating to his left arm for 10 minutes. He had been mowing his lawn when the chest pain occurred. It resolved about 5 minutes after he sat down to rest. He states that he often gets similar symptoms during physical activity. The symptoms resolve with rest. He currently has no medical complaints. His past medical history includes hyperlipidemia and obesity. His physical examination is normal. His vital signs are as follows: BP, 155/91; pulse, 88 beats per minute, pulse oximetry, 98% on room air; and respirations, 16 per minute. Based on his past medical history and physical examination, what is the most likely diagnosis?
    a. Stable angina
    b. Prinzmetal's angina
    c. Variant angina
    d. Aortic aneurysm

116. A 77-year-old female patient comes to your clinic complaining of worsening vision for the past month. She notes that the center of her vision has been deteriorating. It has become incredibly difficult for her to read. Her peripheral vision remains intact. She denies the presence of floaters or flashes of light, photophobia, headache, nausea, vomiting, or trauma. Her past medical history includes osteoarthritis and osteoporosis. She denies trauma or recent illness. What is the most likely diagnosis?
    a. Optic neuritis
    b. Macular degeneration
    c. Glaucoma
    d. Retinal artery occlusion

117. A 42-year-old female comes to the ER for right-sided tinnitus, worsening ataxia, right-sided hearing loss, dizziness, and headache of one month's duration. She denies trauma or recent illness. She has no significant past medical history. The symptoms are not exacerbated or alleviated by motion. Her physical examination is normal. What is the next step in your medical management?
    a. Order an electromyography
    b. Order an ear, nose, and throat (ENT) consult
    c. Perform the Dix–Hallpike maneuver
    d. Order a magnetic resonance imaging (MRI) scan of the brain

118. A four-year-old female child is brought in for persistent coughing. Prior to the coughing episode, the child had been seen playing with a toy car. The toy car cannot be found. The child's oxygen saturation on room air is 91%. Upon physical examination, you do not see an object in the child's oropharynx. Her lungs are diminished on the right. The child has stridor. After administering oxygen, what is the next step in your medical management?
    a. Order stat chest x-ray
    b. Perform a finger sweep to see if you can remove the object
    c. Administer nebulizer treatment
    d. Order a stat bronchoscopy

119. A 76-year-old female comes to the ER with nonproductive cough, chest pain with inspiration, and shortness of breath of two days' duration. Her vital signs are as follows: BP, 144/72; respirations, 25 per minute; pulse, 101 beats per minute; and oxygen saturation on room air, 93%. On physical examination, she has diminished breath sounds on the right side. She has dullness to percussion and decreased tactile fremitus on the right side. She has a known history of tobacco abuse and chronic obstructive pulmonary disease (COPD). Based on your physical examination, what is the most likely diagnosis?
- a. Asthma
- b. Pleural effusion
- c. Pneumothorax
- d. Influenza

120. A patient comes to your office complaining of progressive knee pain of one month's duration. You suspect a meniscus tear. Which of the following maneuvers would you do to help confirm the diagnosis?
- a. Obturator test
- b. McMurray test
- c. Murphy test
- d McBurney point tenderness

121. You are evaluating an x ray of a patient who fell; it shows a bone fragment separated from the bone. What kind of fracture is this?
- a. Avulsion fracture
- b. Greenstick fracture
- c. Comminuted fracture
- d. Oblique fracture

122. A 65-year-old male comes to your office with worsening cough and dyspnea of two months' duration. He has no other medical problems. He states that he had worked in a coal mine for 30 years, but he has recently retired. His lungs on chest x ray show a honeycomb pattern. Based on your findings, what is the most likely diagnosis?
- a. Pneumoconiosis
- b. Schistosomiasis
- c. Coccidioidomycosis
- d. Tuberculosis

123. A 21-year-old male comes to your office after finding a hard, fixed, painless lump on his testicle. He's never had testicular lesions before. He has no past medical history. You shine a penlight at the lesion; it does not transmit light. Based on your physical examination, what is the most likely diagnosis?
- a. Hydrocele
- b. Testicular carcinoma
- c. Varicocele
- d. Testicular torsion

124. A patient comes to your office complaining of persistent unilateral shoulder pain that started after his wrestling match at school. You suspect a rotator cuff tear. Which of the following tests would you perform to help confirm the diagnosis?
    a. Anterior drawer test
    b. Lachman test
    c. McMurray test
    d. Drop-arm test

125. A mother brings her six-year-old daughter to the ER for left-sided ear pain of three days' duration associated with mild hearing loss, swelling, and fever. She states that her daughter had been recently treated for an inner ear infection one week prior. The child has no ataxia, vertigo, lymphadenopathy, tinnitus, nausea, or vomiting. Her temperature in the ER is 102.1° F. On physical examination, you notice mild displacement of the ear caused by swelling of the posterior ear. Her tympanic membrane is erythematous. Based on her medical history and physical examination, what is the most likely diagnosis?
    a. Acoustic neuroma
    b. Cholesteatoma
    c. Mastoiditis
    d. Ménière's disease

126. A 51-year-old HIV patient presents with fever, headache, nausea, and vomiting. His complete blood count (CBC) shows a leukocytosis with bandemia. A lumbar puncture is performed, and cultures are sent to the lab. His India ink stain is positive. What is the most likely organism causing his meningitis?
    a. *Histoplasma*
    b. *Neisseria*
    c. *Cryptococcus*
    d. *Haemophilus*

127. A five-year-old child is brought to the ER by his father for an acute asthma exacerbation. Which of the following would NOT be a treatment of choice in an acute asthma exacerbation?
    a. Singulair
    b. Xopenex
    c. Ventolin
    d. Proventil

128. A mother brings her toddler into your office for a multitude of symptoms. Her daughter has been developing nausea, vomiting, fever, and abdominal pain for the past several weeks. During the child's physical examination, you notice that the child has a nontender abdominal mass. The patient also has no right iris (aniridia) and has unilateral swelling on one side of her body. The mother states that she has a family history of cancer, but she can't remember what kind. Based on the child's medical history and physical examination, what kind of tumor is most likely responsible for the child's symptoms?
    a. Hodgkin's lymphoma
    b. Lipoma
    c. Wilms' tumor
    d. Kaposi sarcoma

129. A mother gives birth to her baby at 28 weeks of gestation. Immediately after labor, the child goes into respiratory distress. No complications have occurred during the pregnancy prior to labor. The mother has no relevant past medical history. What is the most likely diagnosis for the child's respiratory symptoms?
    a. Respiratory syncytial virus (RSV)
    b. Hyaline membrane disease
    c. *Pneumocystis* pneumonia
    d. Pneumoconiosis

130. A 21-year-old male presents to the ER with right-sided eye pain after being involved in a physical altercation. His right conjunctiva has a medial well-circumscribed erythematous area. His extraocular muscles (EOMs) are intact, and his pupils are equal and reactive. He has no vision loss or periorbital swelling. Based on his medical history and physical examination, what is the most likely diagnosis?
    a. Blepharitis
    b. Hordeolum
    c. Hyphema
    d. Optic neuritis

131. You are examining a patient in the ER for acute alcohol intoxication. He is well known to the ER for his chronic alcoholism. During your physical examination, you notice that he has white patches on his tongue that cannot be scraped off. This condition is called
    a. Leukoplakia
    b. Oral thrush
    c. Parotitis
    d. Gingivostomatitis

132. A cardiologist is examining the chest x ray of a child with a known cyanotic heart defect. He mentions that the child has a "boot-shaped heart." What heart defect does the child most likely have?
    a. Ventricular septal defect
    b. Patent ductus arteriosus
    c. Atrial septal defect
    d. Tetralogy of Fallot

133. A patient presents to your office with various symptoms. Based on the patient's medical history and physical examination, you suspect sarcoidosis. Which of the following tests would you order to confirm the diagnosis?
    a. Computed tomography (CT) scan of the chest
    b. Bronchoscopy with biopsy
    c. Lumbar puncture
    d. Serum phosphorus

134. A 28-year-old female comes to your clinic concerned because she has been developing multiple painful breast lumps over the past several months. They enlarge and shrink in size during the month. During your physical examination, you find multiple bilateral soft, painful breast masses. There is no erythema, skin changes, nipple discharge, or lymphadenopathy. What is the most likely diagnosis?
    a. Breast cancer
    b. Fibroadenoma
    c. Fibrocystic breast disease
    d. Gynecomastia

135. A 26-year-old patient has just been diagnosed with a fibroadenoma via biopsy. What is the next step in your medical management?
    a. Monitor for now; no further intervention is needed
    b. Recommend birth control pills
    c. Repeat biopsy in two months
    d. Recommend surgical consultation for a mastectomy

136. Which of the following is NOT a treatment for active tuberculosis?
    a. Clindamycin
    b. Amikacin
    c. Streptomycin
    d. Ethambutol

137. Which of the following remedies would NOT help alleviate the effects of barotrauma?
    a. Chew gum
    b. Suck on candy
    c. Yawn
    d. Ascend quickly

138. A father brings his one-year-old daughter in for mild respiratory distress of one day's duration. Originally, her symptoms started out like a common cold, but then she developed a noisy, nonproductive cough and low-grade fever. On physical examination, you notice intercostal retractions. Her temperature is 100.5° F; otherwise, her vitals are normal. Based on her medical history and physical examination, what is the most likely diagnosis?
    a. Hyaline membrane disease
    b. Bronchiolitis
    c. Tuberculosis
    d. Cystic fibrosis

139. Which of the following is a first-line treatment for Hashimoto's thyroiditis?
    a. Lantus
    b. Levothyroxine
    c. Lanoxin
    d. Lamisil

140. A 45-year-old man with no history of medical problems has developed worsening, unpredictable mood changes and a decline in cognitive function. He has recently developed an ataxic gait and uncoordinated, jerky body movements. What is the most likely diagnosis?
    a. Tourette syndrome
    b. Guillain–Barré syndrome
    c. Cerebral palsy
    d. Huntington's disease

141. A patient presents with myalgias, fatigue, and diffuse bony pain. Further workup reveals the presence of osteoporosis and nephrolithiasis. What is the most likely diagnosis?
    a. Hyperthyroidism
    b. Hypoparathyroidism
    c. Hyperparathyroidism
    d. Hypothyroidism

142. What is the first-line treatment for a scabies infection?
    a. Permethrin
    b. Olanzapine
    c. Phenergan
    d. Ondansetron

143. A patient with a known history of gout comes to your clinic asking about what he can do to reduce the occurrence of his gout attacks. Which of the following dietary recommendations would you NOT recommend?
    a. Reduce red meat intake
    b. Reduce seafood intake
    c. Reduce calcium intake
    d. Reduce alcohol intake

144. A 25-year-old female is admitted to the hospital for fever of unknown origin. She has a temperature of 102.3° F and is complaining of fever, chills, and diaphoresis. She has a known history of intravenous (IV) drug abuse. The attending physician notes that the patient has Janeway lesions. Based on her medical history and physical examination, the most likely diagnosis is
    a. Pneumonia
    b. Meningitis
    c. Endocarditis
    d. *Clostridium difficile* colitis

145. Which of the following medications would you NOT use in a patient with restrictive cardiomyopathy?
    a. Furosemide
    b. Metoprolol
    c. Aspirin
    d. Epinephrine

146. A patient with *Clostridium difficile* colitis has been experiencing worsening abdominal pain and fever. An abdominal x ray shows colonic distension. What is the most likely diagnosis based on symptoms and x-ray findings?
    a. Ogilvie's syndrome
    b. Toxic megacolon
    c. Intussusception
    d. Hirschsprung's disease

147. A patient with a known history of alcoholism comes to the ER with left-upper quadrant pain radiating to his back for the past day. He's had this pain previously after an alcohol binge, but this episode is much more painful. What is the most likely diagnosis?
    a. Cholangitis
    b. Mallory–Weiss tear
    c. Pancreatitis
    d. Hepatitis

148. Family members bring a 61-year-old man to your office for the first time for a wellness checkup. As they are filling out paperwork, you notice that he has a resting tremor, slow movements, rigidity, and shuffling gait. What is the most likely diagnosis?
    a. Huntington's disease
    b. Alzheimer's dementia
    c. Parkinson's disease
    d. Guillain–Barré syndrome

149. A 42-year-old female with a known history of systemic lupus erythematous comes to your office with a myriad of complaints including unintentional weight gain, increase in body hair, acne, stretch marks, and muscle weakness. She takes prednisone and nonsteroidal anti-inflammatory drugs (NSAIDs) to help control her lupus symptoms. What is the most likely diagnosis?
    a. Cushing's syndrome
    b. Addison's disease
    c. Acromegaly
    d. Hashimoto's disease

150. A 21-year-old female comes to the ER complaining of a blistering rash and facial swelling that started in the morning. She has never had this rash before. She has no significant past medical history. The only medication she is currently taking is penicillin for streptococcal pharyngitis. On physical examination, you notice diffuse dark reddish purple papular rash on her trunk, face, and extremities with extensive blister formation. Her temperature is 99.9° F; otherwise, her vitals are normal. Based on her medical history and physical examination, what is the most likely diagnosis?
    a. Turner syndrome
    b. Stevens–Johnson syndrome
    c. Cushing's syndrome
    d. Guillain–Barré syndrome

151. A mother brings her six-year-old son in for his annual wellness visit. The child has no past medical history. During the examination, his mother states that about three weeks ago, the child had a viral infection. Following the viral infection, she noticed pinpoint reddish-purple dots on his extremities that appeared and spontaneously disappeared. Currently, the child's examination and vital signs are normal. Based on his medical history and physical examination, what was the most likely diagnosis causing his dermal symptoms?

    a. Idiopathic thrombocytopenic purpura

    b. Stevens–Johnson syndrome

    c. Von Willebrand disease

    d. Glucose-6-phosphate dehydrogenase (G6PD) deficiency

152. A couple brings their three-year-old daughter to the ER for worsening cough, fever, and sore throat. The child has no past medical history; however, the parents admit that they did not have their daughter vaccinated. On physical examination, you notice that the child is slightly cyanotic. You also see a grayish-black, tough, fiberlike covering of her oropharynx. Based on her medical history and physical examination, what is the most likely diagnosis?

    a. Cryptococcosis

    b. Shigellosis

    c. Cholera

    d. Diphtheria

153. A mother brings her 16-year-old daughter to the ER complaining of fever, sore throat, lethargy, and swollen cervical lymph glands. The child's temperature is 100.1° F; her other vital signs are normal. The child is mildly lethargic but easily aroused and does not appear to be dehydrated. Her physical examination is essentially normal other than her cervical lymphadenopathy. A monospot test is positive. What is the next step in your medical management?

    a. Prescribe amantadine

    b. Prescribe Augmentin

    c. Recommend computed tomography (CT) scan of the abdomen

    d. Recommend rest and fluids

154. A 71-year-old male comes to your office with a history of multiple, nontraumatic fractures for the past six months. Blood work reveals hypercalcemia and anemia, and his BUN/creatinine are 36/1.7. Urine studies reveal the presence of the Bence Jones protein. What is the most likely diagnosis?

    a. Acute myelogenous leukemia (AML)

    b. Multiple myeloma

    c. Acute lymphocytic leukemia (ALL)

    d. Paget's disease

155. Which of the following would be the LEAST helpful diagnostic test in diagnosing hemolytic anemia?

    a. International normalized ratio (INR)

    b. Coombs' test, direct

    c. Complete blood count (CBC)

    d. Lactate dehydrogenase (LDH) test

156. An infant is born with microcephaly, deafness, chorioretinitis, hepatosplenomegaly, and thrombocytopenia. Which of the following diseases would NOT be a likely cause?
    a. Influenza
    b. Rubella
    c. Toxoplasmosis
    d. Cytomegalovirus

157. A patient is diagnosed with mild iron-deficiency anemia. Which of the following foods would you NOT recommend your patient to increase his iron intake?
    a. Spinach
    b. Eggs
    c. Pasta
    d. Oranges

158. A 45-year-old patient comes to your clinic with an itchy, purplish rash on her wrists and ankle of five days' duration. She's had this rash before, but it usually resolves on its own. Other than the rash, she generally feels well. She has a history of hepatitis C. On physical examination, you notice that her vitals are normal. You note well-defined, pruritic, planar, purple, polygonal papules and plaques on her ankles and wrists. Based on her medical history and physical examination, what is the most likely diagnosis?
    a. Leukoplakia
    b. Impetigo
    c. Psoriasis
    d. Lichen planus

159. All of the following are treatments for dyshidrosis EXCEPT:
    a. Antibiotics
    b. Emollients
    c. Steroids
    d. Diphenhydramine

160. A 10-year-old patient has just been diagnosed with diabetes mellitus type 1. What is the first-line medication that you would prescribe?
    a. Metformin
    b. Lantus
    c. Glimepiride
    d. Glyburide

161. A 58-year-old male with a known history of alcohol abuse is brought to the ER for altered mental status. He is oriented to person only, he is vomiting, he is diaphoretic, and you notice a fine tremor. His pupils are dilated, but they are briskly reactive. His vital signs are as follows: BP, 166/89; respirations, 25 per minute; pulse, 119 beats per minute; and pulse oximetry, 95%. He states that he has not had a drink in two days. He denies drug abuse. Based on his medical history and physical examination, what is the most likely diagnosis?
    a. Delusional disorder
    b. Alcohol intoxication
    c. Alcohol withdrawal
    d. Dysthymic disorder

162. A mother brings her 13-year-old son to your office. He has been complaining of persistent unilateral knee pain for several weeks. The pain is exacerbated by movement. The child denies a history of trauma. A prior knee x ray taken in the ER is negative. On physical examination, you notice a painful bony bump just below the affected knee. There is no sign of infection. There is no joint laxity. The child has no medical problems. Based on his medical history and physical examination, what is the most likely diagnosis?
    a. Anterior cruciate ligament (ACL) disruption
    b. Polymyositis
    c. Ganglion cyst
    d. Osgood–Schlatter disease

163. You have a patient that has just been diagnosed with polyarteritis nodosa. What is the next step in your medical management?
    a. Start prednisone
    b. Start clindamycin
    c. Start permethrin
    d. Start amantadine

164. Which of the following is NOT a risk factor for developing condyloma acuminata?
    a. Birth control pills
    b. Late coital age
    c. Smoking
    d. Multiple sex partners

165. An adult patient has an excess of human growth hormone. Which of the following will be the most likely diagnosis?
    a. Gigantism
    b. Dwarfism
    c. Cushing's syndrome
    d. Acromegaly

166. A 35-year-old woman comes to your office with a myriad of complaints. She has noticed fatigue, progressive ataxia, muscle spasms, dizziness, and difficulty with coordination of fine motor movements. She states that she has recently been diagnosed with optic neuritis. What is the most likely diagnosis?
    a. Alzheimer's disease
    b. Meningitis
    c. Multiple sclerosis
    d. Huntington's disease

167. A woman comes to the ER complaining of dry mouth, drooling, right-sided facial swelling, and pain inside of her right cheek. Chewing aggravates the pain. She has had no vocal changes or difficulty with swallowing. Her only medical history is Sjögren's syndrome. What is the most likely diagnosis?
    a. Epiglottitis
    b. Parotitis
    c. Peritonsillar abscess
    d. Oral leukoplakia

168. A five-year-old boy is brought in by his mother to your clinic complaining of sores inside his mouth of three days' duration. She denies fever, discharge from lesions, or trauma. She admits that he's had these lesions before, but they went away on their own. He has no past medical history, and his vitals are normal. On physical examination, you notice two ulcers inside of his lower lip that have a grayish-yellow base and an erythematous halo. What is the next step in your medical management?

    a. Recommend nonsteroidal anti-inflammatory drugs (NSAIDs)
    b. Prescribe oral antiviral medication
    c. Prescribe oral antibiotics
    d. Recommend a decrease in folic acid intake

169. A 13-year-old male patient is brought to the ER with sudden-onset unilateral testicular pain following a trauma that occurred four hours previously. What is the next step in your medical management?

    a. Recommend warm compresses
    b. Stat surgery consult
    c. Order pain medication to see if it alleviates symptoms
    d. Order intravenous (IV) antibiotics

170. A patient is admitted to the ICU with a traumatic head injury. Other than the head injury, the patient has no past medical history. The nurse calls you with the morning labs to let you know that the patient's serum sodium is 150 and the serum potassium is 3.2. The serum glucose and urine glucose are normal. The nurse notes that the patient's urine output has increased to over 300 mL per hour. The urine specific gravity is <1.005. The patient has been drinking profusely throughout the night, but she is still complaining of thirst. Based on the lab results and the patient's medical history, what is the most likely diagnosis?

    a. Hypothyroidism
    b. Diabetes mellitus
    c. Hyperthyroidism
    d. Diabetes insipidus

171. A 35-year-old female comes to your clinic complaining of a painful sore on her neck of several weeks' duration. It keeps changing in appearance. On physical examination, you notice an asymmetric 9 mm papule on the right side of the patient's neck that has mixed areas of brown, blue, and black. It is moderately tender. No discharge can be expressed. There are no other lesions on her body. Based on the patient's medical history and physical examination, what is the most likely diagnosis?

    a. Impetigo
    b. Basal-cell carcinoma
    c. Melanoma
    d. Squamous-cell carcinoma

172. A 61-year-old male comes to the ER with a five-day history of worsening dysuria, hematuria, abdominal pain, and urinary incontinence. He has had an unintentional 15-pound weight loss over the past 30 days. He has a history of smoking one pack of cigarettes per day for 25 years, but he quit smoking five years ago. He has mild tenderness of the bilateral lower quadrants and suprapubic area. Based on his medical history and physical examination, what is the most likely diagnosis?
    a. Wilms' tumor
    b. Prostatitis
    c. Orchitis
    d. Bladder carcinoma

173. A 25-year-old with no past medical history is diagnosed with a corneal abrasion after she tried to remove her contact lens. What is the next step in her medical management?
    a. Gentamicin eyedrops for seven days
    b. Xalatan eyedrops for seven days
    c. Lumigan eyedrops for seven days
    d. Timoptic eyedrops for seven days

174. A patient has just been diagnosed with diabetes insipidus. What is your drug of choice for treating this condition?
    a. Depakote
    b. Decadron
    c. Desmopressin
    d. Detrol

175. A four-year-old child is brought to the ER for the fourth time for first-degree burns. Her right hand and foot have first-degree burns in a "glove and stocking" distribution. The child's prior visits document burns that presented the same way. The mother's explanation is that the child grabbed a hot pan off of the stove. Your next step is to
    a. Call child protective services prior to discharge
    b. Discharge the patient with Silvadene
    c. Discharge the child with Silvadene and po antibiotics
    d. Admit the patient for monitoring

176. Which of the following would NOT be a medical treatment of schizophrenia?
    a. Haldol
    b. Zyprexa
    c. Zofran
    d. Seroquel

177. A patient comes to your office and explains that he has recently been diagnosed with actinic keratosis. What should you advise him to do?
    a. Use antifungal cream
    b. Stay out of the sun
    c. Use steroid cream
    d. Recommend washing all linens in hot water

178. A patient comes to the ER complaining of swelling and pain of the nail bed on her finger for the past several days. The patient states that she had cut her finger several days ago before the symptoms appeared. On physical examination, you notice erythema, tenderness, and swelling of the medial aspect of her nail bed. Scant purulent discharge can be expressed. The patient has no past medical history. What is the most likely diagnosis?

    a. Scabies
    b. Paronychia
    c. Onychomycosis
    d. Condyloma acuminata

179. A patient comes to your clinic with widespread symmetrical loss of pigmentation of his or her skin. What is the most likely diagnosis?

    a. Lipoma
    b. Xanthelasma
    c. Mongolian spots
    d. Vitiligo

180. Which of the following medications would NOT be recommended in a patient with a history of fecal impaction?

    a. Colace
    b. Senna
    c. Morphine
    d. Milk of Magnesia

181. Which of the following medications may be administered to a patient who is having an episode of supraventricular tachycardia?

    a. Atropine
    b. Allopurinol
    c. Atorvastatin
    d. Adenosine

182. A patient presents with shortness of breath, dizziness, and chest pain. An electrocardiogram (EKG) shows sinus bradycardia. The patient's vital signs are as follows: BP, 101/55; pulse, 31 beats per minute; respirations, 18 per minute; and oxygen saturation, 96% on room air. What is the next step in your medical management?

    a. Give atropine
    b. Give amiodarone
    c. Give vasopressin
    d. Give adenosine

183. A patient in your office had blood drawn as part of her annual visit. On her blood work, you notice her HBsAg is negative, her anti-HBc is negative, and her anti-HBs is positive. Based on her lab values, what is the diagnosis?

    a. She is susceptible to being infected with hepatitis B
    b. She is chronically infected with hepatitis B
    c. She is immune due to hepatitis B due to prior vaccination
    d. She is acutely infected with hepatitis B

184. You are seeing a patient with suspected giant-cell arteritis. What is the next step in your management?
   a. Start on po antibiotics
   b. Recommend oncology referral for chemotherapy
   c. Monitor for now
   d. Recommend vascular surgery referral for biopsy

185. A patient in your office had blood drawn as part of her annual visit. You notice that her thyroid-stimulating hormone (TSH) level is high, her T3 level is normal, and her T4 level is low. Based on her lab values, what is the diagnosis?
   a. Addison's disease
   b. Hypothyroidism
   c. Hyperthyroidism
   d. Graves' disease

186. Which of the following medications may be useful in shortening the course of influenza if given early enough in the course of infection?
   a. Oseltamivir
   b. Acyclovir
   c. Famciclovir
   d. Augmentin

187. A patient is ambulating with physical therapy in the ICU when one of the therapists tells you that the patient's blood pressure went from 155/88 in the supine position to 131/70 in the sitting position. The other vital signs are as follows: pulse, 99; respirations, 18 per minute; and oxygen saturation, 97% on room air. The patient is now complaining of dizziness and headache. The patient's electrocardiogram (EKG) is normal. What is the most likely diagnosis?
   a. Sick sinus syndrome
   b. Angina
   c. Orthostatic hypotension
   d. Atrial fibrillation

188. A 68-year-old male presents to the ER with headache and nausea. A computed tomography (CT) scan of his head, electrocardiogram (EKG), and troponin level are normal. The urinalysis shows proteinuria. The patient's vital signs are as follows: pulse, 98 beats per minute; respirations, 16 per minute; and BP, 205/121. What is the most likely diagnosis?
   a. Stage 2 hypertension
   b. Hypertensive crisis
   c. Prehypertension
   d. Stage 1 hypertension

189. A 27-year-old obese female comes to your clinic complaining of worsening fatigue and frequent urination of several weeks' duration. Her urinalysis is positive for glucose and yeast. Her vital signs are normal. What is the next step in your medical management?
   a. Order ciprofloxacin and Pyridium
   b. Order a urine culture and blood cultures
   c. Order a repeat urinalysis in two weeks
   d. Order a hemoglobin A1C (HA1C) test, complete blood count (CBC), and basic metabolic panel (BMP)

190. A 21-year-old male comes to the ER with worsening left-sided testicular pain and swelling of three days' duration. He denies trauma. He has no past medical history. His vitals are normal. On physical examination, you palpate his scrotum, which feels like there's a mass of worms inside. Based on his medical history and physical, the most likely diagnosis is
    a. Hydrocele
    b. Varicocele
    c. Testicular torsion
    d. Testicular carcinoma

191. A patient comes to your clinic complaining of worsening diaphoresis, palpitations, and generalized tremor for several weeks. On physical examination, you notice that the patient has exophthalmos. What is the most likely diagnosis?
    a. Graves' disease
    b. Addison's disease
    c. Cushing's disease
    d. Hashimoto's disease

192. A 24-year-old male comes to the ER complaining of fever, chills, groin pain, dysuria, painful ejaculation, and testicular swelling of two days' duration. He denies trauma. What is the most likely diagnosis?
    a. Pyelonephritis
    b. Epididymitis
    c. Prostatitis
    d. Cystitis

193. A patient comes to your clinic for his annual purified protein derivative (PPD) injection. The patient works as a nurse at a local hospital. What is the minimum diameter of induration for a positive PPD test in this patient?
    a. 2 mm
    b. 5 mm
    c. 10 mm
    d. 15 mm

194. You have just examined a patient and suspect that she has Graves' disease. What is the next step in your medical management?
    a. Order thyroid function tests
    b. Order a complete endocrine panel
    c. Order a cortisol level
    d. Order a hemoglobin A1C (HA1C)

195. A woman with a history of bipolar disorder presents to the ER with altered mental status. She was intubated by emergency medical services (EMS) when she was found to be unconscious by the team. Her family notes that she was on lithium for her bipolar disorder. Her lithium level is high. Her blood urea nitrogen (BUN) and creatinine are 96/3.2. The patient is anuric. What is the immediate next course of medical action?
    a. Dialysis
    b. Fluid hydration
    c. Repeat lithium level in 12 hours
    d. Repeat BUN/creatinine in 12 hours

196. Which of the following groups is NOT recommended to get the flu vaccine?
    a. Adults age 50 and older
    b. Pregnant women
    c. Children less than 6 months old
    d. Health-care workers

197. A 44-year-old female presents to the ER with worsening nausea, vomiting, and diarrhea. She notes that she's been craving salty foods recently. Her vital signs are as follows: BP, 88/55; pulse, 66 beats per minute; respirations, 14 per minute; pulse oximetry, 98% on room air; and temperature, 98.9 °F. You notice that her skin has patchy areas of hyperpigmentation, which appear as if she had gone tanning. What is the most likely diagnosis?
    a. Hashimoto's disease
    b. Graves' disease
    c. Cushing's disease
    d. Addison's disease

198. A patient comes to your office complaining of headache, persistent urinary tract infections, unintentional weight loss, and fatigue. His fasting serum glucose is 161. His hemoglobin A1C (HA1C) is 6.2. His vitals are normal. His body mass index (BMI) is normal. He has no past medical problems. What is your medical recommendation to this patient?
    a. Lose weight
    b. Modify diet
    c. Start metformin
    d. Start insulin

199. A patient comes to your office complaining of erectile dysfunction. Which of the following medications would you NOT prescribe for this condition?
    a. Cialis
    b. Levitra
    c. Viagra
    d. Propecia

200. A patient with no past medical history had a purified protein derivative (PPD) shot three days ago and now has an induration of 5 mm. She works as a librarian. What is the next step in your medical management?
    a. Order a chest x ray
    b. Order a repeat PPD in one month
    c. No intervention for now
    d. Start tuberculosis medications

201. A 24-year-old male comes to your clinic complaining of having epididymitis. He states that he's had several prior epididymitis infections. He notes that he is sexually active and occasionally does not use protection. He denies other medical problems. What would you advise this patient?
    a. Increase fluid intake
    b. Avoid red meat, seafood, and alcohol
    c. Use protection when having intercourse
    d. Recommend urology referral

202. During a colonoscopy, it is discovered that a patient has multiple areas of outpouching along the colonic wall. What is the most likely diagnosis?
    a. Intussusception
    b. Diverticulosis
    c. Mallory–Weiss tear
    d. Celiac sprue

203. You suspect that a patient has septic arthritis. Which of the following would NOT be part of your medical management?
    a. Prescribe colchicine
    b. Perform a joint aspiration
    c. Order blood cultures
    d. Prescribe nonsteroidal anti-inflammatory drugs (NSAIDs)

204. You have just diagnosed a patient with celiac disease. What is the next step in your medical management?
    a. Prescribe antibiotics
    b. Order blood cultures
    c. Surgery referral
    d. Recommend dietary modifications

205. A 40-year-old male patient comes to the ER complaining of left-lower extremity pain. He is diagnosed with a blood clot in his left soleal vein. He has a past medical history of hypertension and hyperlipidemia. What is the next step in your medical management?
    a. Discharge home and get follow up Doppler ultrasound in two weeks
    b. Start Coumadin as an outpatient
    c. Admit the patient and start a Heparin infusion and Coumadin
    d. Surgery consult for placement of an inferior vena cava (IVC) filter

206. A mother brings her three-year-old son to the ER, stating that he fell on the playground earlier and then he stopped using his left arm. On physical examination, the child is holding his left arm flexed and pronated. He is not in any pain or distress as long as his arm is maintained in that position. There is no swelling, deformity, or discoloration of the extremity. Based on his medical history and physical examination, what is the most likely diagnosis?
    a. Lisfranc fracture
    b. Colles' fracture
    c. Nursemaid's elbow
    d. Greenstick fracture

207. A one-month-old baby girl born full term is diagnosed with patent ductus arteriosus (PDA). Her vital signs and physical examination are normal. What is the next step in your medical management?
    a. Recommend cardiology evaluation for possible surgical closure
    b. No intervention for now
    c. Prescribe aspirin 81 mg
    d. Prescribe indomethacin

208. A patient has just been diagnosed with benign prostatic hypertrophy. Which of the following medication would you NOT prescribe for this condition?
    a. Proscar
    b. Cardura
    c. Rapaflo
    d. Ramipril

209. You are seeing a 58-year-old patient in the ER who you think may be having an acute cerebral vascular accident. His symptoms started 30 minutes ago. His past medical history includes hypertension, obesity, and hyperlipidemia. His vital signs are normal. What is the next step in your medical management?
    a. Start a heparin infusion
    b. Reassess his examination in 30 minutes
    c. Administer tissue plasminogen activator (tPA)
    d. Order a computed tomography (CT) scan of the brain

210. A patient is diagnosed with *Clostridium difficile* colitis. The patient has no allergies to medication. Which of the following medications would you prescribe?
    a. Vancomycin po
    b. Clindamycin po
    c. IV azithromycin
    d. IV vancomycin

211. Which of the following medications would help treat a patient in status epilepticus?
    a. Levetiracetam and linezolid
    b. Phenylephrine and Lomotil
    c. Phenytoin and lorazepam
    d. Phenytoin and linezolid

212. Which medical triad includes three factors thought to contribute to thrombosis?
    a. Beck's triad
    b. Virchow's triad
    c. Charcot's triad
    d. Cushing's triad

213. A patient comes to the ER with right-sided foot pain after accidentally striking his foot against a baseboard. He has moderate pain at the first and second metatarsals with mild swelling with palpable deformity. Based on his medical history and physical, what is the most likely diagnosis?
    a. Le Fort fracture
    b. Lisfranc fracture
    c. Monteggia fracture
    d. Colles' fracture

214. A patient with cystic fibrosis asks you what medications she can take to help decrease her risk of secondary infection. Which of the following medications would you NOT advise this patient to take?
    a. Motrin
    b. Amiodarone
    c. Mucinex
    d. Albuterol

215. Which of the following is a complication of pulmonary tuberculosis?
    a. Parkinson's disease
    b. Hashimoto's disease
    c. Cushing's disease
    d. Pott's disease

216. A patient comes to your clinic complaining of pains all over her body. Multiple lab tests and scans have been negative for acute pathology. She has a history of depression. What is the most likely diagnosis?
    a. Fibromyalgia
    b. Polyarteritis nodosa
    c. Osteoarthritis
    d. Polymyalgia rheumatica

217. Which of the following medications would be used for a person diagnosed with generalized anxiety disorder?
    a. Prednisolone
    b. Promethazine
    c. Permethrin
    d. Paroxetine

218. A 68-year-old woman comes to your clinic complaining of decreasing vision in her left eye for the past several weeks. She noticed that she has problems differentiating between contrasts and identifying colors. She denies headache, trauma, and eye pain or discharge from the eye. She has no significant past medical history. She has a clouding of her left lens. What is the most likely diagnosis?
    a. Hyphema
    b. Blepharitis
    c. Cataract
    d. Conjunctivitis

219. You suspect a patient has a deep venous thrombus. Which of the following tests should you initially order?
    a. X ray
    b. Doppler ultrasound
    c. Computed tomography (CT) scan
    d. Magnetic resonance imaging (MRI)

220. A bleeding defect is seen in the distal esophagus of a patient during an esophagogastroduodenoscopy. The patient has a known history of alcoholism. What is the most likely diagnosis?
    a. Mallory–Weiss tear
    b. Crohn's disease
    c. Ulcerative colitis
    d. Whipple's disease

221. A 66-year-old female comes to the ER complaining of right calf pain and swelling of 12 hours' duration. She has a past medical history of arthritis and osteoporosis. She states that she had a right hip replacement four days ago. On physical examination, you note that she has a positive Homan's sign. Based on her medical history and physical examination, what is the most likely diagnosis?
    a. Septic arthritis
    b. Osgood–Schlatter disease
    c. Osteomyelitis
    d. Venous thrombus

222. While reviewing a two-dimensional echocardiography (2D echo) with a cardiologist, you both see that there is backflow of blood from the left ventricle into the left atrium. What is this condition called?
    a. Mitral regurgitation
    b. Pulmonic regurgitation
    c. Tricuspid regurgitation
    d. Aortic regurgitation

223. A patient in the intensive care unit (ICU) suddenly goes into pulseless ventricular tachycardia. What is one of the first medications you would administer?
    a. Magnesium sulfate
    b. Lidocaine
    c. Epinephrine
    d. Amiodarone

224. Parents bring their 13-year-old son into your clinic for his annual physical evaluation. They have expressed concern because they have noticed that the child has been developing breasts over the past year, which has been a source of anxiety and distress for their son. On physical examination, you notice that the child has enlarged mammary glands bilaterally. The child has no past medical history. The rest of his physical examination is normal. Based on the medical history and physical examination, what is the most likely diagnosis?
    a. Fibrocystic breast disease
    b. Gynecomastia
    c. Fibroadenoma
    d. Carcinoma

225. Parents bring in their two-year-old child to your clinic. They note that he has been tugging on his ears for the past two days. He has been getting over a viral upper respiratory infection, but he is otherwise healthy. Upon physical examination, you notice that his left tympanic membrane is erythematous and bulging. His physical examination is otherwise normal. Based on the medical history and physical examination, what is the most likely diagnosis?
    a. Otitis media
    b. Mastoiditis
    c. Otitis externa
    d. Acoustic neuroma

226. A 45-year-old male with a known history of human immunodeficiency virus (HIV) is brought to the ER with sudden onset of confusion, nausea, vomiting, neck pain, headache, and photophobia. There is no history of trauma. A computed tomography (CT) scan without contrast of the head and neck is negative for acute pathology. Upon physical examination, you note that the patient has a positive Kerning's sign. Based on the medical history and physical examination, what is the most likely diagnosis?
   a. Guillain–Barré syndrome
   b. Meningitis
   c. Huntington's disease
   d. Schistosomiasis

227. A patient with an unknown infection undergoes a lumbar puncture. The lumbar puncture results show an elevated opening pressure, elevated white blood cell count, elevated neutrophil count, and decreased glucose level. Based on the results, what is the most likely diagnosis?
   a. Huntington's disease
   b. Bacterial meningitis
   c. Viral meningitis
   d. Myasthenia gravis

228. A blood gas shows the following results: pH, 7.31; $PaCO_2$, 50; HCO_3, 25; and PaO_2, 94. Which of the following is the most likely diagnosis?
   a. Metabolic alkalosis
   b. Respiratory alkalosis
   c. Metabolic acidosis
   d. Respiratory acidosis

229. A 26-year-old patient is brought to the ER by his family for sudden onset of dementia, ataxia, and urinary incontinence of four days' duration. He has recently recovered from a cerebral aneurysm rupture. A computed tomography (CT) scan shows distended ventricles. A lumbar puncture is performed, but the results are normal. What is the most likely diagnosis?
   a. Medulloblastoma
   b. Intraventricular hemorrhage
   c. Normal pressure hydrocephalus (NPH)
   d. Hygroma

230. A 15-year-old female is brought to your clinic by her mother, who states that her child has not been eating. The girl has no past medical history. Upon further discussion, the child confides in you that she purposely has been skipping meals so she can lose weight. What is the most likely diagnosis?
   a. Anorexia nervosa
   b. Bulimia nervosa
   c. Generalized anxiety disorder
   d. Bipolar disorder

231. A 40-year-old male comes to your clinic and reports that he feels nervous all of the time. He has no history of personal loss, disturbing life event, or illness. His physical examination and vital signs are normal. He has no medical problems. What is the most likely diagnosis?
    a. Dysthymic disorder
    b. Generalized anxiety disorder
    c. Posttraumatic stress disorder
    d. Phobia

232. A patient in the intensive care unit has the following blood gas: pH, 7.47; $PaCO_2$, 39; HCO_3, 29. What is the most likely diagnosis?
    a. Respiratory acidosis
    b. Respiratory alkalosis
    c. Metabolic alkalosis
    d. Metabolic acidosis

233. A patient with normal pressure hydrocephalus undergoes a lumbar puncture. The patient's symptoms improve. What is the next step in this patient's management?
    a. Obtain a magnetic resonance imaging (MRI) scan of the brain
    b. Repeat the lumbar puncture in 48 hours
    c. Ventricular peritoneal shunt
    d. Perform an electroencephalogram (EEG)

234. A patient comes to your clinic for an annual physical examination. The patient confesses to you that she has a hard time coming to your clinic, or being outside in general, because of her fear of being outdoors. She reports feelings of extreme anxiety once she leaves her house. She denies any reason for her to be nervous of crowds of people. What is the most likely diagnosis?
    a. Generalized anxiety disorder
    b. Posttraumatic stress disorder
    c. Dysthymic disorder
    d. Phobia disorder

235. A patient has hypertrophic cardiomyopathy. What is the most common cause for this condition?
    a. Genetic mutation
    b. Disease
    c. Infection
    d. Cancer

236. Parents bring their child into the ER stating that the child has developed rapid, uncontrolled body movements and a fever of 102° F at home. You notice these body movements during your physical examination as well. You draw blood for lab work, which shows that the patient has a white blood cell count of 17,000 as well as an elevated erythrocyte sedimentation rate (ESR). Which of the following signs/symptoms is not part of the minor manifestations of rheumatic fever according to the Jones criteria?
    a. Fever
    b. Chorea
    c. Leukocytosis
    d. Elevated ESR

237. You are reviewing a two-dimensional echocardiogram when you notice backflow of blood from the right ventricle into the right atrium. The most likely diagnosis is
    a. Aortic regurgitation
    b Mitral regurgitation
    c. Pulmonic regurgitation
    d. Tricuspid regurgitation

238. Which of the following medications should NOT be given in a patient with pulseless ventricular fibrillation?
    a. Amiodarone
    b. Lidocaine
    c. Vasopressin
    d. Atropine

239. A nurse hands you the following arterial blood gas results: pH, 7.49; $PaCO_2$, 20; and HCO_3, 23. Which of the following is the most likely diagnosis?
    a. Metabolic alkalosis
    b. Respiratory alkalosis
    c. Metabolic acidosis
    d. Respiratory acidosis

240. A patient is brought to the ER for acute alcohol intoxication. As the patient begins to wake up, you notice persistent, involuntary, horizontal eye movements of both eyes. What is the most likely diagnosis?
    a. Conjunctivitis
    b. Nystagmus
    c. Entropion
    d. Exotropia

241. A patient arrives in the ER complaining of chest pain, dizziness, and shortness of breath. An electrocardiogram (EKG) shows a secondary R wave in lead V1 and a widened QRS complex. What is this conduction disorder called?
    a. Torsades de pointes
    b. Right bundle branch block
    c. Atrial fibrillation
    d. Sinus tachycardia

242. A 65-year-old male patient presents to the ER with dysarthria, ataxia, and left-sided weakness, which occurred for about 30 minutes and then spontaneously resolved. His physical examination is normal. A computed tomography (CT) scan of the brain is normal. What is the most likely diagnosis?
    a. Transient ischemic attack
    b. Cerebral aneurysm rupture
    c. Cerebral vascular accident
    d. Migraine

243. A patient with a known history of anxiety and depression is in your clinic for a routine physical examination and confides in you that he wants to commit suicide. He tells you how and when he plans to do it. Which of the following is NOT an appropriate action as a medical professional?
   a. Advise the patient to call a suicide hotline
   b. Obtain a stat psychiatric referral
   c. Do not report the patient's actions
   d. Advise the patient's spouse or parents of his intent

244. A patient comes to your clinic complaining of persistent right-eye irritation. The conjunctiva is normal. You note that the patient's right lower lid is turned inward. What is this condition called?
   a. Entropion
   b. Exotropia
   c. Ectropion
   d. Esotropia

245. Parents bring in their five-year-old son for his annual physical examination. The parents state that their son has been having trouble at school and at home for frequent temper tantrums, angry outbursts, short temper, and hostility toward others. He hasn't gone through any life-threatening situations, suffered personal losses, or had any recent changes in his life. His physical examination and vital signs are normal. He has no past medical history. What is the most likely diagnosis?
   a. Adjustment disorder
   b. Dysthymic disorder
   c. Attention-deficit hyperactivity disorder
   d. Oppositional-defiant disorder

246. One of your patients has been diagnosed with phlebitis. Which of the following would NOT be a part of your medical management?
   a. Prescribe Colchicine
   b. Recommend compression stockings
   c. Prescribe analgesics
   d. Recommend warm compresses

247. A patient comes to the ER with palpitations, chest pain, dizziness, and shortness of breath. An electrocardiogram (EKG) shows a heart rate of 120 beats per minute. The EKG shows irregular QRS complexes and no P waves. What is the most likely diagnosis?
   a. Right bundle branch block
   b. Sinus tachycardia
   c. Atrial fibrillation
   d. Sinus bradycardia

248. A 16-year-old female patient arrives in the ER complaining of headache, nausea, and photophobia. She is diagnosed with a migraine headache. Which of the following medications would you prescribe for this patient to help prevent and treat future episodes?
   a. Fluvastatin
   b. Frovatriptan
   c. Fluoxetine
   d. Fexofenadine

249. A patient is diagnosed with Guillain–Barré syndrome. Which of the following is NOT a method to reduce symptoms, prevent complications, and speed up recovery?
   a. Plasmapheresis
   b. Intubation
   c. Immunoglobulin therapy
   d. Lumbar puncture

250. A 21-year-old male patient arrives in your office for the first time for a routine physical examination. While talking to him, you note that he has involuntary facial tics. His cognitive function is normal. What is the most likely diagnosis for his behavior?
   a. Huntington's disease
   b. Tourette disorder
   c. Alzheimer's disease
   d. Multiple sclerosis

251. You are examining a patient with suspected chronic obstructive pulmonary disease (COPD). Which of the following is the best test to help aid your diagnosis?
   a. Spirometry
   b. Chest x ray
   c. Auscultation with a stethoscope
   d. Electrocardiogram (EKG)

252. Which of the following tests is the most sensitive for detecting cystic fibrosis?
   a. Chest x ray
   b. Fecal fat test
   c. Sweat chloride test
   d. Computed tomography (CT) scan of the chest

253. A patient arrives in the ER complaining of worsening hemoptysis, fever, chills, and weakness for the past week. This patient has a history of human immunodeficiency virus (HIV). A chest x ray is ordered, which shows a fungal ball in the right lung. What is the most likely diagnosis?
   a. Cystic fibrosis
   b. Pneumoconiosis
   c. Sarcoidosis
   d. Aspergillosis

254. A mother brings in her 18-month-old son to your clinic, noting that he has been displaying progressively deteriorating social and communication skills and repetitive behaviors. This triad of symptoms best defines which of the following disorders?
   a. Oppositional-defiant disorder
   b. Attention-deficit hyperactivity disorder
   c. Autism disorder
   d. Adjustment disorder

255. A mother pregnant with her first child is Rh-positive. The child is Rh-positive. What is the next step in medical management?
    a. Prescribe antibiotics
    b. Order an ultrasound
    c. No intervention
    d. Prescribe RhoGAM

256. A woman who is 36 weeks pregnant develops eclampsia. Her liver function tests and complete blood count are normal. What would be the next step in medical management?
    a. Observe on telemetry monitor
    b. Discharge home and monitor as an outpatient
    c. Induce labor
    d. Order a stat blood transfusion

257. A 56-year-old man with a history of chronic obstructive pulmonary disease (COPD) comes to the ER complaining of worsening shortness of breath and chest pain. A chest x ray shows blunting of the right costophrenic angle. What is the most likely diagnosis?
    a. Pleural effusion
    b. Aspergillosis
    c. Pneumoconiosis
    d. Pneumothorax

258. Which of the following chest x-ray findings is most consistent with the diagnosis of a pneumothorax whose size is approximately 5%?
    a. Honeycomb appearance of the lungs
    b. Granulomas
    c. Area on chest x ray with no lung markings
    d. Normal chest x ray

259. Which of the following conditions would NOT be a contributing factor to the development of obesity?
    a. Graves' disease
    b. Hypothyroidism
    c. Cushing's syndrome
    d. Menopause

260. Which of the following is NOT a treatment for allergic rhinitis?
    a. Decongestants
    b. Antihistamines
    c. Antibiotics
    d. Corticosteroids

261. Which of the following would NOT be used in the treatment of a patient with a phobia disorder?
    a. Xanax
    b. Metoprolol
    c. Lexapro
    d. Ritalin

262. Which of the following treatments is NOT an intervention for a patient going through withdrawal from alcohol?
   a. Zofran
   b. Narcan
   c. Thiamine
   d. Ativan

263. A 37-year-old female patient comes to the ER complaining of worsening fever, dysphonia, and dysphagia of three days' duration. She notes recently having a tooth infection, but she did not seek medical attention for it. While you are talking to the patient, her family member says, "she sounds like she has a hot potato in her mouth." Her tongue is swollen and out of place, and she has swelling and erythema of her proximal neck. What is the most likely diagnosis?
   a. Oral leukoplakia
   b. Acute pharyngitis
   c. Ludwig's angina
   d. Aphthous ulcers

264. A patient being seen in the ER is diagnosed with a blowout fracture. Which of the following would NOT be an intervention for this patient?
   a. Irrigation
   b. Antibiotics
   c. Steroids
   d. Surgery

265. A patient comes to the ER complaining of facial pain and swelling after being physically assaulted. A computed tomography (CT) scan reveals a fractured maxilla. What is the most likely diagnosis?
   a. Boxer's fracture
   b. Lisfranc fracture
   c. Colles' fracture
   d. Le Fort fracture

266. What is the most common preventable cause of pelvic inflammatory disease?
   a. Appendicitis
   b. Ectopic pregnancy
   c. Childbirth
   d. Venereal disease

267. A patient is diagnosed with gastroesophageal reflux disease. Which of the following medications is the most appropriate treatment for this condition?
   a. Ketoconazole
   b. Metronidazole
   c. Fluconazole
   d. Esomeprazole

268. Which of the following statements is FALSE regarding Meckel's diverticulum?
   a. It is more common in females than males
   b. It is usually found about two feet from the ileocecal valve
   c. Initial presentation is more common in toddlers than adults
   d. It affects approximately 2% of the population

269. A patient comes to your clinic complaining of worsening gastroesophageal reflux symptoms as well as abdominal pain and hematemesis. A serum gastrin level is high. A computed tomography (CT) scan of the abdomen shows multiple small tumors in the head of the pancreas and the duodenum. What is the most likely diagnosis?
    a. Celiac disease
    b. Zollinger–Ellison syndrome
    c. Whipple's disease
    d. Crohn's disease

270. A patient comes to the ER with increasing left shoulder pain and decreased range of motion after a heavy box fell on his shoulder. On physical examination, he has limited abduction. A shoulder x ray is negative for fracture or dislocation. What is the next step in your medical management?
    a. Order a repeat x ray in two weeks
    b. Order a magnetic resonance imaging (MRI) scan of the shoulder
    c. No intervention
    d. Administer electromyography (EMG)

271. A patient is admitted to the hospital for multiple right leg fractures following a motor vehicle accident. The leg is casted, and the patient is sent to the intensive care unit (ICU) for monitoring. A nurse calls you later on that day to tell you that the patient's right foot has become pale and cold. An arterial ultrasound shows no flow. His creatine phosphokinase (CPK) level is 14,000. What is the most likely diagnosis?
    a. Osgood–Schlatter disease
    b. Deep venous thrombosis
    c. Compartment syndrome
    d. Septic arthritis

272. A patient is diagnosed with trichomoniasis. What is the next step in your medical management?
    a. Rocephin
    b. Metronidazole
    c. Azithromycin
    d. Fluconazole

273. A patient comes to your clinic stating that she has noticed skin changes over her right breast. During the physical examination, you note that her skin has a swollen, pitted surface. What is the most likely diagnosis?
    a. Carcinoma
    b. Abscess
    c. Gynecomastia
    d. Fibroadenoma

274. Which of the following will not help alleviate the symptoms of premenstrual syndrome?
    a. Exercise
    b. Dietary modifications
    c. Birth control pills
    d. Caffeine

275. Which of the following will NOT help prevent cervical cancer?
    a. Regular Pap smears
    b. Limit tobacco abuse
    c. Cease having children
    d. Limit the number of sexual partners

276. Which of the following is the best way to prevent beriberi?
    a. Increase calcium intake
    b. Increase thiamine intake
    c. Increase folate intake
    d. Increase iron intake

277. Which of the following is the best way to prevent osteoporosis?
    a. Increase calcium intake
    b. Increase thiamine intake
    c. Increase folate intake
    d. Increase iron intake

278. A friend is telling you about a family member who suffers from a disease resulting is misshapen bones and persistent pathologic fractures. The most likely diagnosis for this condition is
    a. Septic arthritis
    b. Paget's disease
    c. Osteosarcoma
    d. Wilms' tumor

279. A woman who is 35 weeks pregnant presents to the ER with continuous contractions, abdominal pain, back pain, and bright-red vaginal bleeding. What is the most likely diagnosis?
    a. Endometriosis
    b. Premature rupture of the membranes
    c. Placental abruption (abruptio placentae)
    d. Placenta previa

280. A 23-year-old male complaining of right knee pain after a football injury two days ago comes to the ER. His right knee is diffusely swollen, and he has difficulty putting weight on his right leg. The patient has a positive Lachman test. What is the most likely diagnosis?
    a. Posterior cruciate ligament tear
    b. Lateral collateral ligament tear
    c. Medial collateral ligament tear
    d. Anterior cruciate ligament tear

281. A patient comes to the ER complaining of left wrist pain after falling on an outstretched hand. An x ray shows a fracture of the distal radius and a dislocation at the radioulnar joint. What is the most likely diagnosis?
    a. Le Fort fracture
    b. Colles' fracture
    c. Galeazzi fracture
    d. Monteggia fracture

282. An x ray shows a transverse and mildly displaced fourth metacarpal fracture. The patient had come to the ER complaining of hand pain after being involved in a physical altercation. What is the most likely diagnosis?
    a. Colles' fracture
    b. Lisfranc fracture
    c. Hangman's fracture
    d. Boxer's fracture

283. A 24-year-old female who is 12 weeks pregnant comes to the ER complaining of sudden-onset abdominal pain and vaginal bleeding. She has had a prior transvaginal ultrasound, which showed an intrauterine pregnancy (IUP). An ultrasound cannot visualize the IUP. A urine pregnancy test is negative. What is the most likely diagnosis?
    a. Threatened abortion
    b. Missed abortion
    c. Completed abortion
    d Dysmenorrhea

284. A patient comes to the ER with nausea, vomiting, and constipation for two days. The patient was discharged from the hospital a week before after having a laparoscopic appendectomy. An abdominal x ray shows a distended bowel without evidence of obstruction. What is the most likely diagnosis?
    a. Gastroesophageal reflux disease
    b. Ileus
    c. Toxic megacolon
    d. Irritable bowel syndrome

285. Which of the following would NOT be an appropriate treatment for giardiasis?
    a. Furosemide
    b. Ondansetron
    c. Loperamide
    d. Metronidazole

286. Which of the following tests is NOT appropriate in the workup of lactose intolerance?
    a. Lactose tolerance test
    b. Lactose-hydrogen breath test
    c. Serum calcium
    d. Stool pH

287. Which of the following tests is the most diagnostic for monitoring the course of choriocarcinoma and its response to therapy?
    a. Complete blood cell count
    b. Bence Jones protein
    c. Computed tomography (CT) scan of the abdomen and pelvis
    d. Beta human chorionic gonadotropin (hCG)

288. All of the following are therapies used to treat leiomyomas EXCEPT
    a. Nonsteroidal anti-inflammatory drugs (NSAIDs)
    b. Birth control pills
    c. Antibiotics
    d. Iron supplements

289. A 16-year-old female comes to the office with worsening pelvic pain, dysmenorrhea, throbbing pain that radiates down her legs, and dysuria for several weeks. She is not sexually active. She has no past medical history. Abdominal and pelvic ultrasounds are negative. A urine pregnancy test is negative. She undergoes a laparoscopy, which shows multiple dark-colored lesions on the ovaries, outside of the uterus, and on the abdominal wall. What is the most likely diagnosis?
    a. Dystocia
    b. Leiomyoma
    c. Choriocarcinoma
    d. Endometriosis

290. Which of the following would NOT be a treatment for sciatica?
    a. Nonsteroidal anti-inflammatory drugs (NSAIDs)
    b. Corticosteroid injections
    c. Surgery
    d. Physical therapy

291. A 17-year-old female is brought to your clinic for worsening pain and swelling of her knees, elbows, and hips. She has recently developed a butterfly-shaped rash that covers the bridge of her nose and her cheeks. There is no history of trauma. She has no significant past medical history. X rays of the knees, elbows, and hips are normal. What is the most likely diagnosis?
    a. Systemic lupus erythematous
    b. Paget's disease
    c. Polymyositis
    d. Huntington's disease

292. Which of the following is NOT an appropriate intervention for a partial small-bowel obstruction?
    a. Antibiotics
    b. Intravenous (IV) fluids
    c. Nasogastric tube
    d. Antiemetic medications

293. A patient comes to your office complaining of alternating episodes of diarrhea and constipation that get worse after eating. Her lab tests are normal, her colonoscopy is normal, and a computed tomography (CT) scan of the abdomen and pelvis is normal. The symptoms are not caused by one particular type of food. She has a known history of anxiety and depression. What is the most likely diagnosis?
    a. Irritable bowel syndrome
    b. Crohn's disease
    c. Ulcerative colitis
    d. Toxic megacolon

294. A patient is diagnosed with pelvic inflammatory disease. Which of the following is the most appropriate treatment for this condition?
    a. Antifungal medications
    b. Antibiotics
    c. Antiviral medications
    d. No treatment is necessary

295. A patient is diagnosed with polymyositis. Which of the following is the most appropriate treatment for this condition?
a. Antibiotics
b. Nonsteroidal anti-inflammatory drugs (NSAIDs)
c. Antiviral medications
d. Corticosteroids

296. What is the primary underlying cause of spondylolisthesis?
a. Incorrect alignment of the disc
b. Insufficient calcium
c. Unknown cause
d. Infectious etiology

297. Which of the following is the least effective method of preventing unwanted pregnancy?
a. Intrauterine device
b. Birth control pills
c. Withdrawal method
d. Condoms

298. Which of the following medications is the most appropriate in treating rheumatoid arthritis?
a. Metronidazole
b. Meropenem
c. Metformin
d. Methotrexate

299. Which of the following is a major contributing factor to the development of osteoarthritis?
a. Immune disorder
b. Degenerative disease
c. Congenital disorder
d. Infectious etiology

300. An 82-year-old male with a known history of osteoarthritis comes to your clinic complaining of worsening back pain. During the examination, you notice he has a C-shaped curvature of his spine, causing him to look like a hunchback. What is the most likely diagnosis for this condition?
a. Kyphosis
b. Cauda equina syndrome
c. Avascular necrosis
d. Sciatica

Answers and Explanations

1. C: Cushing's triad is a clinical <u>triad</u> defined as hypertension, bradycardia, and irregular respirations. It suggests rising intracranial pressure due to intracranial pathology such as hemorrhage.

Beck's triad is the combination of distended jugular veins, hypotension, and muffled heart sounds. It occurs as a result of pericardial effusion.

Charcot's triad is the combination of <u>jaundice</u>, <u>fever</u>, and right-upper quadrant <u>abdominal pain</u>. It occurs as a result of <u>ascending cholangitis</u>.

Bergman's triad is the combination of dyspnea, petechiae, and mental status changes. It occurs when a patient has a fat embolism.

2. A: **Major manifestations of acute rheumatic fever include the following:**
Erythema marginatum: raised, nonpruritic, pink rings on the trunk and inner surfaces of the limbs
Carditis: inflammation of the heart muscle
Chorea: rapid, uncontrolled body movements
Subcutaneous nodules: painless, firm collections of collagen fibers over bones or <u>tendons</u>
<u>Polyarthritis</u>: temporary migrating inflammation of the large joints

Minor manifestations of acute rheumatic fever include the following:
1) <u>Fever</u> (101 °F to 102 °F)
2) Arthralgia: joint pain without swelling
3) Elevated erythrocyte sedimentation rate (ESR) or C-reactive protein (CRP)
4) Leukocytosis
5) Prior episode of rheumatic heart disease
6) Heart block seen on an electrocardiogram (EKG)

3. D: Psoriasis causes cells to build up rapidly on the surface of the skin, forming itchy, dry, red, raised patches covered with grayish silvery lesions that are easily friable. Psoriasis is sometimes painful. Plaques frequently occur on the skin of the <u>elbows</u> and knees, but they can affect any area. This is a chronic condition.

Impetigo is a bacterial infection that is most commonly caused by *Staphylococcus aureus* or *Streptococcus pyogenes*. It causes lesions that can occur anywhere on the body. They are small, red, and pus-filled and can crack open and form a yellow or honey-colored, thick crust. They occur most commonly in young children.

Tinea corporis, also known as "ringworm," is a fungal infection that develops on the superficial layer of the skin, occurring anywhere on the body. It is characterized by an itchy, red, circular rash with a central clearing.

Rosacea is a chronic inflammatory skin condition characterized by redness of the face, most commonly on the cheeks, nose, and forehead.

4. B: In Crohn's disease, the colon wall may have a "cobblestone" appearance due to the intermittent pattern of affected and nonaffected colonic tissue.

Celiac sprue is an immune reaction that damages the lining of the small intestine and prevents it from absorbing important nutrients. A diagnosis can be made by an upper <u>endoscopy</u> with biopsy.

Ulcerative colitis usually affects continuous stretches of the colon and rectum.

Whipple's disease is rare chronic disease caused by a bacterial infection. The affected bowel is usually swollen with raised, yellowish patches.

5. C: A positive Murphy's sign aids in the diagnosis of acute cholecystitis.

The Brudziński sign is positive when flexion of the neck usually causes flexion of the hip and knee. This maneuver is used to help diagnose meningitis.

The psoas sign is positive when a patient experiences abdominal pain when he or she actively flexes the leg at the hip and knee. This maneuver is used to help diagnose appendicitis.

The Levine sign is positive when a patient is holding a clenched fist over his or her chest to describe dull, pressing chest pain consistent with the discomfort of angina pectoris.

6. B: Vicryl sutures are absorbable. They take anywhere from 40 to 70 days to absorb. Other examples of absorbable sutures include Monocryl and chromic gut. Prolene, silk, and nylon sutures are all nonabsorbable sutures. Other examples of nonabsorbable suture materials include polyester sutures and stainless steel sutures. Dermabond is a type of skin adhesive meant for superficial skin lacerations; it should never be used on any other surface besides the skin.

7. C: Esophageal achalasia is when the lower esophageal sphincter does not relax properly. This impairs the smooth passage of food from the lower esophagus into the stomach. Acid reflux, dysphagia, and chest pain are symptoms of esophageal achalasia. Hematochezia is when a person has bright-red blood coming from the rectum. This occurrence is commonly associated with gastrointestinal (GI) bleeding.

8. C: CREST syndrome includes five main features: **c**alcinosis, **R**aynaud's syndrome, **e**sophageal dysmotility, **s**clerodactyly, and **t**elangiectasia. The CREST syndrome is part of the immune disorder scleroderma. This immune disorder causes skin and body tissues to improperly tighten.

Solar urticaria is the development of hives when the skin is exposed to sunlight; it is not related to CREST syndrome.

9. B: Reiter's syndrome causes inflammation of the urinary tract, eyes, skin, mucous membranes, and joints. Chlamydia is the most common cause of Reiter's syndrome.

Sjögren's syndrome is a disorder of the immune system that causes a decrease in the production of mucus and moisture.

Turner syndrome is a genetic condition in which females are missing all or part of an X chromosome. Some of the symptoms may include infertility, amenorrhea, short stature, and webbed neck.

Down syndrome is a genetic condition in which there is a chromosomal abnormality on chromosome 21. Some signs of Down syndrome may include broad forehead and tongue, slanted eyes, small ears, and cognitive and cardiac defects.

10. D: Ceftriaxone 250 mg IM injection in a single dose plus azithromycin 1 gm PO in a single dose or doxycycline 100 mg PO BID for seven days is the recommended regimen for treating gonorrhea (GC)/chlamydia infections. Clindamycin and Maxipime are not given as treatment for either gonorrhea or chlamydia. The patient should be treated in the ER for suspected GC/chlamydia infection to prevent the patient from potentially spreading the disease.

11. B: Naloxone (Narcan) is an opiate antidote to treat potential or confirmed narcotic overdoses. Oxycodone is an opiate.

Prednisolone is a corticosteroid drug. It is useful for the treatment of a wide range of inflammatory and autoimmune conditions.

Buspirone is used in the short-term relief of anxiety symptoms. Although this may be useful as a maintenance drug for the patient's history of anxiety, he is not anxious during the examination.

12. D: Augmentin is a penicillin, and cefepime and cephalexin are cephalosporins. Approximately 10% of patients with a penicillin reaction will also have an allergy to the cephalosporins. In patients with a documented allergy to pencillins, the use of cephalosporins is contraindicated. Clarithromycin is a macrolide and may be safely administered to a patient with a penicillin allergy.

13. A: Pegged teeth, also known as Hutchinson's teeth; swollen joints; deafness; blindness; and other nervous-symptom abnormalities are characteristic of congenital syphilis.
Down syndrome patients have a myriad of physical signs such as broad forehead and tongue, eyelid creases, small ears, short stature, and a flat head. They do not have pegged teeth and generally have unusually flexible joints.
Osgood–Schlatter disease is characterized by chronic knee pain in young children and adolescents.
Turner syndrome is a genetic condition in which females are missing all or part of an X chromosome. Some of the symptoms may include infertility, amenorrhea, short stature, and a webbed neck.

14. B: A hordeolum appears as a red, swollen, tender pimple on the edge of the eyelid. It is caused by an oil gland that has become blocked.
Xanthelasma are raised, yellow patches on the eyelids. The incidence of occurrence increases with age. They are common in patients with hyperlipidemia.
Mongolian spots are nonraised, grayish-blue skin lesions most commonly seen on the sacrum or buttocks.
A felon is an infection inside the fingertip that can expand and spread if left untreated.

15. D: Xanthelasma are raised yellow patches on the eyelids. The incidence of occurrence increases with age. They are common in patients with hyperlipidemia.
Dermoid cysts are skin growths or outpouchings that may contain miscellaneous structures such as skin, hair, or teeth. They are not skin lesions that develop over time; they are seen at birth.
Impetigo is a bacterial infection that is most commonly caused by *Staphylococcus aureus* or *Streptococcus pyogenes*. It causes lesions that can occur anywhere on the body. They are small, red, and pus-filled and can crack open and form a yellow or honey-colored, thick crust. They occur most commonly in young children.
Mongolian spots are flat, blue, or blue-gray skin markings near the buttocks that commonly appear at birth or shortly thereafter.

16. C: Medulloblastomas are the most common malignant brain tumor and are significantly more common in children than in adults. They usually occur in the cerebellum.
A hygroma is a collection of cerebrospinal fluid in the subdural space. Acute hygromas are usually caused by head trauma or a recent neurosurgical procedure.
Schistosomiasis is a chronic parasitic infection due to eating improperly cooked pork. On a magnetic resonance imaging (MRI) scan of the brain, it can appear as multiple enhancing nodules occurring on bilateral cerebral hemispheres.
Melanoma is a malignant skin cancer.

17. A: Charcot's triad is the combination of <u>jaundice</u>, <u>fever</u>, and right-upper quadrant <u>abdominal pain</u>. It occurs as a result of <u>ascending cholangitis</u>.
Acute appendicitis usually presents as periumbilical, epigastric, or right-lower quadrant abdominal pain, fever, nausea, vomiting, and extreme sensitivity to movement called the jar sign.
Choledocholithiasis is the presence of stones within the common bile duct without infection. Patients do not usually display symptoms.

Acute pyelonephritis usually presents as fever, shaking chills, epigastric or left-sided abdominal pain, nausea, vomiting, urinary tract infection (UTI) symptoms, and back pain.

18. C: In early pregnancy, high levels of estrogen cause increased venous pressure, causing the mucosal surfaces of the genitals to turn a purplish or bluish color.
The obturator sign is positive when abdominal pain is elicited with the internal rotation of the flexed right leg. This maneuver helps diagnose appendicitis.
The Levine sign is positive when a patient is holding a clenched fist over his or her chest to describe dull, pressing chest pain consistent with the discomfort of angina pectoris.
Kerning's sign is positive when a patient is unable to extend his or her leg when the hip is flexed. This maneuver helps diagnose meningitis.

19. A: Colchicine is used only in acute gout attacks.
Allopurinol (Zyloprim) is used for the treatment of chronic gout and is used to prevent rather than treat gout attacks. Other treatments for gout include nonsteroidal anti-inflammatory drugs (NSAIDs) and steroids. Tetracycline is an antibiotic and is not used to treat gout.
Amantadine has been used in the treatment of the influenza virus and for Parkinson's disease.

20. A: The Dix–Hallpike test involves a patient sitting upright with his or her head laterally rotated to one side. The patient is asked to lie down quickly with his or her head slightly extended. The test is considered positive if this maneuver reproduces symptoms.
An electroencephalogram (EEG) helps diagnose seizures or abnormal brain activity.
The **transcranial Doppler ultrasound (TCD)** measures the presence of vasospasm in the brain's blood vessels.
Phalen's maneuver is a diagnostic tool used to help diagnose carpal tunnel syndrome.

21. B: This child has Down syndrome, which is caused by a defect of chromosome 21.
Chromosome 23 is the sex chromosome.
Turner syndrome is a genetic condition in which females are missing all or part of an X chromosome. Some of the symptoms may include infertility, amenorrhea, short stature, and webbed neck.
Klinefelter's syndrome patients have an extra Y chromosome, leading to poor muscle strength, decreased fertility or infertility, gynecomastia, and low testosterone levels.
There is no chromosome 24. All humans have 23 chromosomal pairs, totaling 46 chromosomes.
Patients with abnormalities on chromosome 13 (also known as Patau's syndrome) usually have serious brain, pulmonary, and circulatory defects that are often fatal. Few patients survive infancy. Those that survive have severe intellectual and physical disabilities.

22. A: Electrical alternans is the alternation of the QRS complex between beats, most commonly seen with pericardial tamponade or severe pericardial effusion. Given the patient's history of recent surgery and his diagnosis of pericardial tamponade, this patient most likely has Dressler's syndrome. This can occur days to months after a cardiac injury when the body mistakenly attacks healthy heart tissue.

23. C: Severe ischemia can result in electrocardiogram (EKG) changes within minutes of the occurrence. Other helpful diagnostic aids would include troponin level, creatine phosphokinase-MB (CPK-MB) level, and a two-dimensional echocardiogram (2D echo). These aids can be more diagnostic than an EKG, but an EKG result is obtained much quicker than blood work or a 2D echo. It takes a minimum of three hours for a cardiac insult to be reflected in blood tests.
Choice a would show an anterior myocardial infarction (MI).

Choice b would show a lateral-wall MI.
Choice d would show a posterior-wall MI.

24. B: There are two types of second-degree heart block. (1) Mobitz type I (Wenckebach block) is characterized by progressive prolongation of the PR interval on beats followed by a blocked P wave/dropped QRS complex. The PR interval resets, and the cycle repeats.
(2) Mobitz type II heart block is characterized by intermittently nonconducting P waves. The PR interval remains unchanged.
In first-degree heart block, there is a prolonged PR interval that regularly precedes a QRS complex.
In third-degree heart block (complete heart block), there is no apparent relationship between P waves and QRS complexes.
Asystole is a state of no cardiac electrical activity.

25. A: The other modalities would be used if the patient had symptomatic bradycardia. Symptoms of bradycardia may include pallor, weakness, dizziness, altered mental status, fatigue, and shortness of breath. If the patient had been symptomatic, atropine is the first-line agent used. In the event that atropine is ineffective, epinephrine and dopamine may be used. If the patient displays signs of poor perfusion, he or she may be a candidate for transcutaneous pacing.

26. D: Hypertension is not a factor in Beck's triad. Beck's triad is the combination of distended jugular veins due to increased venous pressure, hypotension due to low arterial pressure, and muffled heart sounds due to excessive fluid on the heart. It occurs as a result of pericardial effusion. Aside from physical examination findings, an electrocardiogram (EKG) and/or a two-dimensional echocardiogram may help diagnose this condition.

27. C: Warm air does not commonly cause an asthma exacerbation, although extreme heat or humidity may cause an asthma attack. Cold air usually triggers an asthma attack because it can irritate the airways.
Sinusitis or any upper respiratory infection that affects breathing can cause irritation and induce an asthma attack.
Cigarette smoke is a common trigger that can cause irritation and inflammation in the airways, which can aggravate asthma. Patients who live around tobacco smokers are predisposed to developing asthma.
Allergens such as dust and pollen can aggravate the airways, which can induce an asthma attack.

28. B: The beta cells, which are located in the islets of Langerhans in the pancreas, secrete insulin. Insulin stimulates the cells to store glucose, lowering the blood sugar levels.
The alpha cells produce glucagon, which stimulates cells to break down their glucose reserves to raise the serum glucose level.
The gamma cells of the pancreas secrete a specialized type of peptide, which reduces one's appetite.
The delta cells of the pancreas secrete somatostatin, which plays a role in food absorption by the small intestine.

29. D: Diabetics are at risk for hypertension, not hypotension. Diabetics have higher levels of blood sugar because the pancreas produces insufficient or no insulin. High levels of blood glucose stimulate systemic inflammation and atherosclerosis formation, causing a multitude of other pathologies.
Atherosclerotic plaques decrease the lumen of blood vessels, causing hypertension. Excessive deposits in the renal tubules can cause chronic renal insufficiency and potentially renal failure. The systemic inflammation caused by diabetes can also lead to neuropathy.

30. D: The most effective treatment of *Helicobacter pylori* is the combination of two antibiotics (amoxicillin, clarithromycin, metronidazole, and tetracycline) and a proton pump inhibitor. Two antibiotics are recommended due to potential antibiotic resistance. It is recommended that the patient be treated for 7 to 14 days to increase the chances of complete recovery.

31. A: Obesity is not a major risk factor.
More than half of the diagnosed cases of peptic ulcers are caused by *Helicobacter pylori*.
H. pylori may be diagnosed with a stool antigen test, a blood antibody test, and a carbon urea breath test, as well as other modalities.
Major risk factors include smoking, alcohol consumption, and nonsteroidal anti-inflammatory drug (NSAID) use.

32. D: <u>Parkinson's disease</u> destroys dopamine-producing neurons in the substantia nigra and causes motor symptoms (<u>dyskinesia</u>, <u>tremor</u>, rigidity) as well as cognitive symptoms. Approximately 80% of the substantia nigra is destroyed prior to the onset of symptoms. Norepinephrine and epinephrine are major components in the body's fight-or-flight response. Serotonin is involved with a multitude of functions including mood, cell growth, and hemostasis.

33. C: <u>Parkinson's disease</u> destroys dopamine-producing neurons in the substantia nigra and causes motor symptoms (<u>dyskinesia</u>, <u>tremor</u>, rigidity) as well as cognitive symptoms. Approximately 80% of the substantia nigra is destroyed prior to the onset of symptoms.
The medulla oblongata helps control the sympathetic and parasympathetic nervous systems, respirations, and basic reflexes.
The hippocampus plays a major role in storing old memories and the formation of new ones.
The pituitary gland controls major endocrine functions, pain relief, temperature regulation, and water balance. It is sometimes called the "master gland," because it is responsible for regulating so many important body functions.

34. C: Left bundle branch block acts as a red flag for four conditions: severe aortic valve disease, ischemic heart disease, chronic hypertension, and cardiomyopathy.
Pericardial tamponade generally has abnormalities with QRS complexes on electrocardiogram (EKG).
Pulmonary emboli are generally diagnosed by ventilation-perfusion (VQ) scan or computed tomography (CT) angiogram of the chest. In some patients with a pulmonary embolus, the EKG may be normal. The most common EKG findings are T-wave abnormalities.
Mitral valve prolapse is generally not diagnosed on an EKG. It is usually diagnosed by the patient's history, auscultation with a stethoscope, and two-dimensional echocardiogram.

35. B: This patient may have a pulmonary embolus, which is best diagnosed with a computed tomography (CT) angiogram of the chest. Sickle-cell disease increases the risk of pulmonary embolus, stroke, heart attack, pulmonary hypertension, skin ulcers, priapism, as well as other health problems.
A CT scan of the chest without contrast would most likely be nondiagnostic. Waiting for a troponin level or an arterial blood gas (ABG) would increase the risk of mortality in this patient.

36. A: The classic four features of tetralogy of Fallot include ventricular septal defect, narrowing of the pulmonary outflow tract, right ventricular hypertrophy, and an overriding aorta. Tetralogy of Fallot is the most common cyanotic heart defect. The reason why cyanosis occurs is due to the mixing of oxygen-rich and oxygen-poor blood through the ventricular septal defect.

37. A: The most common congenital heart defect is ventricular septal defect. The hole may be small and may spontaneously close on its own. If the hole is small but remains patent, the patient may be asymptomatic. If the hole is large enough to cause symptoms, it may warrant surgical intervention. The occurrence of aortic stenosis increases with age, but it is not the most common heart defect. Tricuspid atresia is one of the most uncommon cyanotic congenital heart defects. Tetralogy of Fallot is the most common type of cyanotic congenital heart defect.

38. D: A persistent, dry cough is the most common side effect of taking angiotensin-converting enzyme (ACE) inhibitors. The development of a cough is not serious and does not have any long-term health complications. In the event that the cough persists, the patient should be placed on a different medication regimen. Switching to another ACE inhibitor would not be helpful because if one ACE inhibitor causes a cough, all medications of this class would likely cause the same symptom.

39. C: *Staphylococcus aureus* is a gram-positive coccus that is responsible for common skin infections as well as other illnesses.
Staphylococcus pseudintermedius is a gram-positive coccus. It is very common in animals, especially dogs, but it is rare in humans.
Haemophilus influenzae is a gram-negative coccobacillus. It is a main cause of pneumonia, meningitis, as well as other pathologies. It does not commonly cause skin infections.
Streptococcus pneumoniae is one of the main causative organisms in pneumonia, meningitis, as well as other pathologies. It is much less common in skin infections.

40. D: Addison's disease is caused by a lack of cortisol. Giving cortisol exogenously helps alleviate the disease's symptoms.
Diabetes is caused by insufficient or complete lack of insulin production. Many diabetic patients depend on insulin injections in order to help control their disease.
Patients with insufficient growth hormone depend on somatropin injections to help alleviate their disease's symptoms.
Synthroid (levothyroxine) is a medication taken by patients with hypothyroidism.

41. C: Hypotension plays no role in the pathology of chronic obstructive pulmonary disease (COPD). Because the lungs are chronically damaged, the patient is more predisposed to pulmonary infections such as pneumonia.
Cor pulmonale is right-sided heart failure caused by pulmonary hypertension. Because COPD is an obstructive disease that occurs in the lungs, it increases the right ventricle's afterload, which causes the ventricle to swell and become dilated. Perfusion becomes more strenuous, and the blood pressure increases to keep pace.
The risk of myocardial infarction increases in the presence of COPD because COPD causes heart failure, which can lead to a heart attack and potentially cardiac arrest.

42. B: Symptoms of cystic fibrosis (CF) may include abdominal discomfort from chronic constipation, salty-tasting skin, poor appetite, fatigue, fever, and pancreatitis. There are a myriad of signs and symptoms in patients with CF. A physical examination and medical history of both the child and the parents are important in making the diagnosis. The sweat chloride test is the standard diagnostic test for cystic fibrosis, but there are other modalities to test for CF, including genetic testing, stool tests, computed tomography (CT) scan of the chest, or a chest x ray.

43. B: Sickle-cell disease is an autosomal-recessive genetic blood disorder caused by a defect on chromosome 11. Patients who have only one recessive allele have sickle-cell trait; they are usually asymptomatic and do not suffer the same medical complications as those with the disease. Sickle-cell disease increases the risk of stroke, heart attack, pulmonary hypertension, skin ulcers, priapism, as well as other health problems. Sickle-cell disease does not increase the risk for diabetes.

44. D: The patient has a urinary tract infection and needs an antibiotic to cover gram-negative organisms. The most common cause of urinary tract infections is *Escherichia coli*. Augmentin would not provide sufficient coverage. Choices a and b would be used to treat potential gonorrhea (GC)/chlamydia infections. Patients with urinary tract infections should be treated for a minimum of three days and up to seven days.

45. A: Macrobid is a category B medication, which are generally considered safe for use in pregnant women. The other choices are category C medications. Category C medications have shown potential adverse effects in prior research studies, but they may sometimes be used depending on the importance of the indication. Because the patient has a urinary tract infection (UTI), which is important, but not life-threatening, plus, she has no drug allergies, there are safer alternatives to use besides category C medications.

46. A: You should advise all patients with presumed or confirmed venereal disease to inform their partner(s) as soon as possible so they can also get tested. This helps to prevent others from spreading the disease and potentially infecting more people. As a medical provider, you cannot tell the patient's family or loved ones without permission without breaking *Health Insurance Portability and Accountability Act* (HIPAA) privacy laws.

47. B: Bipolar disorder is generally described as intermittent periods of mania and depression. Dysthymic disorder is a milder form of depression; there are no periods of mania. Posttraumatic stress disorder is described as feelings of stress, anger, anxiety, or depression after witnessing or experiencing a traumatic event.
An adjustment disorder is described as having feelings of stress, anger, anxiety, or general emotional lability after experiencing a major life change such as moving away from home or starting a new school.

48. D: Pyridium is often given in conjunction with an antibiotic to help alleviate dysuria. The most common side effect of Pyridium is bright-orange urine. Other common side effects may include headache and rash. Although the decision to discontinue the medication must be based on the severity of the side effects, a change in urine color should not be the reason to discontinue the medication. The urine will go back to its normal color once the medication course has been completed.

49. C: Increasing one's fluid intake is the most important way to help prevent kidney stones. Kidney stones are usually made up of calcium oxalate, which can be found in dairy, fruits such as apples and grapes, vegetables such as broccoli and turnips, beer, as well as several other foods. Those who suffer from kidney stones may find it advisable to limit foods high in calcium oxalate.

50. B: Escitalopram is a serotonin reuptake inhibitor (SSRI) commonly used to treat anxiety and depression.
Levothyroxine is a synthetic thyroid hormone medication used for those with hypothyroid disease.

Amiodarone is used to treat cardiac arrhythmias such as atrial fibrillation and ventricular fibrillation.

Haloperidol is an antipsychotic medication that can also be used to treat drug or alcohol withdrawal symptoms. Because this woman is not intoxicated and has no history of substance abuse or psychotic episodes, this medication would not be appropriate.

51. A: Von Willebrand disease is a hereditary bleeding disorder caused by factor VIII clotting deficiency. It is a much milder form of hemophilia.

Thalassemia is a genetic disorder that causes an inadequate level of hemoglobin to be produced in the body, causing chronic anemia.

Myeloma is a cancer of the plasma cells. It may present with anemia, but also with bone pain, infection, fatigue, and loss of bowel or bladder function. It is not affected or controlled by factor VIII.

52. C: Cauda equina syndrome can be caused by disease, trauma, or infection. It affects the nerve roots from L1 to L5 and S1 to S5, which can cause motor dysfunction, urinary retention, and saddle anesthesias, among other neurological issues. It can be diagnosed with a computed tomography (CT) scan or magnetic resonance imaging (MRI) scan. A spine surgeon will decide whether or not the patient needs surgical decompression based on the presentation and radiological findings.

Kyphosis is a degeneration of the thoracic spine, causing a "hunchback" appearance.

Fibromyalgia is a disease causing chronic pain, which is potentially due to oversensitive nerves.

A Greenstick fracture is most commonly seen in children due to the flexibility of their bones. It occurs when the bony cortex bends abnormally, causing a partial break.

53. C: Slipped capital femoral epiphysis is when the femoral head is displaced from the acetabulum, causing hip and knee pain as well as gait disturbances. Once diagnosed, it is usually surgically corrected to prevent avascular necrosis of the femoral head. It is usually seen in prepubescent and pubescent children who are going through a growth spurt.

Osteitis pubis is a noninfectious inflammation of the pubic symphysis, causing lower abdominal or groin pain. This condition is normally seen in athletes.

Developmental dysplasia of the hip is when a child is born with one or both femoral heads spontaneously displaced from the acetabulum. This is diagnosed when the child is a toddler or when a young child is learning to walk.

Paget's disease is the abnormal formation and degeneration of bone usually in a localized area in the body. It is extremely uncommon in children.

54. D: Bisphosphonates such as Fosamax, nonsteroidal anti-inflammatory drugs (NSAIDs), and calcitonin are the mainstays of treatment for Paget's disease. Paget's disease is the abnormal formation and degeneration of bone, usually in a localized area of the body. Alkaline phosphatase is found in bone; after bony destruction or injury, it is released into the blood, increasing serum levels. It is one way to diagnose this disease. The diagnosis can also be made on CT scan, magnetic resonance imaging (MRI), or bone scan. Colchicine would provide little value because it is used to treat acute gout exacerbations.

55. B: Retinal artery occlusion is commonly caused by a clot that blocks the blood flow to the eye; it is very common in patients with coagulopathy disorders, hypertension, diabetes, or advanced atherosclerosis. The most common presentation is unilateral vision loss.

Conjunctivitis is the bacterial, viral, or allergy-induced inflammation of the conjunctiva, which may cause a foreign-body sensation, redness, visual disturbances, itching, tearing, and discharge. It does not cause sudden, painless blindness.

Acute angle closure glaucoma occurs when the intraocular pressure is so high that it damages the optic nerve, which could impair vision and cause severe eye pain. Patients usually note visual disturbances prior to actually losing their vision, such as seeing halos around objects. They may also present with headache on the same side as the vision loss, orbital or periorbital pain, nausea, and vomiting.

Retinal detachment is commonly caused by trauma, but it can also be caused by advanced age or disease processes such as diabetes. Immediately prior to losing vision, patients usually have partial vision loss or visual disturbances such as the appearance of flashes and floaters.

56. B: Using a tongue depressor to directly visualize the oropharynx is contraindicated in epiglottitis because this may induce airway spasm.
Direct visualization can be performed by an ear, nose, and throat (ENT) doctor after the patient is intubated and in the OR, so that the patient's airway is protected.
A lateral cervical spine x-ray may help confirm the suspected diagnosis; a thickened epiglottis often appears on x-ray as a "thumbprint sign."
Administration of penicillins, cephalosporins, or clindamycin is recommended.

57. B: Bacteria are the most common cause of otitis externa, or swimmer's ear. There are many bacterial pathogens, but *Pseudomonas aeruginosa* is the most common cause. *Staphylococcus aureus* and *Haemophilus influenzae* cause otitis externa as well, but they are not as common. *Aspergillus* is one of the most common fungal pathogens of otitis externa, along with *Candida albicans*. Fungal pathogens are more common in diabetic patients or those who are immunocompromised.

58. B: Antibiotic ear drops and pain medications are the mainstays of medical management of otitis externa.
Oral antibiotics are generally not prescribed.
Imaging of the brain or the ears is generally not indicated unless abscess or osteomyelitis is suspected; these complications are very rare.
An ear, nose, and throat (ENT) consult is not necessary for otitis externa. It is a very common condition, which usually resolves with antibiotics.

59. A: Labyrinthitis is the most likely diagnosis. It usually follows a viral infection such as the flu or the common cold, although it can occur after trauma or because of substance abuse. It differs from Ménière's disease because hearing and balance do not deteriorate after each episode. In cases of labyrinthitis, inner ear functions return to baseline after every episode. In Ménière's disease, there is a chronic deterioration of inner ear function.
Due to the patient's normal physical examination and vital signs, infectious processes such as otitis media and mastoiditis should be ruled out.

60. D: The patient has benign prostatic hypertrophy, which becomes more common in men as they age. Tamsulosin is an alpha-blocker, which improves urinary retention caused by benign prostate enlargement.
Terbinafine is used for tinea unguium.
Tramadol is an opiate medication used to alleviate pain.
Tegretol is used for the medical management of seizures.

61. A: The thiazolidinediones such as pioglitazone and sulfonylurea medications such as glimepiride and glyburide are pregnancy category C medications. Category C medications have shown potential adverse effects in prior research studies, but they may sometimes used depending on the importance of the indication. Medications such as Novolin are pregnancy category B medications,

which should be used before trying a pregnancy category C medication, if possible. Because this patient has not yet had any medications for her diabetes, Novolin is the most preferable.

62. B: Although the patient is at risk for developing diabetes, his fasting blood sugar and hemoglobin A1C are normal. Medications at this point are unnecessary. Rechecking the hemoglobin A1C in one week would be useless because it is a calculation of an average blood sugar level over a three-month period. This patient's hemoglobin A1C doesn't need to be checked for at least another three months.

63. B: This woman should be checked when she is 38 years old. The current recommendation in the United States is to get screened 10 years prior to the age of a first-degree relative who was diagnosed with colon cancer. If no risk factors are present, then it is recommended to obtain a colonoscopy by 50 years of age. Because her father was 48 years old when he was diagnosed, she should get screened at age 38. If she had no significant family history, then her first colonoscopy should be when she is 50 years old.

64. C: Erythromycin helps shorten the course of the illness. It may also help prevent the child from spreading it to others if administered early enough. If erythromycin is given too late in the course of the disease, it is ineffective. Augmentin, clindamycin, and *guaifenesin* play no role in the treatment or prevention of pertussis. The most important way to prevent pertussis is to get vaccinated.

65. C: The patient has respiratory syncytial virus (RSV). It is an acute, self-limiting, usually non-life-threatening virus that most commonly presents with a barking, or "seal-like," cough. It is more prevalent in children who attend day care, small children who live with school-aged children, and children who live in a home in which someone smokes.
The patient's fever and other presenting symptoms make asthma a less likely diagnosis. Pneumonia usually presents with a high fever (above 101.5° F), productive cough, myalgias, shortness of breath, as well as a myriad of other symptoms. A barking cough is usually not present. Patients with cystic fibrosis display signs and symptoms very early in life such as abdominal discomfort from chronic constipation, poor weight gain, steatorrhea, salty-tasting skin, poor appetite, fatigue, fever, and pancreatitis. It would not develop suddenly in a three-year-old child with no prior symptoms.

66. D: A primary, or spontaneous, pneumothorax occurs in the absence of underlying pulmonary pathology. The patient has no past medical history such as lung cancer or cystic fibrosis. A secondary, or complicated, pneumothorax occurs due to underlying pulmonary disease such as lung cancer, cystic fibrosis, chronic obstructive pulmonary disease (COPD), or other diseases. Trauma, such as a stab wound or a gunshot wound, can cause a pneumothorax, but there was no trauma noted in the physical examination or the medical history. Pneumonia may cause chest pain and shortness of breath, but there would not be an absence of lung markings on the chest x-ray. Lung cancer would show up as a radio-opaque mass or masses on chest x-ray.

67. B: This patient most likely has tuberculosis. Other symptoms of tuberculosis may include nausea, vomiting, anorexia, and fatigue.
Bronchitis and pneumothoraces do not present with cavitary lesions on chest x-ray.
Lung cancer may present with cavitary lesions on x-ray, but the acute onset of symptoms and type of symptoms that he has points more toward an infectious etiology.

68. A: <u>Oxymetazoline hydrochloride</u> is a nasal decongestant that may cause rhinitis medicamentosa or rebound nasal congestion. Patients should be advised to discard the medication after three to five days to prevent this from happening.

Benzonatate is an antitussive that does not cause rhinitis medicamentosa.

Ofloxacin are antibiotic eardrops used to treat infections of the ear canal.

Guaifenesin is an expectorant used to treat cough and chest congestion.

69. D: This patient should be given a baby aspirin for prophylaxis against potential future heart attacks and simvastatin for his hyperlipidemia. It is recommended that one's LDL level should be 100 to 130 if no risk factors are present and less than 100 if risk factors are present. His blood pressure, heart, rate, two-dimensional echocardiogram, and stress test are normal: prescribing antihypertensive medications such as metoprolol and amlodipine is unnecessary.

70. C: Pyloric stenosis commonly presents in neonates, but presentation of symptoms may start when the child is several months old. The chief symptoms are abdominal pain, dehydration, swollen abdomen, and, most notably, projectile vomiting. The narrowed pylorus may feel like a small mass in the epigastrium.

A Mallory–Weiss tear in the esophageal junction is usually seen in alcoholic patients. It is caused by persistent episodes of vomiting; however, any pathological process that causes forceful coughing or vomiting may cause a Mallory–Weiss tear.

Gastroesophageal reflux disease (GERD) and gastritis may cause abdominal discomfort and occasionally vomiting, but they would not cause projectile vomiting, failure to thrive, or be associated with an abdominal mass.

71. C: A Mallory–Weiss tear in the esophageal junction is usually seen in alcoholic patients caused by persistent episodes of vomiting; however, any pathological process that causes forceful coughing or vomiting may cause a Mallory–Weiss tear.

Pyloric stenosis commonly presents in neonates, but presentation of symptoms may start when the child is several months old. It does not suddenly present in the sixth decade of life.

Celiac sprue is an immune reaction that damages the lining of the small intestine and prevents it from absorbing important nutrients. It presents with nausea, vomiting, diarrhea, and abdominal pain, which occur after ingesting gluten products.

Whipple's disease is a bacterial infection of the bowel. It is a rare infection that presents with fever, abdominal pain, nonbloody vomiting, diarrhea, and arthralgias.

72. C: Esotropia is a condition in which one eye is normal and the other deviates medially.

Exotropia is a condition in which one eye is normal and the other eye deviates laterally.

Hypertropia is a condition in which one eye is normal and the other eye deviates upward.

Hypotropia is a condition in which one eye is normal and the other eye deviates downward. All of these conditions fall under the general term "strabismus," which means an abnormal alignment of the eyes.

73. B: Bacterial conjunctivitis is an infection of the conjunctiva, causing one or both eyes to have a pinkish or reddish appearance. It is usually associated with fever, purulent discharge, and yellow-gold crusting of the eyelids and lashes. It is common among children and is highly contagious.

Viral conjunctivitis usually presents with clear discharge. Fever and crusting around the lids and lashes are much less common.

Allergic conjunctivitis presents with itchy watery eyes, sneezing, sniffling, clear rhinorrhea, and other allergy symptoms.

Dacryoadenitis is an infection of the eye due to a clogged tear duct, which can present with red eyes, pain, swelling of the medial aspect of the upper eyelid, and lymphadenopathy.

74. A: Erythromycin ointment is the drug of choice in a child with bacterial conjunctivitis. Ciprofloxacin ointment can also be used to treat bacterial conjunctivitis, but the use of fluoroquinolones is contraindicated in children.
Trifluridine is used to treat keratitis caused by herpes simplex.
Famciclovir is used to treat keratitis caused by herpes zoster.

75. D: Niacin's most common side effect is flushing, which may be associated with pruritus. If these symptoms develop, the dosage may need to be adjusted, but the drug does not have to be discontinued. Simvastatin, atorvastatin, and rosuvastatin may cause pruritus, but they generally cause jaundice, not flushing. Other side effects of statin medications may include fever, abdominal pain, and arthralgias.

76. A: The patient is not in any respiratory distress, and he is not hypoxic. He most likely has a bacterial pneumonia, which requires po antibiotics.
The chest x-ray shows the infiltrate: a computed tomography (CT) scan of the chest exposes the patient to more radiation that he does not need.
If he had significant past medical problems or appeared toxic, then hospitalization and intravenous (IV) antibiotics may be needed. The diagnosis of pneumonia can be made based on physical examination, medical history, and possibly a chest x ray.
The patient does not need an arterial blood gas (ABG) because he is saturating 98% on room air.

77. A: Niacin may cause flushing or pruritus, but it should not be discontinued unless symptoms are severe. Niacin should originally be prescribed at the lowest dose possible to help prevent these symptoms; if the patient tolerates the dosage, it can always be titrated up. If flushing and pruritus do occur, patients can take medications such as Decadron and/or Benadryl. Nonsteroidal anti-inflammatory drugs (NSAIDs) taken prior to the niacin dose can help to minimize flushing.

78. A: The child has croup, which is most commonly caused by the parainfluenza virus. Antibiotics would be of little value. Steroids and/or epinephrine would be prescribed if the patient was in respiratory distress or had a prolonged course of illness. The mainstays of therapy in uncomplicated cases of croup are humidified air, rest, and maintaining adequate hydration.

79. B: Trimethoprim-sulfamethoxazole is the first-line treatment in patients with *Pneumocystis* pneumonia (PCP). Augmentin and gentamicin play no role in the treatment of this disease. Corticosteroids may be used in conjunction with an antibiotic to treat PCP, but they are not to be used as the sole treatment. Patients with a CD4 count of less than 200 are at risk for contracting PCP. PCP is one of the leading causes of death in acquired immunodeficiency syndrome (AIDS) patients.

80. D: Dietary restrictions are an important part of controlling the neurological complications that phenylketonuria (PKU) may cause. Patients with PKU are unable to break down phenylalanine, a common amino acid found in foods. Patients with PKU must strictly adhere to diets low in phenylalanine. If the diagnosis is not made early or if patients are not compliant with their dietary restrictions, complications such as hyperactivity, seizures, and intellectual disability may occur. Ritalin and antiseizure medications such as Dilantin will be used after sequelae develop.
Routine blood work is of little value: once the diagnosis is made via blood test, there is no need to do routine blood work.

81. C: Hand washing is the most important measure in preventing communicable diseases. Wearing a face mask may help, but it does not fully prevent against spreading diseases. If someone's hands are contaminated and he or she touches the mouth or eyes, wearing a face mask will not prevent the person from getting ill.
Wearing gloves is important, but the gloves may rip. If the gloves touch a contaminated surface and then touch someone's mouth or face, the gloves will not prevent against getting ill. Maintaining a sterile environment at all times is not plausible.

82. D: Pregnant women may eat fish and seafood as long as they are cooked thoroughly. Listeriosis is spread through contaminated food. Therefore, avoiding unpasteurized milk is recommended. It is also recommended to thoroughly wash produce, cook meat and fish prior to eating it and to limit processed foods such as hot dogs and deli meats during pregnancy. Hot dogs and deli meats may be contaminated after they are cooked and prior to being packaged. Pregnant women infected with *Listeria monocytogenes* may exhibit only mild symptoms, but this may result in the death of the fetus.

83. B: Immediately cleansing the wound is the number-one way to help prevent rabies. The rabies vaccine will prevent rabies, but it usually takes longer to obtain than it does to wash the wound. If the animal is caught, it would have to be tested for rabies prior to subjecting the bite victim to a series of vaccinations.
Administration of antibiotics may be necessary if a secondary infection develops, but this would not be useful in preventing rabies from occurring.

84. A: Lotrimin cream helps treat fungal infections. Mites burrowing underneath the skin cause scabies infections. Topical creams such as permethrin can be used to treat infections. Pills are available for persistent infections refractory to topical treatment. Washing clothing and linens in hot water and avoiding infected people are ways to help prevent the spread of infection.

85. D: The patient most likely has a kidney stone. An abdominal computed tomography (CT) scan or a kidney, ureter, and bladder (KUB) x-ray should be ordered to confirm the diagnosis. Costovertebral angle (CVA) tenderness is usually a sign of a kidney infection.
Hepatitis and cholecystitis are unlikely because they usually present with right-upper quadrant or right epigastric pain. Liver function tests are usually not normal in cases of acute infection. CVA tenderness is not present.
Appendicitis, like nephrolithiasis, presents with nausea, vomiting, fever, and chills, but the abdominal pain is usually present in the right-lower quadrant or right epigastrium. CVA tenderness is not present.

86. B: Hypervolemia is the least likely to cause cardiac arrest. There are 12 main causes of cardiac arrest (six H's and six T's): hypovolemia, hypoxia, hydrogen ions (acidosis), hyperkalemia, hypokalemia, hypothermia, toxins, tamponade, tension pneumothorax, thrombosis, thromboembolism, and trauma. Hypervolemia may increase the heart's preload, which may eventually lead to heart failure, but it is much less likely to cause a myocardial infarction.

87. B: The patient is displaying signs of acute appendicitis. Causing discomfort by shaking the bed or chair in which the patient is positioned is called the jar sign. Causing discomfort by flexing the right leg at the hip and the knee is called the psoas sign. The patient has discomfort during these maneuvers due to peritoneal irritation. These maneuvers help diagnose acute appendicitis and are not present in the other conditions listed.

88. D: The patient has acute meningitis. The triad of meningitis is photophobia, nuchal rigidity, and headache, although fever, nausea, vomiting, anorexia, and flulike symptoms are also common. The patient has a positive Brudziński's sign. The Brudziński sign is positive when flexion of the neck causes flexion of the hip and knee due to inflammation of the meninges.

A subarachnoid hemorrhage or migraine headache may present with headache, nausea, and vomiting, but the Brudziński sign would not be positive in the presence of a subarachnoid hemorrhage or a migraine headache.

Vestibulocerebellar syndrome is a progressive neurological disease in which patients show symptoms in early childhood.

89. A: The patient most likely has a pericardial tamponade. Pericardial tamponade is the abnormal collection of fluid that develops on the heart due to injury or prior disease, although the cause may be idiopathic. The patient's symptoms are consistent with Beck's triad. Beck's triad is the combination of hypotension, muffled heart sounds, and distended jugular veins.

A pneumothorax is much less likely. The patient is saturating 99% on room air, and his lungs sounds are equal bilaterally.

An aortic dissection usually presents with sharp, tearing chest pain that radiates to the back. Auscultation of the heart usually reveals a blowing murmur, not quiet heart sounds.

Stable angina is described as chest pain that is alleviated with rest.

90. A: In first-degree heart block, there is a prolonged PR interval that regularly precedes a QRS complex.

There are two types of second-degree heart block. Mobitz type I, or Wenckebach block, is characterized by progressive prolongation of the PR interval on beats followed by a blocked P wave/dropped QRS complex. The PR interval resets, and the cycle repeats.

Mobitz type II heart block is characterized by intermittently nonconducting P waves. The PR interval remains unchanged.

In third-degree (complete) heart block, there is no apparent relationship between P waves and QRS complexes.

91. C: Bulimia nervosa is a psychiatric disorder that usually occurs in female adolescents and young women that consists of forcefully purging after every meal in order to control one's weight. Signs and symptoms of this disorder are varied, but dental problems are most common due to the frequent exposure to stomach acid due to vomiting. Women who have this disorder are usually mildly overweight, or their weight is normal.

Dysthymic disorder is a milder form of depression.

Anorexia nervosa is when someone purposely severely limits his or her food intake in order to control his or her weight.

Panic disorder occurs when someone experiences extreme nervousness or fear that may or may not be connected to a specific trigger.

92. A: Haloperidol is an antipsychotic medication. This patient most likely has schizophrenia. Schizophrenia is a mental disorder that makes it hard for a person to differentiate between what is real and not real. It also affects one's concentration, mood balance, sleep, and ability to maintain appropriate behavior.

Choices b and c are selective serotonin reuptake inhibitors (SSRIs), which are used to treat anxiety, depression, panic disorder, and posttraumatic stress disorder. They may provide some relief of symptoms, but they should be used in conjunction with other antipsychotic medications.

Choice d is a sedative. This may provide some relief of symptoms, but it should not be the only medication used in a schizophrenic patient.

93. C: The child most likely has glucose-6-phosphate dehydrogenase (G6PD) deficiency. It is an <u>X-linked recessive</u> <u>hereditary disease</u> in which the defect of this enzyme causes red blood cells to break down prematurely. It is much more prevalent in males than females. It is the most common enzyme defect in humans. Many types of foods (such as legumes and artificial food coloring), medications (nonsteroidal anti-inflammatory drugs [NSAIDs], aspirin, and sulfa drugs), as well as environmental triggers (mothballs, pollen, and henna), can cause acute exacerbations. The only treatment for this disease is to avoid known triggers as much as possible.
Leukocytosis is the elevation of a person's white blood cell (WBC) count in the presence of infection, disease, or stress. The patient's WBC count is normal.
Thrombocytopenia is the presence of an abnormally low platelet count due to infection, medications (i.e., chemotherapy drugs), disease, or blood loss.
Von Willebrand disease is a hereditary bleeding disorder caused by factor VIII clotting deficiency. It is a much milder form of hemophilia. It doesn't cause jaundice or hemolytic anemia.

94. C: The mainstays of treatment for thalassemia major are folate supplements and regular blood transfusions. In cases of severe disease, chelation therapy (removal of excess iron from the blood) and bone marrow transplants are necessary. Thalassemia major is a rare genetic blood disorder in which the hemoglobin is defective and causes mild to severe hemolytic anemia. Patients with thalassemia should avoid iron because they are already at risk for iron overload in their blood due to regular blood transfusions.
Avoiding legumes, nonsteroidal anti-inflammatory drugs (NSAIDs), and henna would be suggestions for those with G6PD deficiency, not those who have thalassemia major.

95. D: This woman most likely has placenta previa, which commonly presents with painless, bright-red vaginal bleeding in the end of the second trimester or the beginning of the third trimester. It is due to a low-lying placenta. As the uterus enlarges, it may push up against the placenta, causing a small part to tear, and bright-red bleeding occurs.
Placental abruption (abruptio placentae) is the complete separation of the placenta, causing bright-red vaginal bleeding, abdominal and/or back pain, and severe contractions.
Premature rupture of the membranes is when a woman's water breaks prior to the onset of labor. Dystocia is defined as difficult childbirth.

96. B: This woman may have an ectopic pregnancy versus a threatened abortion. Because she is only six weeks pregnant, the intrauterine pregnancy (IUP) may be too small to see. If the repeat beta human chorionic gonadotropin (HCG) increases normally and an IUP is seen after two days, then the diagnosis is most likely threatened abortion. If the beta HCG levels become higher than normal and an IUP still cannot be seen, then methotrexate or a surgical consult may be needed to treat the ectopic pregnancy.

97. A: Impetigo is a bacterial infection that is most commonly caused by *Staphylococcus aureus* or *Streptococcus pyogenes*. It causes lesions that can occur anywhere on the body. They are small, red, and pus-filled and can crack open and form a yellow or honey-colored, thick crust. They most commonly occur in young children. These lesions are contagious, and family members and friends should avoid touching them until they are completely healed. Family members should wash bed linens in hot water and avoid sharing personal-care products such as razors and towels with the patient to prevent the spread of the disease. Hand washing is strongly recommended as well.

98. B: Tinea corporis, also known as "ringworm," is a fungal infection that can occur anywhere on the body. It is usually described as a red, circular lesion with a central clearing with grayish or flesh-toned scales. Ketoconazole is an antifungal medication that is used to treat superficial fungal or yeast infections.
Erythromycin, mupirocin, and metronidazole are all antibiotics used to treat bacterial infections. They are generally ineffective at treating fungal infections.

99. C: Paraphimosis is when the foreskin cannot be brought back to its original position. If it cannot be resolved at the bedside with conservative methods, then surgical intervention may be necessary. Cryptorchidism is a condition in which one or both testicles have not descended into the scrotum. Phimosis is when the foreskin cannot be retracted.
A hydrocele is the collection of fluid around the testicle due to infection or malignancy. Sometimes, the cause can be idiopathic.

100. D: Cryptorchidism usually resolves on its own without treatment. Because the child is so young, no intervention would be necessary at this time. If after one year of age the testicle still has not descended, then hormone injections may be necessary. If that fails, then an orchiopexy is needed. An undescended testicle carries an increased risk of developing testicular cancer and infertility.

101. A: A hydrocele is the collection of fluid around the testicle due to infection or malignancy. Sometimes, the cause can be idiopathic. It is not harmful and has no serious long-term complications.
Testicular torsion is a medical emergency. It occurs when the spermatic cord becomes twisted and blood flow to the testicle is severely diminished or absent. It presents with acute onset of pain and swelling of the affected testicle.
A varicocele is an enlargement of the veins in the scrotum, causing testicular aching and/or swelling to occur. The venous enlargement is usually due to faulty valves in the veins or compression of a neighboring vein disrupting blood flow in nearby veins.
Cryptorchidism is a condition in which one or both testicles have not descended into the scrotum.

102. D: A D-dimer test is a highly sensitive but nonspecific blood test for detecting the presence of clots. If the person is already diagnosed with a pulmonary embolus (PE), then the D-dimer will be positive. It will take weeks to months to get the clot to dissolve. Because the patient has sickle-cell disease and is at high risk for developing future clots, placing her on a heparin infusion, sending her home on warfarin, and placing an inferior vena cava (IVC) filter are viable treatment options. Because the patient has a PE that is causing chest pain, administering analgesics would be appropriate management.

103. C: He should be getting the influenza vaccine every year. Though he is not in a high-risk group (i.e., very young, very old, health-care worker, or immunocompromised), the vaccine still provides modest protection against contracting the influenza virus. Conservative measures such as frequent hand washing are also recommended. His tobacco abuse increases the risk of contracting pulmonary diseases such as influenza and also raises the complication rates in the event that he does contract the disease. Therefore, severely limiting tobacco use or quitting altogether is recommended.

104. B: Furosemide is used to treat congestive heart failure and edema, but it is not a treatment used in atrial fibrillation.
Metoprolol is a beta-blocker that helps slow the heart rate down.

Warfarin is a blood thinner that helps prevent the heart from sending clots to the lungs or brain. Lanoxin reduces strain on the heart and is used to treat hypertension, cardiomyopathy, and atrial fibrillation.

105. D: Coccidioidomycosis, also known as "valley fever," is a self-limiting respiratory infection caused by a fungus endemic to southwestern soil in the United States. It may present with cough with or without hemoptysis and flulike symptoms. It may also present with erythema nodosum, which is painful erythematous lumps.
Pneumocystis pneumonia usually occurs in immunocompromised patients such as those with HIV. Symptoms are similar to the influenza virus. Patients most commonly have a nonproductive cough. The symptoms do not spontaneously resolve; po and sometimes IV antibiotics are needed to treat this opportunistic infection.
Symptoms of tuberculosis may include fever, night sweats, hemoptysis, nausea, vomiting, anorexia, and fatigue. This disease does not go away on its own.
Respiratory syncytial virus (RSV) is an acute, self-limiting, usually non-life-threatening virus that most commonly presents with a barking or "seal-like" cough. It is more prevalent in children who attend daycare, small children who live with school-aged children, and children who live in a home in which someone smokes.

106. A: A two-dimensional echocardiogram can make a definitive diagnosis of ventricular septal defect (VSD). VSD is the most common congenital heart defect. Smaller defects may close spontaneously, and no further treatment is needed. Larger defects can cause heart failure and pulmonary hypertension, as well as other complications.
A chest x-ray may show cardiomegaly, but it is not a definitive test of VSD.
An electrocardiogram (EKG) may show left ventricular hypertrophy, but it is not used as a definitive test for VSD.
Auscultation with a stethoscope may reveal a heart murmur, but it is not a dependable diagnostic aid for VSD.

107. B: Coarctation of the aorta is an acyanotic congenital heart defect commonly associated with Turner syndrome. Generally, it is more common in boys than girls. It involves a narrowing of the aorta, which may cause no symptoms depending on the severity of the narrowing. Symptoms can include syncope, chest pain, shortness of breath, dizziness, cold lower extremities, failure to thrive, and chronic fatigue. A chest x ray may reveal the "figure 3 sign": prestenotic dilatation of the aortic arch and left subclavian artery, indentation at the coarctation, and poststenotic dilatation of the descending aorta.

108. C: Torsades de pointes literally means "twisting of the points." It is a polymorphic ventricular tachycardia that can be caused by congenital disease, electrolyte abnormalities caused by malnourishment or alcoholism, or adverse drug interactions. Administering antiarrhythmic medications and reversing the electrolyte abnormalities, if applicable, are the mainstays of therapy.

109. A: Prinzmetal's angina is a condition that typically occurs in young women. It is much more common in people who smoke cigarettes. It is due to vasospasm of coronary arteries; it spontaneously resolves without treatment. Typically, it will occur at rest, and no electrocardiogram (EKG) changes may be seen unless the test is performed during an acute episode.
Unstable angina is a condition in which chest pain occurs at rest and during activity due to severe atherosclerosis.
Stable angina is chest pain that is alleviated with rest due to mild to moderate atherosclerotic disease.

Costochondritis occurs when the chest wall is strained due to strenuous physical activity, trauma, or idiopathic cause. Palpation reproduces symptoms.

110. D: Small-cell carcinoma is responsible for causing a number of paraneoplastic syndromes such as syndrome of inappropriate antidiuretic hormone (SIADH), Cushing's syndrome, and limbic encephalitis. Paraneoplastic syndromes are a localized or systemic response to the presence of tumor cells in the body. The other three choices are subtypes of non-small-cell carcinoma, which is not commonly a cause of paraneoplastic syndromes.

111. C: A chest x-ray may be ordered in a case of infective endocarditis, but it is one of the least helpful tests compared to the other choices. A chest x ray may show cardiomegaly or a pyogenic abscess, but it can also be normal is some cases.
Blood cultures would be positive, which shows that the patient has bacteremia. An infection needs to be present in order to make the diagnosis of infective endocarditis.
A computed tomography (CT) scan of the chest would show a fluid collection, abscess, or inflammation around the endocardium.
An echocardiogram would show one or more vegetations on the heart; this is the preferred diagnostic aid.

112. C: Limiting one's tobacco use (or preferably quitting smoking altogether), limiting sodium intake, and increasing physical activity are all recommendations a health-care professional should make to a patient with prehypertension. Prehypertension is defined as systolic blood pressure of 120 to 139 and diastolic blood pressure 81 to 89 on three consecutive visits four to six weeks apart. Medication regimens can be avoided if patients take conservative measures to lower their blood pressure.

113. C: No intervention is needed. The patient has mitral valve prolapse, a condition in which the mitral valve does not close completely. In the majority of patients, mitral valve prolapse does not adversely affect their health and no intervention is needed. Some patients may experience chest pain, dizziness, palpitations, and dyspnea, and in these cases, further workup and possible intervention may be warranted.

114. B: The main treatment in the presence of a non-ST segment elevation myocardial infarction (NSTEMI) is oxygen, aspirin, nitroglycerin, and a beta-blocker if hypertension is present. Beta-blockers such as metoprolol decrease the workload of the heart. Antiplatelet medications, such as aspirin, are used to help prevent clot formation. Clopidogrel is used if aspirin is not tolerated, but in most situations, aspirin is the first-line antiplatelet regimen. Nitroglycerin helps increase the serum nitric oxide in the blood, which helps prevent against further cardiac damage. A troponin level, an echocardiogram, and morphine may be administered once the patient has been stabilized.

115. A: This patient has stable angina. Stable angina is present when a patient experiences chest pain that is alleviated with rest. This condition occurs with mild to moderate atherosclerotic disease. A patient may develop chest pain during periods of physical activity caused by cardiac ischemia. During rest, the body's demands on the heart lessen and the blood flow becomes adequate enough to perfuse the heart.
Prinzmetal's angina is a condition that typically occurs in young women in the presence or absence of atherosclerosis. It is much more common in people who smoke. It is due to vasospasm of coronary arteries; it spontaneously resolves without treatment. Typically, it will occur at rest. Unstable/variant angina is a condition in which chest pain occurs at rest and during activity due to severe atherosclerosis.

An aortic aneurysm is an outpouching of part of the vessel wall, or it may be a circumferential outpouching of the vessel wall caused by disease or trauma. Patients may be asymptomatic, but as the aneurysm becomes significantly large or ruptures, the patient will display severe abdominal or back pain. Symptoms do not resolve with rest.

116. B: Macular degeneration is an age-related eye disease that affects central vision, while peripheral vision is preserved. Approximately one-third of patients older than age 75 suffer from this condition. The macula is responsible for central vision; it is located on the center of the retina. Once macular degeneration occurs, there are some medications and dietary modifications that can slow the progression. It generally does not lead to blindness.
Open-angle glaucoma presents with worsening unilateral or bilateral painless blindness.
Acute-angle closure glaucoma occurs when the intraocular pressure is so high that it damages the optic nerve, which could impair vision and cause severe eye pain.
A clot blocking blood flow to the eye causes retinal artery occlusion; it is very common in patients with coagulopathy disorders, hypertension, diabetes, or advanced atherosclerosis.
The most common presentation is sudden unilateral vision loss.
Optic neuritis is the inflammation of the optic nerve due to infectious or immunologic disorders. It presents with sudden onset eye pain and loss of vision.

117. D: The patient may have an acoustic neuroma; a magnetic resonance imaging (MRI) scan of the brain is an essential diagnostic tool. Acoustic neuromas are tumors of the acoustic nerve that may cause facial droop or unilateral facial paresthesias/pain, ataxia, tinnitus, hearing loss, dizziness, and receptive aphasia.
An electromyography (EMG) test might be considered if muscle weakness or facial droop is present to test the activity of muscles and the nerves. This patient's physical examination is normal, so an EMG is of little use.
An ear, nose, and throat (ENT) consult would be appropriate once a workup has been done and tests have been resulted.
The Dix–Hallpike maneuver helps to confirm the diagnosis of benign positional vertigo. Movement does not exacerbate the patient's symptoms, so this condition should not be a differential diagnosis.

118. D: The child has aspirated her toy, and a stat bronchoscopy should be performed to confirm the diagnosis and remove the object.
If the child is stable, a chest x ray should be ordered to help confirm the diagnosis; however, in the presence of stridor and mild hypoxia, a bronchoscopy should be the first choice.
A blind finger sweep should be avoided because it may push the object further into the airway.
Although oxygen administration is recommended, nebulizer treatments would provide little added value; the child's respiratory distress is due to choking, not due to bronchospasm caused by disease.

119. B: The patient has a right-sided pleural effusion, most likely due to her chronic obstructive pulmonary disease (COPD). It is a pathologic fluid collection in the pleura. It may develop postoperatively, but more commonly it is caused by infection or disease. Pleural effusions may present with dyspnea, pleuritic chest pain, fever, and cough. In instances of a large pleural effusion, breath sounds will be diminished due to the fluid collection in the lung. Tactile fremitus is decreased due to the fluid in the pleural space, which decreases the lung's ability to expand. There is dullness to percussion due to the increased fluid and decreased air space.
In cases of a pneumothorax, the symptoms may present the same as those with pleural effusion. On physical examination, tactile fremitus is decreased due to the decreased lung space/size. Percussion is hyperresonant due to the extra air in the pleural space. Breath sounds are diminished.

Acute asthma exacerbation and influenza may present with similar symptoms, but there would be no decreased tactile fremitus or dullness to percussion.

120. B: The McMurray test is a maneuver that can help diagnose a meniscal tear. If you suspect a medial meniscal tear, place one hand on the patient's foot and another on the medial aspect of the affected knee. Flex the knee while internally rotating the leg. If you feel a pop or a click, and the patient experiences pain, the test is positive for meniscal injury. To diagnose a lateral tear, place one hand on the lateral aspect of the affected knee and externally rotate the leg.
The Murphy test helps to diagnose acute cholecystitis.
McBurney point tenderness helps diagnose acute appendicitis.
The obturator test helps diagnose acute appendicitis.

121. A: An avulsion fracture is when one piece of bone is separated from the whole.
A Greenstick fracture is most commonly seen in children due to the flexibility of their bones. It occurs when the bony cortex bends abnormally, causing a partial break.
A comminuted fracture is when the bone is shattered into several pieces.
An oblique fracture is a diagonal break in the bone.

122. A: This patient most likely has pneumoconiosis, also known as "miner's lung" due to a miner's prolonged coal-dust exposure. It presents as an upper respiratory infection that does not resolve. The honeycomb appearance on chest x-ray is a common finding. There is no medical treatment other than to remove the causative agent.
Schistosomiasis is a chronic parasitic infection caused by eating improperly cooked pork. On a magnetic resonance imaging (MRI) scan of the brain, it appears as multiple enhancing nodules occurring in bilateral cerebral hemispheres.
Tuberculosis is a bacterial infection of the lungs, causing symptoms such as night sweats, lymphadenopathy, fever, chills, hemoptysis, nausea, vomiting, anorexia, and fatigue.
Coccidioidomycosis, also known as "valley fever," is a self-limiting respiratory infection caused by a fungus endemic to soil of the southwestern United States. It may present with cough with or without hemoptysis and flulike symptoms. It may also present with erythema nodosum, which is characterized by painful erythematous lumps.

123. B: Testicular carcinomas present as hard, painless, fixed, solid testicular lesions. Your next step should be to order imaging studies and blood work to confirm the diagnosis.
A hydrocele is a soft, painless, fixed testicular mass. It is due to a collection of fluid around the testicle due to infection or malignancy. Sometimes, the cause is unknown. Hydroceles are not harmful and have no serious long-term complications.
A varicocele is an enlargement of the veins in the scrotum, causing testicular aching and/or swelling to occur. The venous enlargement is usually due to faulty valves in the veins or compression of a neighboring vein disrupting blood flow in nearby veins.
Testicular torsion is a medical emergency. It occurs when the spermatic cord becomes twisted, and blood flow to the testicle is severely diminished or absent. It presents with acute onset of pain and swelling of the affected testicle.

124. D: The drop-arm test can help confirm the diagnosis of a rotator cuff tear, although the only way to truly confirm the diagnosis would be a magnetic resonance imaging (MRI) scan. The examiner will have the patient abduct both arms 90° and rotate his arms so that the thumbs are pointing downward. If the patient is unable to keep his affected arm abducted when the examiner applies pressure, the examiner should suspect a rotator cuff tear. The other three maneuvers are helpful in diagnosing meniscus tears.

125. C: Mastoiditis is an infection of the mastoid bone of the skull. It is generally a complication of inner ear infections. Symptoms may include fever, ear pain, ear discharge, fever, swelling behind the ear (where the mastoid bone is located), hearing loss, headache, and erythema. Imaging studies such as magnetic resonance imaging (MRI) and computed tomography (CT) scans can make the definitive diagnosis.

Ménière's disease is a usually chronic disorder of the inner ear, causing a mild to severe sensation of fullness in the affected ear, vertigo, dizziness, and hearing loss. The exact cause is unknown, but it is most likely multifactorial. Ménière's disease is much more common in adults than in children. It does not cause fever or swelling behind the ear.

Acoustic neuromas are tumors of the acoustic nerve. They are much more common in adults than in children. Symptoms include hearing loss, dizziness, headache, tinnitus, facial droop, and ataxia. They do not cause fever or swelling behind the ear.

A cholesteatoma is a fluid-filled cyst, which may or may not be infected, caused by poorly functioning Eustachian tubes. Symptoms may include ear drainage, pain, and tinnitus. If infection is present, fever may occur as well. It does not cause swelling behind the ear.

126. C: *Cryptococcus* is the pathogen causing this patient's meningitis. It is one of the defining opportunistic infections of patients with acquired immunodeficiency syndrome (AIDS); their CD4 count is usually less than 200. It is the most common fungal pathogen in immunocompromised patients, such as those with cancer or AIDS. Diagnosis is made via India ink stain. Treatment includes po and/or IV antifungal medications. The prognosis for AIDS patients with *Cryptococcus* meningitis is very poor. The other choices provided are not diagnosed with an India ink stain.

127. A: Singulair is a leukotriene inhibitor. It is used to help prevent asthma exacerbations and seasonal allergies. It is a preventative medicine, but it should not be used as treatment during acute episodes. Singulair, Xopenex, and Ventolin are short-acting beta-2 bronchodilators. These medications are some of the first-line agents in treating an acute asthma exacerbation.

128. C: Wilms' tumor is the most common renal tumor in pediatric patients. The exact cause is unknown, but incidence does increase with family history, suggesting there is a genetic component. Symptoms may include abdominal pain, abdominal mass, nausea, vomiting, constipation, and changes in urine color. Signs such as hemihypertrophy and aniridia (complete or partial absence of the iris) may be associated with this disease.

Kaposi's sarcoma generally appears as multiple cutaneous lesions, but it may affect the internal organs as well.

Hodgkin's lymphoma is a malignancy of the white blood cells.

A lipoma is a benign tumor created by the overgrowth of fatty tissue.

129. B: Hyaline membrane disease, also known as infant respiratory distress syndrome, is a common cause of respiratory distress in premature infants. It is due to insufficient surfactant. Treatments include supplemental oxygen and the administration of synthetic surfactant.

Pneumocystis pneumonia usually occurs in immunocompromised patients. Symptoms are similar to the influenza virus. Patients most commonly have a nonproductive cough.

Pneumoconiosis, also known as "miner's lung," is a lung disease caused by prolonged dust exposure.

Respiratory syncytial virus (RSV) is an acute, self-limiting, usually non-life-threatening virus that most commonly presents with a barking, or "seal-like" cough. It is prevalent in children who attend daycare, small children who live with school-aged children, and children who live in a home in which someone smokes.

130. C: This patient most likely has a hyphema, considering his symptoms and history of recent trauma. A hyphema is a localized hemorrhage in the eye due to rupture of the blood vessel(s).
A hordeolum appears as a red, swollen, tender pimple on the edge of the eyelid. It is caused by a blocked oil gland.
Optic neuritis is the inflammation of the optic nerve due to infectious or immunologic disorders. It presents with sudden-onset eye pain and loss of vision.
Blepharitis is the inflammation and swelling of the eyelid due to allergies, infection, or underlying conditions such as rosacea.

131. A: Leukoplakia is a condition in which white patches may develop on the tongue or inside the mouth. It is similar in appearance to oral thrush, except that in cases of thrush, the white lesions may be scraped off. The causes of leukoplakia are unknown, but it is commonly seen in alcoholics and those who smoke or chew tobacco.
Thrush is a yeast infection seen in patients who are poorly controlled diabetics, those who have been on long-term steroids or antibiotics, and immunocompromised patients.
Parotitis is an infection of the parotid gland, which can produce facial swelling and pain.
Gingivostomatitis is a yeast infection of the mouth and gums, appearing as painful sores.

132. D: Out of the choices given, tetralogy of Fallot is the only cyanotic congenital cardiac defect. It is the most common congenital cyanotic heart defect, usually associated with chromosomal abnormalities. Tetralogy of Fallot is most commonly caused by infections during pregnancy or by excessive alcohol intake during pregnancy. The radiological sign "boot-shaped heart" or "cœur en sabot" is most commonly associated with tetralogy of Fallot. The heart looks like a boot due to right-ventricular hypertrophy and pulmonary stenosis.

133. B: Bronchoscopy with biopsy would provide definitive confirmation of the diagnosis. Patients with sarcoidosis have multiple granulomas in their lungs as well as other organs. Sarcoidosis is a systemic inflammatory disease that can attack any organ, but it most commonly attacks the lymph nodes and lungs.
A lumbar puncture would provide no diagnostic value.
A computed tomography (CT) scan and serum phosphorus may aid in the diagnosis, but they are not definitive tests.

134. C: This patient most likely has fibrocystic breast disease. It is a benign condition in which singular or multiple breast cysts develop. They can occur right before one's menses begins or may be unrelated to menses. People placed on hormone replacement therapy or birth control pills generally have less severe symptoms.
Breast cancer is unlikely, considering the patient's presentation and physical examination. Malignant breast masses don't shrink in size spontaneously, are generally nontender, and usually do not occur bilaterally.
Fibroadenomas are generally singular, rubbery, nontender breast lesions that are benign in nature.
Gynecomastia is the appearance of breasts in males due to enlarged mammary glands. This may be due to obesity, congenital etiology, endocrine abnormality, or underlying disease. This condition usually resolves on its own in a patient with no significant past medical history.

135. A: A fibroadenoma is a benign breast mass that usually does not cause pain. It can be monitored; no intervention is necessary unless it becomes large and the patient requests removal. Birth control pills are not useful in treating fibroadenomas.

Repeating a biopsy would not be helpful. Fibroadenomas are benign lesions that do not become malignant.
There is no reason for a mastectomy because fibroadenomas are benign lesions.

136. A: Clindamycin is not a medication that would be used in the treatment of tuberculosis. There are a multitude of medications used to treat tuberculosis; they are used in a variety of combination therapies. The more common medications are isoniazid, rifampin, pyrazinamide, and ethambutol. Less common drug remedies include amikacin, ethionamide, moxifloxacin, para-aminosalicylic acid, and streptomycin. Affected patients are usually on multiple medications for six months or longer.

137. D: Ascending or descending quickly will exacerbate the effects caused by barotrauma. Barotrauma is when the pressure in the middle ear is higher than that of the outer ear. Symptoms can include ear pain, hearing loss, and dizziness. The goal of treatment or prevention is to keep the Eustachian tubes open so the pressure between the outer ear and the inner ear remains normalized. Actions such as chewing gum, yawning, or sucking on candy can help keep the pressures normalized.

138. B: Bronchiolitis is a common viral upper respiratory infection in children. It usually starts with mild symptoms similar to those of the common cold and then progresses to wheezing, fever, breathing difficulties causing intercostal retractions, and in extreme cases, cyanosis due to respiratory insufficiency.
Symptoms of tuberculosis may include fever, night sweats, hemoptysis, nausea, vomiting, anorexia, and fatigue.
Cystic fibrosis is a chromosomal disorder that causes the lungs to become chronically plugged with mucus. Symptoms may include abdominal discomfort from chronic constipation, salty-tasting skin, poor appetite, fatigue, fever, delayed growth, poor weight gain, clay-colored stools, and frequent episodes of pneumonia. The diagnosis is usually made before or shortly after the child is born.
Hyaline membrane disease, also known as infant respiratory distress syndrome, is a common cause of respiratory distress in premature infants. It is due to insufficient surfactant. Treatments include supplemental oxygen and the administration of synthetic surfactant.

139. B: Levothyroxine is a synthetic thyroid hormone used to treat Hashimoto's thyroiditis, which causes hypothyroidism.
Lanoxin is an antiarrhythmic agent used to treat conditions such as atrial fibrillation.
Lamisil is medication used to treat fungal infections.
Lantus is a type of exogenous insulin used to treat patients with diabetes.

140. D: Huntington's disease is a progressive neurological disorder caused by an autosomal-dominant chromosomal abnormality. It most commonly occurs in people between 30 and 40 years of age.
Tourette syndrome is first noticed in childhood and is characterized by involuntary verbal sounds or motor movements. It does not cause cognitive impairment, although it may be seen in the presence of cognitive disorders.
Guillain–Barré syndrome is an autoimmune disease that causes muscle weakness or paralysis; it does not cause cognitive impairment.
Cerebral palsy is a neurological disorder that causes motor and cognitive impairment. It is diagnosed in infancy or childhood. It may be caused by infection or trauma, but the most common cause is prenatal hypoxia.

141. C: This patient is suffering from hyperparathyroidism. Elevated serum calcium can cause a multitude of nonspecific symptoms such as weakness and fatigue, depression, bone pain, myalgias, constipation, polyuria, polydipsia, cognitive impairment, kidney stones, and osteoporosis. Hypothyroidism causes a slowing in metabolism and potentially impaired cognitive function, producing symptoms as unintentional weight gain, low blood pressure, bradycardia, weakness, myxedema, and slow speech.

Hyperthyroidism causes an increase in metabolism, producing symptoms such as unintentional weight loss, high blood pressure, tremor, palpitations, and weakness.

Hypoparathyroidism will also cause many nonspecific symptoms; the most common is perioral and extremity paresthesias.

142. A: Permethrin cream is an insecticide used to treat skin infections caused by scabies and lice. Olanzapine is an antipsychotic medication used to treat psychiatric disorders.

Phenergan is an antihistamine used to treat allergic reactions and alleviates pruritis.

Ondansetron is an antinausea medication used to help prevent and/or treat nausea and vomiting due to illness or induced by certain medications such as chemotherapy agents.

143. C: Calcium-rich foods help prevent gout flare-ups. Coffee and foods rich in vitamin C also help reduce a patient's risk. Patients should be counseled to refrain or severely limit their intake of red meat, seafood, alcohol, and fructose. Medications used to prevent gout include allopurinol, nonsteroidal anti-inflammatory drugs (NSAIDs), and steroids. Colchicine is most commonly used to treat acute gout attacks.

144. C: This patient has infective endocarditis caused by her drug use. Endocarditis causes a number of symptoms, but the most classic are fever, chills, and diaphoresis. Common causes are indwelling triple-lumen catheters or peripherally inserted central catheter (PICC) lines, dental procedures, and intravenous (IV) drug abuse with contaminated needles. Janeway lesions indicate a diagnosis of endocarditis. These lesions are painful, erythematous areas on the palms and soles, which are only caused by endocarditis.

145. D: Restrictive cardiomyopathy is the inability of the heart to relax between beats. Epinephrine is a vasoconstrictor, which would increase the workload of a heart that is already impaired.

Furosemide and metoprolol decrease the heart rate as well as decrease the preload and afterload on the heart.

The blood is being squeezed through restricted vasculature, which increases the risk of developing clots. Aspirin helps prevent the formation of clots and is commonly used in the treatment of restrictive cardiomyopathy.

146. B: Toxic megacolon is a complication of *Clostridium difficile* colitis. It is the pathologic distension of the colon caused by *C. difficile*, Crohn's disease, and ulcerative colitis. Signs and symptoms may include tachycardia, abdominal pain, abdominal distension, leukocytosis, and fever. The treatment is to decompress the colon either by rectal tube or by surgical intervention. Ogilvie's syndrome is a condition in which a patient presents with signs and symptoms of intestinal obstruction without actually having an obstruction. The bowel loses its ability to contract and to pass food and waste products along the gastrointestinal (GI) tract; this commonly occurs after surgery or in severely chronically ill patients.

Intussusception is when one part of the bowel folds in on itself and causes an obstruction. This is common in children. Symptoms include nausea, vomiting, lethargy, and "red currant jelly" stools.

Hirschsprung's disease is a congenital condition in which the bowel cannot contract and move food and waste products along the GI tract due to lack of nerve innervation of portions of the bowel.

147. C: This patient has alcohol-induced pancreatitis. Alcohol is the leading cause of acute pancreatitis; stones are the second most common cause. Therapies include cessation of alcohol, rest, intravenous (IV) fluids, pain medications, keeping the patient on nothing-by-mouth (NPO) status, and antibiotics in the presence of a secondary infection.
Hepatitis and cholangitis would present with right-sided abdominal pain, along with fever, chills, nausea, vomiting, and possibly jaundice.
Mallory–Weiss tears may be also caused by alcoholism, but they occur in the esophagus and do not cause abdominal pain.

148. C: This patient most likely has Parkinson's disease. The classic four signs of Parkinson's disease are resting tremor, rigidity, slow movements, and shuffling gait. It is due to the deterioration of the substantia nigra.
Guillain–Barré syndrome is an autoimmune disease causing muscle weakness or paralysis. It does not cause resting tremor or rigidity.
Huntington's disease is a progressive neurological disorder caused by an autosomal-dominant chromosomal abnormality. Signs include progressive decline in cognitive function; ataxic gait; and uncoordinated, jerky body movements.
Alzheimer's disease is the development of progressive cognitive decline; the underlying cause is not known. Motor skills are much less affected until late stages of the disease.

149. A: This patient has an excess of cortisol due to her exogenous steroid use, causing Cushing's syndrome. Cushing's syndrome symptoms include buffalo hump (posterior cervical fat pad), swelling of the face, myalgias, unintentional weight gain, irregular menses, striae, hirsutism, hyperglycemia, and bone loss.

150. B: This patient is most likely suffering from Stevens–Johnson syndrome caused by a reaction she's having to penicillin. It is a reaction of the skin and mucous membranes to medication or to a medical condition. It begins with nonspecific upper respiratory infection symptoms and then progresses to dermal manifestations. It can be life threatening if not treated immediately and adequately.
Cushing's syndrome is caused by too much cortisol, causing symptoms such as buffalo hump (posterior cervical fat pad), swelling of the face, myalgias, unintentional weight gain, irregular menses, striae, hirsutism, hyperglycemia, and bone loss.
Guillain–Barré syndrome is an autoimmune disease causing muscle weakness or paralysis.
Turner syndrome is a genetic condition in which females are missing all or part of an X chromosome. Some of the symptoms may include infertility, amenorrhea, short stature, and webbed neck.

151. A: The child most likely had idiopathic thrombocytopenic purpura (ITP) caused by his viral syndrome. It is characterized by petechiae or a pinpoint rash seen on the extremities. In children, ITP usually resolves on its own without treatment.
Stevens–Johnson syndrome begins with nonspecific upper respiratory infection symptoms and then progresses to dermal manifestations. The rash is a diffuse, dark red macular and papular rash with extensive blistering usually requiring hospitalization. It can be life threatening if not treated immediately and adequately.

Von Willebrand disease is a milder form of hemophilia. It is caused by factor VIII deficiency. Symptoms include prolonged bleeding after dental or surgical procedures, minor injuries, and menorrhagia.

Glucose-6-phosphate dehydrogenase (G6PD) deficiency is an <u>X-linked recessive</u> <u>hereditary disease</u> in which the defect of this enzyme causes red blood cells to break down prematurely. It causes pallor, dark urine, jaundice, and failure to thrive. It is generally diagnosed in infancy. Symptoms do not spontaneously resolve.

152. D: The child has diphtheria. It is a very rare respiratory infection in developed countries due to the diphtheria, tetanus, and pertussis (DTaP) vaccine, but children can still get diphtheria if they are not vaccinated. Signs and symptoms include a grayish-black, tough, fiberlike covering of the oropharynx, fever, chills, sore throat, cyanosis, and in severe cases drooling and stridor.
Cryptococcus infections are generally seen in patients who are immunocompromised. Cryptococcus is a fungus that people with normal immune systems can handle. There is no vaccine to prevent against cryptococcus infections.
Shigella causes bacterial gastroenteritis.
Cholera is a rare bacterial gastroenteritis that may cause severe dehydration and death.

153. D: The child has mononucleosis caused by the Epstein–Barr virus. Conservative treatment such as rest, fluids, and refraining from physical activity to prevent splenic rupture are recommended. Amantadine is an antiviral medication used within one to two days after the onset of flu symptoms to help shorten the duration of the illness.
Augmentin would be used if the child had a bacterial upper respiratory infection.
A computed tomography (CT) scan of the abdomen is not recommended if splenic rupture is not suspected.

154. B: This patient has multiple myeloma, which is a type of cancer of the plasma cells. The most common signs and symptoms are bone pain and pathologic fractures. Multiple myeloma can also cause damage to the kidneys, causing anemia. The presence of the Bence Jones protein in the urine distinguishes this as the most likely diagnosis from Paget's disease, which can also cause bone pain and pathologic fractures.
Acute myelogenous leukemia (AML) is a cancer of the blood and bone marrow, usually presenting with bleeding, bruising, fatigue, and weight loss.
Acute lymphocytic leukemia (ALL) is a cancer of the white blood cells, usually presenting with weight loss, fatigue, petechiae, and fever.

155. A: The international normalized ratio (INR) is generally used to measure bleeding time. This lab test is important in monitoring a patient who is taking Coumadin or for the workup of a bleeding disorder. It is generally not used in the workup of hemolytic anemia.
The Coombs' test looks for antibodies that may attach themselves to red blood cells and cause premature apoptosis.
A complete blood count (CBC) may be able to indicate what type of anemia is present, whether the patient is pancytopenic, or if an underlying infection is present.
Lactate dehydrogenase (LDH) is present in blood cells; increased levels of LDH indicate hemolytic anemia.

156. A: Influenza is not responsible for causing the abnormalities seen in this infant. <u>Microcephaly</u>, deafness, <u>chorioretinitis</u>, hepatosplenomegaly, and thrombocytopenia are common signs and symptoms of TORCH infections. TORCH infections can be caused by **t**oxoplasmosis, **o**ther (syphilis,

varicella, human immunodeficiency virus [HIV]), **r**ubella, **c**ytomegalovirus, and **h**erpes simplex virus – type 2 (HSV-2). Prognosis of the infant depends on which type of infection she has. Some TORCH infections can be prevented with vaccines, and others can be treated with antibiotics, but because most infections are viral, there is no cure.

157. C: Pasta, baked goods, and processed foods lack iron and therefore should be avoided or severely limited in patients who have iron-deficiency anemia. Meat, eggs, and beans are obviously rich in protein and iron, but green, leafy vegetables such as kale and spinach are also good sources of iron. Foods that have high vitamin C content such as oranges increase the body's ability to absorb iron.

158. D: This patient has lichen planus, which is commonly described as well-defined, pruritic, planar, purple, polygonal papules and plaques. It may occur on mucous membranes or on the skin. It is a benign condition. The exact cause is unknown. It is linked to some chronic diseases, such as hepatitis C.
Leukoplakia is a condition in which white patches may develop on the tongue or inside the mouth.
Impetigo is a bacterial infection that is most commonly caused by *Staphylococcus aureus* or *Streptococcus pyogenes*. It causes lesions that can occur anywhere on the body. The lesions are small, red, pus-filled and can crack open and form a yellow or honey-colored, thick crust. They occur most commonly in young children.
Psoriasis causes cells to build up rapidly on the surface of the skin, forming itchy, dry, red, raised patches covered with grayish silvery lesions that are easily friable. Psoriasis is sometimes painful. Plaques frequently occur on the skin of the elbows and knees, but they can affect any area. This is a chronic condition.

159. A: Dyshidrosis is a type of eczema most commonly linked to stress and allergies. It is characterized by pruritic blisters on the palms and soles. No antibiotics are warranted. Conservative measures such as the use of steroids, emollients, and Benadryl are used for symptomatic relief. It is recommended that patients not scratch their lesions because scratching may exacerbate symptoms and cause secondary infection. This is a chronic condition.

160. B: Lantus would be the first-line treatment in a patient with newly diagnosed diabetes mellitus – type 1. Type 1 diabetes is an autoimmune disease in which the body attacks the islets of Langerhans of the pancreas. The islets of Langerhans have beta cells, which produce insulin. Patients who are type 1 diabetics are insulin dependent their whole lives. Although other agents may be added later on to help control hyperglycemia, insulin is the first-choice drug.

161. C: The patient is suffering from acute alcohol withdrawal. He states that he has not had an alcoholic beverage in two days. Symptoms may start as soon as a few hours after the last drink or may take two to three days to appear. Signs and symptoms may include tachycardia, nausea, vomiting, diarrhea, diaphoresis, confusion, headaches, seizures, fine motor tremor, and dilated pupils.
The patient is confused, but he is not delusional.
Dysthymic disorder is a milder form of major depressive disorder.

162. D: The patient has Osgood–Schlatter disease, which is an inflammation of the anterior tibial tubercle due to overuse while the bone is still growing. It is most commonly seen in prepubescent boys. Pain medications may be used, and rest is recommended, but no intervention is warranted. Symptoms will resolve eventually.

An anterior cruciate ligament (ACL) disruption is not likely because there is no history of trauma and there is no joint laxity or instability on physical examination.

Polymyositis is the appearance of bilateral muscle weakness and wasting due to immune disorders or disease.

Ganglion cysts may develop due to trauma, overuse, or idiopathic causes. They most commonly appear on the hands and feet.

163. A: Prednisone is a common medication used to treat polyarteritis nodosa. Polyarteritis nodosa is a vasculitis that affects small and medium-sized arteries, causing a large range of nonspecific symptoms. There is no known cause, but the incidence is higher in men than women, and people with hepatitis B have a higher incidence of developing this disorder. Treatment includes steroids and immunosuppressive drugs such as methotrexate.

Antibiotics such as clindamycin are not warranted.

Permethrin cream is an insecticide used to treat skin infections caused by scabies and lice.

Amantadine is a medication used to treat attention deficit-hyperactivity disorder (ADHD) and has been used to treat Parkinson's disease and influenza.

164. B: Condyloma acuminata, or genital warts, is a sexually transmitted disease. Factors such as birth control use, smoking, early age of first coitus, and multiple sexual partners increase the risk of contracting genital warts. There is no cure; however, there are gels and creams that help with the symptoms and the appearance of the warts. Cryosurgery and laser surgery may be useful for acute exacerbations, but warts may still come back after the procedure. The human papilloma virus (HPV) vaccine is available to help prevent genital warts.

165. D: Acromegaly will result in the presence of excessive growth hormone in an adult patient. Because adult patients have already stopped growing, growth hormone will cause bones to thicken and widen, causing pain, weakness, and deformity. If excessive growth hormone occurs in children, gigantism will occur because bones are still in the process of growing longitudinally.

Dwarfism occurs when there is a deficiency in growth hormone.

Cushing's syndrome occurs in the presence of excessive cortisol.

166. C: This patient most likely has multiple sclerosis (MS). One of the most common presenting symptoms is persistent fatigue. One of the most common signs is optic neuritis. Two-thirds of MS patients will experience optic neuritis during the course of their disease. Patients may also present with progressive ataxia, muscle spasms, dizziness, ataxia, uncoordination of fine motor movements, urinary frequency, incontinence, nystagmus, and depression.

Huntington's disease is a progressive neurological disorder caused by an autosomal-dominant chromosomal abnormality. Signs include progressive decline in cognitive function; ataxic gait; and uncoordinated, jerky body movements.

Alzheimer's disease is a progressive cognitive decline. The underlying cause is not known. Motor skills are much less affected until late stages of the disease.

Meningitis is an infection that classically presents with nuchal rigidity, photophobia, and headache.

167. B: This patient most likely has parotitis. The parotid gland is one of the salivary glands; when they get infected, a patient may display dry mouth, drooling, facial swelling, and pain inside of the cheek. Sjögren's syndrome is an immune disorder in which mucous membranes and moisture-secreting glands produce insufficient tears and saliva. Patients with Sjögren's disease have an increased risk of parotitis.

A peritonsillar abscess is an infection of the tonsils; patients generally do not present with cheek pain. A patient may present with drooling, facial swelling, difficulty swallowing, sore throat, and dysphonia.

Leukoplakia is a condition in which white patches may develop on the tongue or inside the mouth. It is similar in appearance to oral thrush, except that in cases of thrush, the white lesions may be scraped off.

Epiglottitis commonly affects children, but it can occur in adults. It is an infection of the epiglottis. Patients will present with upper respiratory infection (URI) symptoms, drooling, dysphonia, stridor, and fever. Sometimes, a patient will hold his or her head forward with the neck extended to keep the airways open.

168. A: The patient has aphthous ulcers, which are non-life-threatening and do not require antibiotics or antiviral medication.

Nonsteroidal anti-inflammatory drugs (NSAIDs), nonalcoholic mouth wash, and steroids are most commonly used to prevent future sores and alleviate the symptoms of present sores. The cause of aphthous ulcers is unknown, but dietary deficiencies in iron and folic acid, trauma, and emotional stress are thought to be potential triggers.

169. B: If testicular torsion is suspected, a stat surgical consult is warranted because the only correction of torsion is surgery. Surgery should be performed within six hours of the trauma in order to save the testicle. If blood flow is compromised for too long, the testicle may need to be removed.

Pain medications should be given, but a surgical consult should be called first.

The patient may need preoperative antibiotics for prophylaxis, depending on the surgeon's preferences, but it should not be the next step in management because testicular torsion is not due to infection.

Warm compresses would help if the patient had an abscess or testicular swelling without torsion, but they would provide very little benefit in this scenario.

170. D: This patient most likely has diabetes insipidus caused by her traumatic head injury. Diabetes insipidus is caused by insufficient antidiuretic hormone (ADH), which causes the body to conserve little, if any, water. This condition may be caused by trauma, surgery, or infection. In this case, it is most likely caused by the patient's traumatic brain injury.

Diabetes mellitus occurs when the body's insulin production is insufficient to meet a patient's glucose intake. Patients with diabetes mellitus will have high glucose levels in their blood and urine; those with diabetes insipidus do not.

Hypothyroidism causes a slowing in metabolism and potentially impaired cognitive function, producing symptoms such as unintentional weight gain, low blood pressure, bradycardia, weakness, myxedema, and slow speech.

Hyperthyroidism causes an increase in metabolism, producing symptoms such as unintentional weight loss, high blood pressure, tremor, palpitations, and weakness.

171. C: This patient most likely has melanoma. The definitive way to make the diagnosis is via biopsy. The way to help diagnose melanoma on physical examination is to think of the mnemonic ABCDE: **a**symmetry, **b**orders, **c**olor, **d**iameter, and **e**volving over time. Melanoma frequently occurs as asymmetric lesions with irregular borders, with multiple colors within one lesion, with a diameter greater than 6 mm, and whose appearance changes or evolves over time.

Squamous-cell carcinoma is usually described as a light-colored, scaly crust on an erythematous base. It is usually found on sun-exposed areas.

Impetigo is a bacterial infection that is most commonly caused by *Staphylococcus aureus* or *Streptococcus pyogenes*. It causes lesions that can occur anywhere on the body. They are small, red, pus-filled and can crack open and form a yellow or honey-colored, thick crust. They occur most commonly in young children.

Basal-cell carcinoma is the most common type of skin cancer. It is usually described as a pearly pink or flesh-colored lesion that is easily friable and does not heal.

172. D: This patient most likely has bladder carcinoma. The definitive way to diagnose this man is through imaging of his abdomen and pelvis.

Wilms' tumor is a common renal tumor in pediatric patients. The exact cause is unknown, but the incidence does increase with family history, suggesting there is a genetic component. Symptoms may include abdominal pain, abdominal mass, nausea, vomiting, constipation, and changes in urine color. Hemihypertrophy and aniridia may be associated with this disease.

Prostatitis is an infection of the prostate gland, causing similar symptoms to that of a urinary tract infection (UTI). Although this patient does have some symptoms of a UTI, his unintentional weight loss and history of tobacco abuse point to carcinoma rather than infection.

Orchitis is an infection of the testicles, which can cause UTI symptoms, testicular pain and swelling, hematospermia, and painful intercourse.

173. A: A corneal abrasion is a scratch on the cornea of the eye, which causes a foreign-body sensation, pain, and conjunctival erythema. Patients should be prescribed an antibiotic such as erythromycin or gentamicin to prevent infection. Patients who wear contact lenses should also be advised to wear eyeglasses while they are on antibiotics so that their abrasion may heal without further complication. The other three medication choices listed are used to treat glaucoma.

174. C: Desmopressin is another name for antidiuretic hormone (ADH), which is used in treating those who have diabetes insipidus. Diabetes insipidus is caused by insufficient ADH, which causes the body to conserve little, if any, water.

Detrol is used in women who experience urinary urgency and frequency due to an overactive bladder.

Depakote is used to treat neurologic conditions such as seizures and migraines.

Decadron is a steroid used to treat certain types of skin disorders and autoimmune diseases.

175. A: The child is potentially being abused at home either by her mother or another person. When an examiner notices burns in a "glove and stocking" distribution, it usually means that the child's extremity is forcefully being placed into something hot and not that something was accidentally spilled. If an accidental spill occurs, you would see a much more irregular pattern, and it is usually only on one side of the extremity. Calling social services such as the Division of Youth and Family Services (DYFS) would be appropriate considering the appearance of the burns and the fact that this is the fourth occurrence.

176. C: Zofran is used to treat and prevent nausea and vomiting. It does not play a role in the medical management of schizophrenia.

Seroquel is a selective serotonin reuptake inhibitor (SRRI) used to treat anxiety, depression, and schizophrenia.

Haldol is a dopamine antagonist used to treat schizophrenia as well as other psychotic disorders.

Zyprexa is an antipsychotic medication used primarily to treat bipolar disorder and schizophrenia.

177. B: Actinic keratosis can appear as a flesh-toned, pink, gray, or reddish macule or papule with a scaly surface caused by overexposure to the sun. These lesions have a propensity for becoming

squamous cell carcinomas, so it is recommended to patients to avoid prolonged sun exposure and to use sunscreen. They may be removed surgically if they cause cosmetic issues.

178. B: Paronychia is an abscess adjacent to the nail bed. This can occur on the fingers or the toes. The cause may be idiopathic, but there is usually a history of trauma or a break in the skin prior to the onset of symptoms. Treatment includes warm compresses, antibiotics, and sometimes incision and drainage of the wound.
Onychomycosis is a fungal infection of the nail, which causes the nail to thicken, become yellow or gray, and occasionally fall off.
Condyloma acuminata is the appearance of genital or anal warts due to a viral sexually transmitted disease.
Scabies is a skin infection usually occurring in the webs of the fingers and toes due to mites burrowing underneath the skin.

179. D: Vitiligo is the hypopigmentation of the skin that usually occurs symmetrically. It may occur in a localized area or in widespread areas on the body. It is more common in darker skinned people. This is a benign condition.
A lipoma is a benign tumor created by the overgrowth of fatty tissue.
Xanthelasma are raised, yellow patches on the eyelids. The incidence of occurrence increases with age. They are common in patients with hyperlipidemia.
Mongolian spots are flat, blue, or blue-gray skin markings near the buttocks that commonly appear at birth or shortly thereafter.

180. C: Morphine is a narcotic medication that can cause constipation. This medication would not be recommended in a patient with a history of fecal impaction because it may precipitate bowel motility issues.
Senna and Colace are stool softeners that may help make it easier to pass a bowel movement in a patient with a history of constipation.
Milk of Magnesia helps prevent water from being reabsorbed in the intestines. Because it increases the amount of water that remains in the bowels, it helps promote bowel movements.

181. D: Adenosine is a medication that is given to a patient experiencing supraventricular tachycardia. It is an antiarrhythmic agent used to slow down the heart rate. The first dose should be given as a 6 mg bolus. If unsuccessful, a 12 mg dose should follow in one to two minutes. The 12 mg may be repeated once if needed.
Atropine is a medication used to speed up the heart rate; it is given to patients experiencing symptomatic bradycardia.
Allopurinol is a medication given to patients to help prevent gout exacerbations.
Atorvastatin is a medication used to lower serum cholesterol levels.

182. A: Atropine, dopamine, and epinephrine are medications that can be given for a patient experiencing symptomatic bradycardia. The other choices given are antiarrhythmic agents, which are used to slow down a patient's heart rate.
Amiodarone may be given to patients having pulseless ventricular tachycardia/ventricular fibrillation or atrial fibrillation.
Vasopressin, like amiodarone, slows down the heart rate and is given in the presence of ventricular tachycardia or ventricular fibrillation.
Adenosine is given to a patient experiencing supraventricular tachycardia.

183. C: This patient is immune to hepatitis B due to prior vaccination. Hepatitis B surface antigen (HBsAg) is present in active or chronic infections. In this case, it is not present.

Total hepatitis B core antibody (anti-HBc) indicates previous or acute hepatitis B infection. In this case, it is not present.

Hepatitis B surface antibody (anti-HBs) is present is patients who are recovering from an infection or who have been immunized. Because the other two lab values are negative, this could only mean that the patient has been successfully vaccinated.

184. D: You should recommend that the patient see a vascular surgeon for a biopsy to confirm the diagnosis. You may start the patient on a course of low-dose steroids. Because patients with giant-cell arteritis are at risk for development of aneurysms and stroke, starting the patient on baby aspirin is recommended. Giant-cell arteritis is the inflammation of the blood vessels that supply blood flow to the head. Common symptoms include unilateral headache, burning or tingling on one side of the head, hearing loss, jaw pain, and hearing or vision changes.

Because there is no infection involved, starting antibiotics would not be helpful.

Giant-cell arteritis involves inflammation of the blood vessels, not malignancy of the blood vessels, so a referral to an oncologist would be of little value.

Monitoring the situation without starting medications or obtaining a biopsy is inappropriate management because patients with giant-cell arteritis are at risk for development of aneurysms and stroke.

185. B: This patient has hypothyroidism. Her thyroid-stimulating hormone (TSH) is attempting to stimulate the thyroid gland to make more thyroid hormone, but the thyroid is unable to produce sufficient thyroid hormone for the body. The pituitary recognizes that there is insufficient thyroid hormone circulating, so it produces more TSH in hopes of stimulating the thyroid more. The T3 levels may be normal or low normal in hypothyroidism because T4 is the active form of thyroid hormone made available to the body.

186. A: Oseltamivir, or Tamiflu, is an antiviral medication used to lessen the severity of flu symptoms if given early enough during the course of infection.

Acyclovir and famciclovir are also antiviral medications, but they are used primarily to treat acute herpes exacerbations. They may also be used in the treatment of herpes zoster.

Augmentin is an antibiotic used to treat bacterial upper respiratory infections. Because influenza is a viral infection, prescribing an antibiotic would be of little use.

187. C: This patient most likely has orthostatic hypotension, which is defined as a drop in systolic blood pressure by 20 mmHg and a drop of at least 10 mmHg in diastolic blood pressure when a patient moves from a supine to sitting position. Symptoms may include weakness, dizziness, headache, and syncope. Orthostatic hypotension may be caused by medications, or it may be due to prolonged bed rest, especially if it occurs in a hospital setting.

188. B: The patient is in hypertensive crisis. Hypertensive crisis is defined as a systolic blood pressure more than 180 and a diastolic blood pressure more than 120 with evidence of organ damage. The patient has proteinuria, which means that the kidneys are showing signs of damage.

Normal hypertension is defined as a systolic blood pressure less than 120 and a diastolic blood pressure less than 80.

Prehypertension is defined as a systolic blood pressure from 120 to 139 and a diastolic blood pressure from 80 to 89.

Stage 1 hypertension is defined as a systolic blood pressure from 140 to 159 and a diastolic blood pressure from 90 to 99.

Stage 2 hypertension is defined as a systolic blood pressure from 160 to 179 and a diastolic blood pressure of greater than 100.

189. D: The patient is displaying signs and symptoms of diabetes mellitus and needs further workup to confirm the diagnosis. Signs of diabetes include frequent hunger, frequent thirst, unintentional weight loss, numbness or paresthesias in the extremities, frequent urinary tract infections, and visual changes. The hemoglobin A1C (HA1C) test monitors the average serum glucose for the previous three months. If it is above 6.0, then the patient is diagnosed with diabetes. A complete blood count (CBC), basic metabolic panel, and urinalysis should be checked in a patient with suspected diabetes. If glucose is present in the urine, then patient has diabetes. A complete blood count (CBC) and basic metabolic panel (BMP) may show electrolyte abnormalities or show if there is a concurrent infection present.
The patient has a yeast infection, which should be treated with Diflucan; antibiotics won't treat a yeast infection. Pyridium helps alleviate dysuria, which is not one of the patient's symptoms. Blood and urine cultures should be ordered if sepsis is suspected. The patient's vital signs are normal, so sepsis should not be a concern.

190. B: A varicocele is an enlargement of the veins in the scrotum, causing testicular aching and/or swelling to occur. The venous enlargement is usually due to faulty valves in the veins or compression of a neighboring vein disrupting blood flow in nearby veins. Palpation of the affected testicle is often described as feeling like "a bag of worms."
Testicular torsion is a medical emergency. It occurs when the spermatic cord becomes twisted and blood flow to the testicle is severely diminished or absent. It presents with acute onset of pain and swelling of the affected testicle.
Testicular carcinomas present as hard, painless, fixed testicular solid lesions.
A hydrocele is the collection of fluid around the testicle due to infection, malignancy, or unknown cause. It appears as a soft, usually painless mass on the testicle. They are not harmful and have no serious long-term complications.

191. A: Graves' disease is one of the most common causes of hyperthyroidism, causing tremor, unintentional weight loss, palpitations, goiter, hypertension, fatigue, nervousness, increased appetite, and exophthalmos.
Addison's disease is due to insufficient cortisol, causing nausea, vomiting, diarrhea, hypotension, and darkening of the skin color, making the patient look like he or she went tanning.
Cushing's disease is due to the presence of excessive cortisol, causing unintentional weight gain, striae, a fat pad or buffalo hump on the posterior neck, facial swelling, and fatigue.
Hashimoto's disease occurs when the immune system attacks the thyroid gland, causing hypothyroidism. Signs and symptoms of hypothyroidism include bradycardia, unintentional weight gain, puffy face, fatigue, muscle weakness, hair loss, and dry skin.

192. B: This patient is displaying symptoms most consistent with epididymitis. Epididymitis is commonly caused by *Escherichia coli*. In sexually active males, the causative organisms are likely gonorrhea (GC)/chlamydia.
Prostatitis and cystitis usually present with symptoms such as fever, chills, hematuria, dysuria, urgency, and frequency.
Pyelonephritis presents with nausea, vomiting, fever, shaking chills, anorexia, abdominal pain, and back pain. Symptoms are exacerbated when the patient is lying down because the kidneys are retroperitoneal organs.

193. C: Health-care workers or those who work in close contact with people who have tuberculosis would need to have 10 mm or greater induration to have a positive purified protein derivative (PPD) test.

A patient with a normal immune system, no underlying disease, is not a health-care worker, and doesn't have regular contact with tuberculosis (TB)-positive patients would need an induration of 15 mm to have a positive PPD test.

An induration of 2 mm in any patient is considered a negative test.

An induration of 5 mm or more is considered positive in any patient that is immunocompromised.

194. A: Graves' disease is one of the most common causes of hyperthyroidism, causing tremor, unintentional weight loss, palpitations, goiter, hypertension, fatigue, nervousness, increased appetite, and exophthalmos. Tests to confirm the diagnosis include a thyroid function panel and an ultrasound or computed tomography (CT) scan of the thyroid if a goiter is present.

195. A: This patient is in acute renal failure due to her lithium overdose. The patient is anuric, which means that the kidneys aren't working properly and are not able to remove the toxin from her blood. Dialysis will remove the toxin from her body so her kidneys can recover. Although the other choices are not necessarily incorrect, they are not the immediate courses of action needed to help treat this patient's renal failure.

196. C: Children younger than 6 months of age are not recommended to get the influenza vaccine. The vaccine is recommended for children 6 months to 18 years old. It is especially important for health-care workers, immunocompromised individuals, people who are living in close quarters such as assisted living facilities and hospitalized patients, and pregnant women.

197. D: This patient most likely has Addison's disease. Addison's disease is due to insufficient cortisol produced by the adrenal glands, causing nausea, vomiting, diarrhea, hypotension, and darkening of the patient's skin color, making the person look like he or she went tanning. Due to the low cortisol levels, the patient will generally have low sodium levels, causing salty food cravings.

198. B: The patient has diabetes and should be advised to modify his diet and maintain an active lifestyle. A patient without diabetes should have an HA1C of less than 6.0. Because this patient's HA1C is 6.2, his body mass index (BMI) is normal, and he has no other past medical problems, his diabetes may be manageable with dietary modifications.

If his HA1C does not normalize in the next two to three months with dietary modifications, starting antihyperglycemic medications would be recommended.

His BMI is normal, so losing weight would not help.

199. D: Propecia is used to treat benign prostatic hypertrophy and baldness. Levitra, Cialis, and Viagra are all used to treat erectile dysfunction. These three medications increase the level of nitrous oxide, which allows for vasodilatation of the blood vessels. By increasing vasodilatation, the penis will stay erect longer and help reverse the symptoms of erectile dysfunction.

200. C: This patient has a negative purified protein derivative (PPD). No further intervention is required. A patient with a normal immune system, no underlying disease, is not a health-care worker, and doesn't have regular contact with tuberculosis (TB)-positive patients would need an induration of 15 mm to have a positive PPD test. Because the patient has no medical issues and works as a librarian, the size of her induration is considered to be a negative test result.

An induration of 2 mm in any patient is considered a negative PPD test result.

An induration of 5 mm or more is considered positive in any patient that is immunocompromised.

Health-care workers or those who work in close contact with people who have tuberculosis would need to have 10 mm or greater induration to have a positive PPD test.

201. C: In sexually active males, the causative organisms are likely to be gonorrhea (GC)/chlamydia. This patient most likely has been getting epididymitis due to GC/chlamydia from unprotected sex. Epididymitis is also commonly caused by *E. coli*. If he did not have a history of having unprotected sex, *E. coli* would be the more likely causative organism, and a urology referral may be recommended.
Drinking plenty of fluids is general advice given to those who suffer from sickle-cell disease, nephrolithiasis, and those who get persistent urinary tract infections (UTIs). Fluid hydration would not help prevent epididymitis.
Avoiding red meat, alcohol, and seafood are recommendations generally given to those with gout or cardiovascular disease.

202. B: Diverticulosis is the presence of pockets in any organ or fluid-filled cavity. The potential for developing this condition increases with age. Development of these pockets does not cause symptoms. If an infection develops within the diverticula, then this condition is called diverticulitis. Mallory–Weiss tears are usually found in the esophageal junction. They are commonly seen in alcoholic patients caused by persistent episodes of vomiting; however, any pathological process that causes forceful coughing or vomiting may cause a Mallory–Weiss tear.
Celiac sprue is an immune reaction that damages the lining of the small intestine and prevents it from absorbing important nutrients. It presents with nausea, vomiting, diarrhea, and abdominal pain, which occur after ingesting gluten products.
Intussusception is when one part of the bowel folds in on itself and causes an obstruction. This is common in children. Symptoms include nausea, vomiting, lethargy, and "red-currant-jelly" stools.

203. A: Colchicine is used for treatment of acute gout exacerbations. This medication would not be useful in treating septic arthritis. A patient with septic arthritis has an infection in the blood that is attacking a joint or joints. Obtaining blood cultures, lab work, getting a joint aspiration, and prescribing pain medications and intravenous (IV) antibiotics are several ways to help diagnose and treat this infection.

204. D: Celiac disease, or celiac sprue, is an immune reaction that damages the lining of the small intestine and prevents it from absorbing important nutrients. It presents as nausea, vomiting, diarrhea, and abdominal pain that occur after ingesting gluten products. The mainstay of treatment is to maintain a gluten-free diet to help prevent future exacerbations. If the disease is refractory to conservative management, patients may be prescribed corticosteroids.

205. A: This patient has a superficial venous thrombus (SVT), which is a blood clot in the leg below the popliteal vein. A blood clot in the popliteal vein or higher is referred to as a deep venous thrombus (DVT). DVTs have a 30% to 50% chance of migrating to the lung; this is called a pulmonary embolus, which carries a high mortality rate. Patients with SVTs have a much lower risk of complications and can be monitored as an outpatient without being placed on medications. Patients who are at high risk, such as those with cancer, sickle-cell disease, lower extremity trauma or surgery, women who are taking birth control pills, patients who are obese, or persons who are bedridden may be started on Coumadin or have an inferior vena cava (IVC) filter placed if Coumadin is contraindicated.

206. C: Nursemaid's elbow describes the dislocation of the elbow most commonly due to trauma. It most commonly occurs in children under the age of eight due to their hyperflexible joints and

growing bones. Children usually have little to no pain and hold their affected extremity in a flexed and pronated position.

A Greenstick fracture is most commonly seen in children due to the flexibility of their bones. It occurs when the bony cortex bends abnormally, causing a partial break.

A Lisfranc fracture is the fracture and dislocation of one or more of the metatarsals.

A Colles' fracture is a fracture and dorsal displacement of the distal radius. It is commonly referred to as a "dinner-fork deformity" on x-ray.

207. B: In vitro, the ductus arteriosus is a blood vessel in which blood travels from the heart to the lungs. It normally closes a few days after birth, but in patients in which it does not, it is called patent ductus arteriosus (PDA). A heart murmur may be auscultated. Tachypnea, poor feeding, failure to thrive, shortness of breath, and diaphoresis are signs and symptoms in those patients who have moderate-to-severe PDA. If the defect is small, the patient may not have any symptoms and can be monitored as an outpatient without medications.

Aspirin is generally avoided in children younger than age 16 because they have an increased risk of developing Reye's syndrome, which causes swelling of the liver and brain.

Indomethacin is the drug of choice used in patients with symptomatic PDA.

Surgical closure of this cardiac defect is generally reserved for those with large defects.

208. D: Ramipril is an antihypertensive medication and is not used in the treatment of benign prostatic hypertrophy. Proscar, Cardura, and Rapaflo are all medications used to treat benign prostatic hypertrophy. Alpha-blockers such as Cardura and Rapaflo help the muscle in the prostate to relax so it does not impinge on the urethra. Medications such as Proscar, which is a 5-alpha reductase inhibitor, help slow the growth of the prostate.

209. D: In a patient who displays strokelike symptoms, the first thing you should do is order a computed tomography (CT) scan of the brain without contrast. If the CT scan is negative, tissue plasminogen activator (tPA) may be started in this patient because he has no contraindications. Tissue plasminogen activator or a heparin infusion should never be started in a suspected stroke case without ordering a CT scan first; if the patient has a hemorrhagic stroke, these medications can exacerbate the bleed and potentially kill the patient. Although the patient's neurological examination should be continually reassessed, treatment should not be postponed.

210. A: *Clostridium difficile* (*C. difficile*) colitis is a common nosocomial (hospital-acquired) infection. It is caused by the alteration of one's normal gastrointestinal (GI) flora, usually caused by long-term antibiotic usage. Vancomycin by mouth is one of the treatments for *C. difficile* colitis. The other medication used is po Flagyl. Vancomycin IV cannot be used in the treatment of *C. difficile* because insufficient amounts of it reach the colon to have any effect. Azithromycin and clindamycin play no role in the treatment of *C. difficile* colitis. Clindamycin is one the antibiotics that runs an increased risk of causing *C. difficile* colitis.

211. C: Status epilepticus describes a patient who continuously seizes. Phenytoin is an antiseizure medication, and lorazepam is used for sedation; both medications are used to help treat status epilepticus. Levetiracetam is also used for the treatment of seizure disorders. Lomotil helps to treat diarrhea. Linezolid is an antibiotic. Neither Lomotil nor linezolid plays any role in the treatment of status epilepticus.

212. B: Virchow's triad includes hypercoagulability, endothelial injury, and hemodynamic changes that increase one's risk of thrombosis.

Charcot's triad is the combination of <u>jaundice</u>, <u>fever</u>, and right-upper quadrant <u>abdominal pain</u>. It occurs as a result of ascending cholangitis.

Cushing's triad is a clinical <u>triad</u> defined as hypertension, bradycardia, and irregular respirations. It suggests rising intracranial pressure due to intracranial pathology such as hemorrhage.

Beck's triad is the combination of distended jugular veins, hypotension, and muffled heart sounds. It occurs as a result of pericardial effusion.

213. B: This patient may have a Lisfranc fracture. A Lisfranc fracture is the fracture and dislocation of one or more of the metatarsals.

Monteggia's fracture is a fracture of the ulna and dislocation of the radius.

A Colles' fracture is a fracture and dorsal displacement of the distal radius. It is commonly referred to as a "dinner-fork deformity" on x-ray.

A Le Fort fracture is a fracture of the maxilla; this type of fracture has four categories based on the severity of the fracture.

214. B: Amiodarone is an antiarrhythmic medication used for diseases such as atrial fibrillation. It plays no role in the treatment of cystic fibrosis nor does it prevent complications that may be associated with cystic fibrosis.

Mucinex helps thin out the copious mucus that collects in the airways of those with cystic fibrosis. By thinning out the mucous, the patient is able to expectorate it more easily, which helps prevent infection.

Albuterol is a bronchodilator that opens up the airways and makes it easier to breathe for those with pulmonary diseases such as cystic fibrosis, asthma, and chronic obstructive pulmonary disease (COPD).

Nonsteroidal anti-inflammatory drugs (NSAIDs) such as Motrin help decrease inflammation, which can help with infections and prevent airway damage.

215. D: Pott's disease is caused by the spread of tuberculosis to the spine. Signs and symptoms may include night sweats, anorexia, back pain, and lower extremity weakness.

<u>Parkinson's disease</u> destroys dopamine-producing neurons in the substantia nigra, and it causes motor symptoms (<u>dyskinesia</u>, <u>tremor</u>, and rigidity) as well as cognitive symptoms.

Hashimoto's disease occurs when the immune system attacks the thyroid gland, causing hypothyroidism. Signs and symptoms of hypothyroidism include bradycardia, unintentional weight gain, puffy face, fatigue, muscle weakness, hair loss, and dry skin.

Cushing's disease is due to the presence of excessive cortisol, causing unintentional weight gain, striae, a fat pad or buffalo hump on the posterior neck, facial swelling, and fatigue.

216. A: Fibromyalgia is a diagnosis of exclusion. Patients often complain of generalized body aches and pains with no known cause found during a workup. It is linked to anxiety and depression in many cases.

Polyarteritis nodosa is a type of vasculitis with unknown cause. Signs and symptoms of this disease may include painful red bumps on the skin, myalgias, fever, arthralgias, and weakness. It is diagnosed through a variety of lab tests and a biopsy.

Osteoarthritis is the degeneration of one or more joints usually diagnosed by x ray.

Polymyalgia rheumatica is a type of rheumatoid disease, which usually affects the larger joints such as the shoulders and hips. It is diagnosed by a variety of lab tests, which show the presence of inflammation, as well as by physical examination.

217. D: Paroxetine is used to treat generalized anxiety disorder, depression, posttraumatic stress disorder, as well as other psychiatric conditions.

Prednisolone is a type of steroid used to treat inflammatory reactions, such as localized skin reactions and asthma.

Promethazine is used to treat and prevent nausea and vomiting. It is also used for motion sickness.

Permethrin is used to treat infections caused by scabies.

218. C: This patient has cataracts, which are sclerotic lesions on the lens that slowly obstruct vision. They become more common with age. Surgical intervention alleviates symptoms.

Conjunctivitis is an infection of the clear portion of the eye called the conjunctiva, which may present with conjunctival erythema, pain or discomfort, itching, discharge, and crusting of the lids or lashes.

A hyphema is a hemorrhage in the anterior portion of the eye, which can be due to inflammation or trauma. It may cause pain or visual disturbances.

Blepharitis is inflammation of the eyelids, causing them to become red and painful. This condition is caused by localized trauma or irritation.

219. B: Doppler ultrasound is the treatment of choice in diagnosing deep venous thromboses. It is very sensitive and exposes the patient to the least amount of radiation.

Computed tomography (CT) and magnetic resonance imaging (MRI) scans are usually reserved for tissue, muscular, or ligamentous injuries or pathologies. They are also good in diagnosing infections or fluid collections.

X rays are not used because they only show bones. They do not show muscles, ligaments, tissues, or blood vessels.

220. A: Mallory–Weiss tears occur in the esophageal junction and are usually seen in alcoholic patients caused by persistent episodes of vomiting. However, any pathological process that causes forceful coughing or vomiting may cause a Mallory–Weiss tear.

In Crohn's disease, the colon wall may have a "cobblestone" appearance due to the intermittent pattern of affected and nonaffected colonic tissue.

Ulcerative colitis usually affects continuous stretches of the colon and rectum.

Whipple's disease is a rare, chronic disease caused by bacterial infection. The affected bowel is usually swollen with raised, yellowish patches.

221. D: This patient most likely has a venous thrombus caused by her recent hip surgery. Patients with venous thromboses have a positive Homan's sign in approximately one-third of the cases. A positive Homan's sign may be elicited if a patient has pain with dorsiflexion of his or her foot while the leg is extended.

Osteomyelitis and septic arthritis are unlikely because they are involved with infection of a joint or joints rather than presenting with muscular pain and swelling.

Osgood–Schlatter disease is the swelling of the tibial tubercle, which commonly occurs in pubescent and prepubescent children.

222. A: Mitral regurgitation is occurring on the two-dimensional echocardiography (2D echo). The mitral valve permits blood flow from the left atrium into the left ventricle. If the valve does not close properly, mitral regurgitation will occur.

Pulmonic regurgitation is the backflow of blood from the pulmonary artery into the right ventricle.

Tricuspid regurgitation is the backflow of blood from the right ventricle into the right atrium.

Aortic regurgitation is the backflow of blood from the aorta into the left ventricle.

223. C: You would give 1 mg of epinephrine, or you could give 40 units of vasopressin. Because vasopressin is not an option, epinephrine would be the drug of choice, according to Advanced

Cardiovascular Life Support (ACLS) protocol. Amiodarone, lidocaine, and magnesium sulfate could be given during a code involving a patient with pulseless ventricular tachycardia, but they would be given after the administration of vasopressin or epinephrine.

224. B: This patient most likely has gynecomastia, which is the appearance of breasts in males due to enlarged mammary glands. This may due to obesity, congenital etiology, endocrine abnormality, or underlying disease. This condition usually resolves on its own in a patient with no significant past medical history.
Fibroadenomas are generally singular, rubbery, nontender breast lesions that are benign in nature. Malignant breast masses are generally nontender breast lesions and usually do not occur bilaterally.
Fibrocystic breast disease is a benign condition in which singular or multiple breast cysts develop. They can occur right before one's menses begins, or they may be unrelated to menses. People placed on hormone replacement therapy or birth control pills generally have less severe symptoms.

225. A: The child has otitis media, which is an infection of the inner ear.
Mastoiditis is an infection of the mastoid bone of the skull. It is generally a complication of inner ear infections. Symptoms may include fever, ear pain, ear discharge, swelling behind the ear (where the mastoid bone is located), hearing loss, headache, and erythema. Imaging studies such as magnetic resonance imaging (MRI) and computed tomography (CT) scans can make a definitive diagnosis.
Acoustic neuromas are tumors of the acoustic nerve. They are much more common in adults than in children. Symptoms include hearing loss, dizziness, headache, tinnitus, facial droop, and ataxia.
Otitis externa is an infection of the outer ear. Signs and symptoms may include pain with palpation of the tragus, otorrhea, fever, and ear tugging.

226. B: This patient has meningitis. Meningitis is an infection that classically presents with nuchal rigidity, photophobia, and headache. The patient has a history of human immunodeficiency virus (HIV); being immunocompromised can predispose a person to developing meningitis. Kerning's sign is positive when a patient is unable to extend his or her leg when the hip is flexed. This maneuver helps diagnose meningitis.
Huntington's disease is a slow, progressive neurological disorder caused by an autosomal-dominant chromosomal abnormality. Signs include progressive decline in cognitive function; ataxic gait; and uncoordinated, jerky body movements.
Schistosomiasis is a chronic parasitic infection due to eating improperly cooked pork. On magnetic resonance imaging (MRI) or computed tomography (CT) scan of the brain, it can appear as multiple enhancing nodules occurring in bilateral cerebral hemispheres.
Guillain–Barré syndrome is an autoimmune disorder in which the body attacks its own nervous system. The cause is generally unknown, but being immunocompromised or getting over a viral infection such as mononucleosis increases the risk of developing this disorder. Signs and symptoms may include numbness, weakness, paresthesias of the extremities, ataxia, dysphagia, and muscle spasms.

227. B: This patient most likely has bacterial meningitis. Neutrophil counts are elevated in patients with bacterial meningitis. Their glucose levels are low because bacteria use glucose. The level of protein in the spinal fluid goes up due to an increase in the presence of bacteria, which have a high composition of protein. Also, there is an increase in the presence of cells that fight infection, which are also composed of protein. When bacteria destroy the body's cells (or vice versa), the protein is released, causing protein levels to rise.
In viral meningitis, the neutrophil count may be elevated, but usually lymphocytes are the predominant cells. The glucose level is normal because viruses do not use glucose. The protein level

is near normal because viruses do not have a high composition of protein. The white blood cell (WBC) count may be normal or elevated.

Myasthenia gravis is an autoimmune disorder in which the body attacks the voluntary muscles, causing facial droop or asymmetry, ataxia, muscle spasms, dysphagia, and airway difficulties. A lumbar puncture would be normal in a patient with myasthenia gravis.

Huntington's disease is a slow, progressive neurological disorder caused by an autosomal-dominant chromosomal abnormality. Signs include progressive decline in cognitive function; ataxic gait; and uncoordinated, jerky body movements. A lumbar puncture would be normal.

228. D: This patient has a respiratory acidosis. The pH is low (normal value 7.35 to 7.45), and the $PaCO_2$ is high (normal value 35 to 45). To interpret an arterial blood gas, first look at the pH. If it is low, acidosis is present. If the pH is high, alkalosis is present.

Next look at the $PaCO_2$; if it is low, alkalosis is present. If it is increased, acidosis is present. If the $PaCO_2$ explains the change of pH, then it is respiratory disorder. If it does not, look at the HCO_3. The normal range is 22 to 26. If the HCO_3 is increased and the pH is high, then you have metabolic alkalosis. If the pH is low and the HCO_3 is low, then you have metabolic acidosis.

229. C: This patient has normal pressure hydrocephalus (NPH). The common triad seen with NPH patients is ataxia, urinary incontinence, and dementia. The opening pressure of a lumbar puncture is normal (hence, "normal pressure" hydrocephalus). The ventricles, however, are enlarged on computed tomography (CT) or magnetic resonance imaging (MRI) scan. The treatment is to perform a lumbar puncture to determine if the symptoms resolve or improve. If they do, then the patient will most likely need a ventricular peritoneal shunt (VPS). NPH can occur without a cause, or it may be due to trauma such an aneurysm rupture, infection, or postsurgical complication.

A hygroma is a collection of cerebrospinal fluid in the subdural space. Acute hygromas are usually caused by head trauma or recent neurosurgical procedure.

Medulloblastomas are the most common malignant brain tumor and are significantly more common in children than in adults. They usually occur in the cerebellum.

An intraventricular hemorrhage is the presence of blood within the ventricles, most commonly due to hypertension. On this patient's CT scan, hydrocephalus, not blood, was noted.

230. A: This patient has anorexia nervosa. It is an eating disorder much more common in girls than boys, and it is most common in adolescents. It is characterized by purposely starving oneself in order to lose weight.

Bulimia nervosa is an eating disorder much more common in girls than boys and most common in adolescents. It involves periods of bingeing followed by periods of fasting in order to lose weight.

Generalized anxiety disorder is a psychiatric disorder in which a person feels anxious or nervous most or all of the time with no known cause.

Bipolar disorder is a psychiatric disorder in which a person has episodes of mania, or extreme happiness and energy, followed by periods of depression.

231. B: This patient has generalized anxiety disorder. Generalized anxiety disorder is a psychiatric disorder in which a person feels anxious or nervous most or all of the time with no known cause.

Posttraumatic stress disorder (PTSD) is when a person feels nervous or anxious all or most of the time due to a known cause, such as the death of a loved one, rape, near-death experience or being involved in a disturbing event such as a school shooting or terrorist attack.

A phobia is feeling extremely nervous or scared about a particular stimulus that is usually nonthreatening to most people (i.e., being afraid to go outside or being afraid of water).

Dysthymic disorder is a milder form of major depressive disorder.

232. C: This patient has metabolic alkalosis. The pH is high, the $PaCO_2$ is normal, and the HCO_3 is high. To interpret an arterial blood gas, first look at the pH. If it is low, acidosis is present. If the pH is high, alkalosis is present. Next look at $PaCO_2$; if it is low, acidosis is present. If it is increased, alkalosis is present. If the $PaCO_2$ explains the change of pH, then it is respiratory disorder. If not, look at the HCO_3. The normal range is 22 to 26. If the HCO_3 is increased and the pH is high, then it indicates metabolic alkalosis. If the pH is low and the HCO_3 is low, it is metabolic acidosis.

233. C: This patient has normal pressure hydrocephalus (NPH) and should undergo a ventricular peritoneal shunt (VPS) if he or she is not a high-risk patient. There is no other way to correct NPH. Performing an electroencephalogram (EEG) may help rule out other etiologies that are causing the patient's symptoms, but it is not a treatment of NPH.
A magnetic resonance image (MRI) scan of the brain may help diagnose NPH and reveal its cause, but it is not a treatment of NPH.
A repeat lumbar puncture is not useful. Once a patient has one lumbar puncture and his or her symptoms improve, the diagnosis is made.

234. D: This patient has a phobia disorder; she has anthropophobia, which is a fear of people. A phobia is feeling extremely nervous or scared about a particular stimulus that is usually nonthreatening to most people (i.e., being afraid to go outside or being afraid of water). Generalized anxiety disorder is a psychiatric disorder in which a person feels anxious or nervous most or all of the time with no known cause.
Posttraumatic stress disorder (PTSD) is when a person feels nervous or anxious all or most of the time due to a known cause such as the death of a loved one, rape, or near-death experience or being involved in a disturbing event such as a school shooting or terrorist attack.
Dysthymic disorder is a milder form of major depressive disorder.

235. A: Genetic mutations are the most common cause of hypertrophic cardiomyopathy. Hypertrophic cardiomyopathy is an abnormal thickening of the cardiac fibers. The thickening of these fibers impairs the heart from filling with blood and its ability to pump out blood to the rest of the body. This condition is diagnosed by an echocardiogram. Surgery, implantation of a pacemaker, and medications may help alleviate the complications this condition may cause.

236. B: Chorea is not a minor manifestation of acute rheumatic fever according to the Jones criteria.
Major manifestations of acute rheumatic fever include the following:
Erythema marginatum: raised, nonpruritic, pink rings on the trunk and inner surfaces of the limbs
Carditis: inflammation of the heart muscle
Chorea: rapid, uncontrolled body movements
Subcutaneous nodules: painless, firm collections of collagen fibers over bones or <u>tendons</u>
Polyarthritis: temporary migrating inflammation of the large joints

Minor manifestations of acute rheumatic fever include the following:
1) <u>Fever</u> (101 °F to 102 °F)
2) <u>Arthralgia</u>: joint pain without swelling
3) Elevated erythrocyte sedimentation rate (ESR) or C-reactive protein (CRP)
4) Leukocytosis
5) Prior episode of rheumatic heart disease
6) Heart block seen on an electrocardiogram (EKG)

237. D: Tricuspid regurgitation is the backflow of blood from the right ventricle into the right atrium.

Aortic regurgitation is the backflow of blood from the aorta into the left ventricle.

The mitral valve permits blood flow from the left atrium into the left ventricle. If the valve does not close properly, mitral regurgitation will occur.

Pulmonic regurgitation is the backflow of blood from the pulmonary artery into the right ventricle.

238. D: Atropine, epinephrine, dopamine, and transcutaneous pacing are used for patients with symptomatic bradycardia.

Atropine is used to increase the heart rate; in ventricular fibrillation, the heart rate is already abnormally fast, so atropine would only exacerbate this arrhythmia.

Vasopressin, epinephrine, lidocaine, magnesium sulfate, and amiodarone are all medications that may be used in pulseless ventricular fibrillation or pulseless ventricular tachycardia.

239. B: This patient has a respiratory alkalosis. To interpret an arterial blood gas, first look at the pH. If it is low, acidosis is present. If the pH is high, alkalosis is present.

Next look at $PaCO_2$; if it is low, alkalosis is present. If it is increased, acidosis is present. If the $PaCO_2$ explains the change of pH, then it is respiratory disorder. If it does not, look at the HCO_3. The normal range is 22 to 26. If the HCO_3 is increased and the pH is high, then it indicates metabolic alkalosis. If the pH is low and the HCO_3 is low, it is metabolic acidosis.

240. B: The patient has horizontal nystagmus, which is common after acute drug or alcohol intoxication. It is an involuntary, oscillating eye movement that occurs bilaterally and resolves once the toxins are out of the body.

Entropion is the inward turning of the upper or lower lid toward the eye.

Exotropia is a condition in which one eye is normal and the other eye deviates laterally.

Conjunctivitis is the infection of the cornea causing pain, blurry vision, conjunctival erythema, and crusting of the lids and/or lashes.

241. B: This patient has right bundle branch block. This conduction arrhythmia has a widened QRS complex and two R waves best seen in V1.

Atrial fibrillation is a type of tachycardia with irregularly irregular QRS complexes and no P waves.

Sinus tachycardia is defined as a heart rate greater than 100 beats per minute with regular QRS complexes preceded by P waves.

Torsades de pointes means "twisting of the points" around the isoelectric baseline of an electrocardiogram (EKG), which describes this polymorphic ventricular tachycardia.

242. A: This patient had a ministroke, or transient ischemic attack (TIA). A TIA is a temporary lack of or insufficient blood flow to the brain, causing strokelike symptoms that resolve on their own once the blood flow is restored. There is no permanent brain damage and no acute findings on radiological studies.

A cerebral vascular accident (CVA) is a stroke. A CVA occurs when there is prolonged lack of or insufficient blood flow to a part of the brain leading to brain cell death, or infarction. There is no way to revive dead blood cells. Complications of a stroke depend on the size of and the location of the infarct. Complications may range from minimal neurological deficits (if any) to significant neurological deficits, or death.

243. C: Although all medical professionals are bound by the Health Insurance Portability and Accountability Act (HIPAA), which ensures patient privacy, there are instances in which a medical professional may share a patient's information. If a patient threatens to injure themselves or others, a medical professional may reach out to local authorities or family members to warn them of the patient's potential plans in order to ensure the safety of the patient and others.

244. A: The patient has entropion, or the inward turning of the lid toward the eye. This may cause excessive tearing or irritation of the eye; if it is severe enough, the patient may develop a corneal abrasion.

Ectropion is the outward turning of the lid away from the eye.

Exotropia is the lateral deviation of the eye.

Esotropia is the inward deviation of the eye.

245. D: This patient has oppositional-defiant disorder (ODD), which is an emotional and psychiatric disorder that causes patients to have labile moods and have problems getting along with and listening to others. There is no one cause; sometimes it runs in families, sometimes it is seen in children of parents who abuse alcohol or drugs, and sometimes it is seen in children whose parents have psychiatric disorders. In some cases, there is no known cause.

Adjustment disorder is when a patient has a problem adjusting to or getting used to new life events or circumstances.

Dysthymic disorder is a milder form of major depressive disorder.

Attention-deficit hyperactivity disorder is when a patient has high level of energy and a short attention span.

246. A: Colchicine is used for the treatment of acute gout.

Phlebitis is the presence of a superficial clot in an extremity (most commonly in the leg), which can cause pain, swelling, and erythema. Patients may be given antibiotics if a secondary infection is present. They may be given anticoagulation medications depending on their risk factors and past medical history. Typically, phlebitis can be treated on an outpatient basis, using analgesics such as nonsteroidal anti-inflammatory drugs (NSAIDs), warm compresses, and compression stockings.

247. C: This patient has atrial fibrillation, which is a type of tachycardia with irregularly irregular QRS complexes and no P waves.

Sinus bradycardia is a heart rate less of than 60 beats per minute. It has regular QRS complexes preceded by P waves.

Right bundle branch block has a widened QRS complex and two R waves best seen in lead V1.

Sinus tachycardia is defined as a heart rate of greater than 100 beats per minute with regular QRS complexes preceded by P waves.

248. B: Frovatriptan is a tryptamine-based medication that helps prevent and treat migraine headaches. Other medications that may be used to treat migraines include nonsteroidal anti-inflammatory drugs (NSAIDs), aspirin, narcotics, and beta-blockers.

Fluoxetine is used to treat anxiety and depression.

Fexofenadine is an antihistamine used to treat seasonal allergy exacerbations.

Fluvastatin is part of the statin drug class that is used to treat hyperlipidemia.

249. D: A lumbar puncture may help aid in the diagnosis of this syndrome, but it is not used as a therapeutic aid, a preventative aid, or as a way to speed up recovery.

Guillain–Barré syndrome is an autoimmune disorder in which the body attacks its own nervous system. The cause is generally unknown, but being immunocompromised or getting over a viral infection such as mononucleosis increases the risk of developing this disorder. Signs and symptoms may include numbness and weakness of the extremities, respiratory distress, paresthesias of the extremities, ataxia, dysphagia, and muscle spasms.

Intubation is used in cases of respiratory distress to help maintain an open airway. Plasmapheresis and immunoglobulin therapy are methods used to help speed recovery.

250. B: Tourette disorder is first noticed in childhood and is characterized by involuntary verbal sounds and/or motor movements. It does not cause cognitive impairment, although it may be seen in the presence of cognitive disorders.

Alzheimer's disease is a progressive cognitive decline; the underlying cause is not known. Motor skills are much less affected until late stages of the disease.

Multiple sclerosis is a demyelinating disease, which may present with progressive ataxia, muscle spasms, dizziness, trouble with coordination of fine motor movements, urinary frequency, incontinence, nystagmus, and depression.

Huntington's disease is a progressive neurological disorder caused by an autosomal-dominant chromosomal abnormality, which usually occurs in the third or fourth decade of life. Signs include progressive decline in cognitive function; ataxic gait; and uncoordinated, jerky body movements.

251. A: Spirometry is the best test to aid in the diagnosis of chronic obstructive pulmonary disease (COPD). Spirometry measures airflow by testing lung volume and lung capacity.

A chest x ray may show pathological changes that accompany COPD, but the x ray may be normal. It is not a diagnostic test for COPD.

Auscultation with a stethoscope may reveal diminished breath sounds, but they can occur with many different conditions. Breath sounds may even be normal in someone with COPD.

An electrocardiogram (EKG) is the least helpful diagnostic aid; it generally is used to help diagnose cardiac-related abnormalities.

252. C: The sweat chloride test is the standard diagnostic test for cystic fibrosis.

A physical examination and past medical history of both the child and the parents are also important in making the diagnosis.

A chest x ray or a computed tomography (CT) scan of the chest may reveal pathologies such as pleural effusions, pneumonia, or bronchiectasis, but it is not diagnostic for cystic fibrosis.

A fecal fat test may help diagnose cystic fibrosis because complications with digestive fluids and pancreatitis are common in this patient population; however, there are other disease states in which a fecal fat test may be abnormal.

253. D: Aspergillosis is a fungal pneumonia commonly occurring in those who are immunocompromised. The classic radiological finding is a fungus ball seen on chest x ray or a computed tomography (CT) scan of the chest.

Sarcoidosis is a disease with an unknown cause in which granulomas can form in the organs or the skin. It is not a fungal disease.

Cystic fibrosis is an autosomal-recessive lung disorder in which mucus in the lungs and digestive tract becomes abnormally thick, causing chronic lung infections and gastrointestinal (GI) complications.

Pneumoconiosis, or "miner's lung," is a lung disease caused by long-term exposure to coal or coal-related products. A fungus ball is not seen on chest x ray because this is not a fungal disease.

254. C: Autism is a neurodevelopmental disorder affecting cognition and social skills. Signs may appear as early as a few weeks of life to as late as two or three years of age. Classic signs of this disorder are cognitive and social impairment and persistent repetitive behaviors. There is no known cause or cure. Speech therapy, behavioral therapies, psychiatric medications, and special education programs are the mainstays of treatment.

Adjustment disorder is when a patient has a problem getting used to new life events or circumstances.

Oppositional-defiant disorder (ODD) is an emotional and psychiatric disorder causing patients to have labile moods and have problems getting along with and listening to others. There is no one cause; sometimes it runs in families, sometimes it is seen in children of parents who abuse alcohol or drugs, and sometimes it is seen in children whose parents have psychiatric disorders. In some cases, there is no known cause.

Attention-deficit hyperactivity disorder is when a patient has high level of energy and a short attention span.

255. C: No intervention is needed if both the mother and baby are Rh-positive. The Rh factor is an antigen that may or may not be attached to one's blood cells. People with a positive blood type (A+, B+, O+, AB+) have the antigen. People with a negative blood type do not have the antigen and are Rh negative. If a mother is Rh negative and a child is Rh positive, RhoGAM needs to be administered. RhoGAM is an injection that suppresses the mother's immune response to the Rh-positive baby, which can help prevent hemolytic disease of the newborn or miscarriage.

Antibiotics are unnecessary because it is a blood incompatibility not an infection.

An ultrasound would be ineffective regarding Rh factor.

256. C: You should advise the patient that labor should be induced immediately. Eclampsia is the development of hypertension, proteinuria, and seizures during the second or third trimester. If the patient is at least 32 weeks pregnant, then she should be induced. The only cure for eclampsia is delivery. If the patient is less than 32 weeks pregnant, she may be managed on anticonvulsants and placed on a telemetry monitor for observation.

Blood transfusions play no role in the treatment or cure of eclampsia if the complete blood count is normal.

257. A: This patient has a pleural effusion, which is a pathologic fluid collection due to his chronic obstructive pulmonary disease (COPD). If the effusion is large enough, it will present with blunting of the costophrenic angle on chest x ray.

Aspergillosis is a fungal pneumonia commonly occurring in those who are immunocompromised. The classic radiological finding is a fungus ball seen on chest x ray or a computed tomography (CT) scan of the chest.

Pneumoconiosis, or "miner's lung," is a lung disease caused by long-term exposure to coal or coal-related products. The classic chest x-ray findings are small cystic radiolucencies that look like honeycombs on chest x ray.

Pneumothoraces will appear as a black space on a chest x ray with no lung markings. If they are small enough, the chest x ray may be normal.

258. D: A moderate-sized pneumothorax (typically one that is larger than 10% in size) will appear as a black space on chest x ray with no lung markings. If it is small (typically less than 10%), the chest x-ray may be normal.

Sarcoidosis is a disease with an unknown cause in which granulomas can form in one's organs or the skin.

Pneumoconiosis, or "miner's lung," is a lung disease caused by long-term exposure to coal or coal-related products. The classic chest x-ray findings are small cystic radiolucencies that look like honeycombs on chest x ray.

259. A: Graves' disease is an autoimmune disease that causes hyperthyroidism, which would promote weight loss, not weight gain.

Untreated hypothyroidism may contribute to obesity because the thyroid plays a role in metabolism. If the thyroid is functioning more sluggishly than normal, weight gain may occur due to the slowing down of metabolism.

Cushing's disease is due to the presence of excessive cortisol, causing unintentional weight gain, striae, a fat pad or buffalo hump on the posterior neck, and facial swelling.

Women going through menopause are at an increased risk for gaining weight due to the various hormonal changes they are going through as well as a redistribution of body fat that commonly occurs during this time.

260. C: Allergic rhinitis is caused by a sensitivity or allergy to something in the environment. It is not a bacterial infection. Antibiotics are not prescribed for allergic rhinitis unless there is a secondary infection present.

Corticosteroids help treat inflammation commonly caused by an overactive immune system as well as help reduce swelling.

Decongestants help reduce the amount of fluid and mucus that accumulate in the airways.

Antihistamines are used to alleviate inflammation and pruritis.

261. D: Phobia disorder is a specific type of anxiety disorder. Although general anxiety disorder may not have a particular trigger or reason for the onset of symptoms, phobias are caused by a particular person, place, or thing. A phobia is feeling extremely nervous or scared about a particular stimulus that is usually nonthreatening to most people (i.e., being afraid to go outside or being afraid of water).

Ritalin is a psychostimulant used to help increase attention span and concentration; it is commonly used in patients who suffer from attention-deficit and hyperactivity disorder. It does not play a role in someone who suffers from phobias.

Xanax is a benzodiazepine, which will cause mild sedation. It is commonly used in those with schizophrenia, anxiety, and depression.

Metoprolol helps to lower blood pressure and heart rate. It is most commonly used in the treatment of hypertension and cardiac arrhythmias, but it may also be used in patients who suffer from phobias and stage fright.

Lexapro is a selective serotonin reuptake inhibitor (SSRI) used in the treatment of anxiety and depression.

262. B: Naloxone (Narcan) is an opiate antidote used to treat potential or confirmed narcotic overdoses. It is not used in the treatment of alcohol withdrawal.

There is no one treatment for alcohol withdrawal. Treatment is based on the symptoms displayed by the patient. Thiamine, magnesium, and folic acid are frequently administered to alcoholic patients because they are usually chronically malnourished and suffer from electrolyte imbalances due to their addiction.

Zofran is an antiemetic medication that prevents and alleviates nausea and vomiting.

Ativan is a benzodiazepine that causes mild sedation. It is usually given to alleviate symptoms such as delirium tremens.

263. C: This patient has a type of peritonsillar abscess called Ludwig's angina. It involves a bacterial infection under the tongue, causing swelling, erythema, dysphonia, dysphagia, and fever. The classic physical finding is a patient who sounds like he or she has a "hot potato in his or her mouth." It may occur spontaneously, but it is commonly preceded by a dental infection.

Acute pharyngitis is an infection of the pharynx that may cause dysphagia, dysphonia, and fever, but it does not commonly cause neck swelling and erythema and does not cause displacement of the tongue.

Aphthous ulcers are open sores that occur on the lips, gums, or tongue. The cause is unknown. They appear as gray, white, or yellow sores on an erythematous base. They may cause dysphagia, but they do not cause dysphonia, fever, neck swelling, or tongue displacement.

Oral leukoplakia is the presence of white plaques in the mouth caused by chronic irritation such as by chewing tobacco or from chronic disease. It does not cause dysphagia, dysphonia, tongue displacement, neck swelling, or erythema.

264. A: Irrigation of the eye would be generally ineffective and is not used in the treatment of a blowout fracture. A blowout fracture is a fracture of the walls and/or floor of the orbital bone most commonly caused by trauma.

Antibiotics are always warranted as prophylaxis against infection.

Steroids are used to help decrease swelling.

Surgery may be warranted depending on the severity of the fracture.

265. D: A Le Fort fracture is a fracture of the maxilla; this type of fracture has four categories based on severity.

A boxer's fracture is a transverse fracture of the fourth and/or fifth metacarpal bones usually as a result of trauma with a closed fist.

A Lisfranc fracture is the fracture and dislocation of one or more of the metatarsals.

A Colles' fracture is a fracture and dorsal displacement of the distal radius. It is commonly referred to as a "dinner-fork deformity" on x-ray.

266. D: The number-one cause of pelvic inflammatory disease (PID) is venereal disease, most notably, gonorrhea and chlamydia. Untreated sexually transmitted diseases may lead to PID, which is the primary preventable cause of infertility.

Approximately 10% to 15% of PID cases are caused by illnesses such as appendicitis or pelvic procedures such as dilation and curettage, abortion, or childbirth.

PID may be caused by a pelvic procedure, such as the removal of an ectopic pregnancy, or PID may cause an ectopic pregnancy to occur.

267. D: Esomeprazole is a proton pump inhibitor that causes the stomach to produce less acid. The reduction of acid production means that less acid is released into the esophagus, which will alleviate or partially alleviate symptoms and the damage done to the esophageal mucosa.

Metronidazole is an antibiotic used in treating anaerobic bacterial infections; it is also an amebicide and antiprotozoal medication.

Ketoconazole and fluconazole are antifungal medications.

268. A: A diverticulum is an outpouching of an organ or fluid-filled cavity. Meckel's diverticulum is two times more prevalent in boys than in girls. Meckel's diverticulum is usually two inches long and found approximately two feet from the ileocecal valve. Two years of age is the most common presentation for those with a complication involving Meckel's diverticulum. Approximately 2% of the population has this condition, although the majority of patients are asymptomatic.

269. B: Zollinger–Ellison syndrome is caused by tumors in the small intestine and pancreas that secrete gastrin, which can cause gastroesophageal reflux disease (GERD)-like symptoms, abdominal pain, hematemesis, and diarrhea.

Celiac sprue is an immune reaction that damages the lining of the small intestine and prevents it from absorbing important nutrients. A diagnosis can be made by an upper endoscopy with biopsy.

Whipple's disease is rare chronic disease caused by a bacterial infection. The affected bowel is usually swollen with raised, yellowish patches. This can usually be seen during sigmoidoscopy or colonoscopy.

In Crohn's disease, the colon wall may have a "cobblestone" appearance due to the intermittent pattern of affected and nonaffected colonic tissue. This can usually be seen during sigmoidoscopy or colonoscopy.

270. B: The patient may have a rotator cuff tear. X rays may be negative because they can only visualize bones, not muscles, ligaments, or tendons. Magnetic resonance imaging (MRI) can definitively determine whether or not a tear is present.

Not treating the patient is not appropriate, especially if he or she has a significantly limited range of motion. Not all rotator cuff tears require surgery, but further evaluation of the injury is warranted because the patient has a significantly decreased range of motion.

Electromyography (EMG) is used to help diagnose the cause of muscle and nerve disorders. It would not be particularly helpful in this case because the patient has a known history of injury. The patient's nerves and muscles are normal; the problem is with the tendon.

271. C: Compartment syndrome involves muscle swelling due to injury, which causes insufficient or complete lack of blood flow to the affected area. The muscles, blood vessels, and tissues of the body are contained into multiple compartments by the fascia. The fascia do not stretch in response to injury, so if the muscle swells, the pressure inside the compartment increases, which can cut off the blood supply to that area. This can cause pallor of the affected area, decreased or absent pulses, and decreased or absent sensation. A creatine phosphokinase (CPK) test might be high due to the muscle damage that is occurring. Compartment syndrome is a surgical emergency. A fasciotomy is performed to allow the muscle to expand without impinging on the blood flow.

Septic arthritis is the infection of a joint or joints due to an infection in the blood. Patients present with a painful, red joint.

Osgood–Schlatter disease is the swelling of the tibial tubercle, which commonly occurs in pubescent and prepubescent children.

Deep venous thrombus is the presence of a clot in the extremity. Patients may be asymptomatic, or they may develop pain and swelling of the affected extremity.

272. B: The patient has trichomoniasis. It is caused by a protozoal infection of the genitourinary tract. It is a sexually transmitted disease that can cause green, frothy discharge from the penis or vagina, dysuria, pain with sexual intercourse, and strong foul vaginal odor. The treatment of choice is metronidazole. Metronidazole is an antibiotic used in treating anaerobic bacterial infections; it is also used in the treatment of some parasitic infections.

Azithromycin and Rocephin are antibiotics used for bacterial infections such as gonorrhea (GC)/chlamydia.

Fluconazole is an antifungal medication used to treat yeast infections.

273. A: This patient is displaying signs of *peau d'orange, a French term meaning "skin of an orange." It is cause by impaired lymphatic drainage and edema caused by advanced inflammatory breast cancer.*

An abscess is a localized area of erythema and tenderness with induration and/or fluctuance caused by a collection of pus underneath the skin.

Gynecomastia is the overgrowth of breast tissue in males, most commonly occurring in adolescence.

A fibroadenoma is a firm, rubbery, benign breast mass. It does not cause overlying skin changes.

274. D: Caffeine can cause insomnia, abdominal cramping, and diarrhea, and it may cause food cravings. It should generally be avoided before and during one's menses.
Exercise has been shown in numerous studies to limit feelings of depression and provide extra energy during the day.
Eating nutritious meals and snacks throughout the day can help regulate blood sugar, which can curb binge eating, food cravings, and mood swings due to hyperglycemia or hypoglycemia.
Birth control pills can better regulate hormones, which may alleviate or at least partially reduce mood swings and depression caused by premenstrual syndrome.

275. C: Ceasing to have children will not help prevent cervical cancer.
Cervical cancer is caused by the human papilloma virus (HPV). Limiting one's sexual partners can decrease the risk of exposure to HPV and decrease the risk of developing cervical cancer.
Regular Pap smears and gynecological examinations can help detect any anomalies early.
Tobacco abuse can increase one's risk of developing cervical cancer by up to five times more than someone who does not smoke.

276. B: Beriberi is caused by a thiamine deficiency primarily seen in developing or underdeveloped countries. Symptoms may include muscle weakness or paralysis due to damaged nerves, heart failure, pleural effusion, encephalopathy, decreased reflexes, as well as a multitude of other complications. Some of these complications may be permanent if the thiamine deficiency is not corrected quickly.

277. A: Osteoporosis is the presence of decreased bone mineral density in the body, which can lead to persistent pathological fractures, depending on the severity of the disease. There are a multitude of factors that can contribute, such as vitamin D deficiency, tobacco abuse, disease, and being immobile for long periods. A diet rich in calcium and vitamin D can help prevent or at least slow the development of osteoporosis.

278. B: Paget's disease is the abnormal formation and degeneration of bone, usually in a localized area in the body. This may cause bony deformities and pathologic fractures. There is no cure, but there are medications that can slow the progression of the disease and help minimize complications.
Wilms' tumor is the most common renal tumor in pediatric patients.
Osteosarcoma is a type of bone cancer commonly occurring in young children and elderly patients. It can cause pathologic fractures, but it does not cause bones to be chronically misshapen.
Septic arthritis is the infection of a joint or joints due to an infection in the blood. Patients present with a painful, red joint.

279. C: Placental abruption (abruptio placentae) is the complete separation of the placenta, causing bright-red vaginal bleeding, abdominal and/or back pain, and severe contractions.
Placenta previa commonly presents with painless, bright-red vaginal bleeding at the end of the second trimester or the beginning of the third trimester. It is due to a low-lying placenta. As the uterus enlarges, it may push up against the placenta, causing a small part to tear and bright-red bleeding occurs.
Endometriosis is the presence of uterine cells/uterine lining in other areas of the body causing dysmenorrhea, pain with intercourse, and infertility.
Premature rupture of the membranes is when a woman's water breaks prior to the onset of labor.

280. D: This patient most likely has an anterior cruciate ligament tear. In the Lachman test, the patient has his knee flexed at 30°, and the examiner pulls on the tibia anteriorly to see if there is any

displacement. If there is anterior displacement, the Lachman test is positive. A magnetic resonance imaging (MRI) scan of the knee is warranted to confirm the diagnosis.

281. C: A Galeazzi fracture is a fracture of the mid or distal radius and dislocation of the radioulnar joint.
A Monteggia fracture is a fracture of the ulna and dislocation of the radius.
A Le Fort fracture is a fracture of the maxilla; this type of fracture has four categories based on severity.
A Colles' fracture is fracture and dorsal displacement of the distal radius. It is commonly referred to as a "dinner-fork deformity" on x-ray.

282. D: A boxer's fracture is the fracture and possible displacement of the fourth or fifth metacarpal, usually following a trauma with a closed fist.
A Colles' fracture is a fracture and dorsal displacement of the distal radius. It is commonly referred to as a "dinner-fork deformity" on x-ray.
A Lisfranc fracture is the fracture and dislocation of one or more of the metatarsals.
A Hangman's fracture is a fracture through the C2, usually following a high-impact trauma or a hanging.

283. C: A completed abortion is when the miscarriage has occurred and the product of conception (POC) has left the body.
Dysmenorrhea is painful or uncomfortable menses.
Abdominal pain and vaginal bleeding may occur in a threatened abortion, but the fetus is still viable. It may be a sign that a miscarriage may occur. However, a woman who experiences a threatened abortion may still deliver a healthy, full-term child.
An incomplete abortion is when the body has expelled only some of the POC. If the patient does not spontaneously expel the POC in the next one to two weeks, medications or dilation and curettage may be performed to remove the rest to prevent infection.

284. B: An ileus is when the bowel has impaired peristalsis. This condition usually occurs after abdominal surgery or disease. The bowel appears to be distended on x ray or computed tomography (CT) scan, but there is no evidence of obstruction.
Toxic megacolon is the pathologic distension of the colon. It is a complication during or following *Clostridium difficile* colitis, although is also may be seen with other diseases such as Crohn's disease.
Irritable bowel syndrome (IBS) is the presence of bowel disturbances without the presence of disease or pathology. Imaging studies are normal. It is commonly linked to anxiety and stress.
Gastroesophageal reflux disease (GERD) is caused by the improper closing of the lower esophageal sphincter, causing chest pain, abdominal pain, burning sensation in the throat, and halitosis.

285. A: Giardiasis, also known as "traveler's diarrhea," is caused by protozoa found in infected water supplies. Signs and symptoms may include profuse watery diarrhea, which may be bloody; nausea; vomiting; abdominal cramping; and fever. The main concern is dehydration, so the patient must be advised to keep hydrated. Other remedies may include ondansetron to prevent nausea, metronidazole to help combat the infection, and loperamide to alleviate the diarrhea.
Furosemide is not an appropriate treatment because as a diuretic its job is to remove fluid from the body, which would only accelerate the development of dehydration.

286. C: Serum calcium is an ineffective test in the workup of lactose intolerance. The test can be normal, and a patient may have lactose intolerance. Lactose intolerance is the body's inability to digest lactose. The undigested lactose can cause flatulence, abdominal cramping, and diarrhea. It is

a largely clinical diagnosis, but the other choices given may be ordered to confirm the suspected diagnosis. It is rarely a serious condition.

287. D: A serum beta human chorionic gonadotropin (hCG) test should be ordered to monitor the progression of choriocarcinoma and its response to therapy. It is an abnormal overgrowth of the cells that normally cover the placenta. It may occur after an ectopic pregnancy, a normal pregnancy, or a planned or spontaneous abortion. Because the placenta produces beta HCG, serial beta HCG levels help monitor the progression or regression of the disease.
A complete blood count is nonspecific and ineffective at monitoring choriocarcinoma.
Bence Jones proteins are found in the urine and may be diagnostic of multiple myeloma.
A computed tomography (CT) scan may help show the size of the tumor and if metastases are present, but ordering several of them would be unwise because it exposes the patient to a significant amount of radiation.

288. C: Antibiotics do not play a role in treating leiomyomas, or uterine fibroids. Fibroids are benign growths that may cause dysmenorrhea, menorrhagia, pain with sexual intercourse, abdominal cramping, and urinary frequency.
Iron supplements help prevent anemia that may be caused by menorrhagia.
Nonsteroidal anti-inflammatory drugs (NSAIDs) can alleviate symptoms of dysmenorrhea and pain with sexual intercourse.
Birth control pills can help regulate hormones and alleviate dysmenorrhea and menorrhagia.

289. D: This patient has endometriosis. Endometriosis is the presence of uterine cells/uterine lining in other areas of the body, causing dysmenorrhea, dysuria, leg cramping, pain with intercourse, and infertility. Imaging studies such as an ultrasound may be normal. Laparoscopy can make the definitive diagnosis.
Dystocia is difficult childbirth.
Fibroids/leiomyomas are benign growths or tumors that may cause dysmenorrhea, menorrhagia, pain with sexual intercourse, abdominal cramping, and urinary frequency. Fibroids large enough to cause symptoms are generally seen on pelvic ultrasound.
Choriocarcinoma is an abnormal overgrowth of the cells that normally cover the placenta. Patients may experience abdominal pain and bleeding. It may occur after an ectopic pregnancy, a normal pregnancy, or a planned or spontaneous abortion. Because the placenta produces beta human chorionic gonadotropin (hCG), a serum HCG or urine pregnancy test will be positive. A mass is usually seen on ultrasound.

290. C: There is no surgery to improve sciatica because the sciatic nerve cannot be removed or resected. The sciatic nerve runs down the lower back and down each of the legs, providing sensation to the lower extremities. The nerve can become inflamed or impinged due to degeneration of the spine, disease, or trauma.
The mainstays of treatment for sciatica are pain medications (such as nonsteroidal anti-inflammatory drugs [NSAIDs], narcotics, and muscle relaxers), ice or heat, and physical therapy.

291. A: Systemic lupus erythematous is an autoimmune disorder that causes inflammation in the joints and organs. There are multiple signs and symptoms, such as polyarthralgia, hair loss, and oral ulcerations, but one of the most unique signs is a malar rash. The malar rash is a butterfly-shaped rash that covers the nose and cheeks.
Paget's disease is the abnormal formation and degeneration of bone, usually in a localized area in the body. This condition may cause bony deformities and pathologic fractures.

Polymyositis is the appearance of bilateral muscle weakness and wasting due to immune disorders or disease.

Huntington's disease is a progressive neurological disorder caused by an autosomal-dominant chromosomal abnormality, which usually occurs in the third or fourth decade of life. Signs include progressive decline in cognitive function; ataxic gait; and uncoordinated, jerky body movements.

292. A: Antibiotics do not play a role in treatment of a small-bowel obstruction. If it is a partial obstruction, conservative management is attempted first. Patients are kept nothing-by-mouth (NPO) status and placed on intravenous (IV) fluid hydration. A nasogastric tube is placed to help decompress the bowel, and antiemetic medications such as Zofran are given as needed for nausea and vomiting.

293. A: Irritable bowel syndrome (IBS) is the presence of bowel disturbances without the presence of disease or pathology. It is commonly linked to anxiety and stress.

In Crohn's disease, the colon wall may have a "cobblestone" appearance due to the intermittent pattern of affected and nonaffected colonic tissue. Ulcerative colitis usually affects continuous stretches of the colon and rectum. The abnormalities of the mucosa can be seen via colonoscopy and imaging studies.

Toxic megacolon is the pathologic distension of the colon seen on CT scan or an x ray of the pelvis. It is a complication during or following *Clostridium difficile* colitis, although it also may be seen with other diseases, such as Crohn's disease.

294. B: Antibiotics are used to treat pelvic inflammatory disease (PID) because it is caused by a bacterial infection. The number-one cause of PID is venereal disease, most notably, gonorrhea and chlamydia. Untreated sexually transmitted diseases may lead to pelvic inflammatory disease, which is the primary preventable cause of infertility. Approximately 10% to 15% of PID cases are caused by illnesses such as appendicitis or pelvic procedures such as dilation and curettage, abortion, or childbirth.

295. D: Corticosteroids are the treatment of choice for polymyositis. Polymyositis is the appearance of bilateral muscle weakness and wasting due to immune disorders or disease. A high creatinine phosphokinase (CPK), a positive muscle biopsy, an elevated white blood cell count, a positive electromyography (EMG), and a history of bilateral muscle weakness with no known cause help confirm the suspected diagnosis. Administration of high-dose steroids may completely reverse the signs and symptoms in most patients.

296. A: Spondylolisthesis is a condition in which the vertebra slips out of place, causing pain or discomfort. The primary cause for this condition is degenerative disease, but it may also be caused by strenuous activity, trauma, or congenital defect. Most treatments include conservative measures such as pain medication, physical therapy, and supportive braces. For severe symptoms or significant disc displacement, surgery may be warranted.

297. C: The withdrawal method involves the male partner pulling out prior to ejaculation. This method has a higher failure rate than the use of intrauterine devices, birth control pills, and condoms, even when it is performed consistently. It is believed that some semen enters the vagina prior to ejaculation, which can result in unwanted pregnancy.

298. D: Methotrexate is an antimetabolite used to treat cancer, autoimmune disorders such as lupus or rheumatoid arthritis, and medical abortions.

Metronidazole is an antibiotic used in treating anaerobic bacterial infections; it is also an amebicide and antiprotozoal medication.

Meropenem is a strong broad-spectrum antibiotic used to treat anaerobic, gram-positive, and gram-negative bacteria.

Metformin is an antihyperglycemic medication used in the treatment of diabetes.

299. B: Though the exact cause of osteoarthritis is unknown, it is related to aging and degenerative disease. Cartilage is a rubbery substance that helps cushion and protect bones. As cartilage gets worn away with age and overuse, the bones begin to rub against each other, causing pain and inflammation. Strenuous activity, multiple fractures, and obesity also play roles in the development of osteoarthritis.

300. A: Kyphosis is an abnormal curvature of the spine, usually due to degenerative disease, but may also be due to trauma, bony diseases such as spina bifida or Paget's disease, and tumors. If the curvature is severe enough, surgery may be warranted, but usually the treatment is conservative management.

Cauda equina syndrome can be caused by disease, trauma, or infection. It affects the nerve roots from L1 to L5 and S1 to S5, which can cause motor dysfunction, urinary retention, saddle anesthesias, among other neurological issues.

Avascular necrosis occurs when there is insufficient or complete lack of blood flow to the bone, causing death of the bone cells. Patients may complain of a painful joint that may or may not be swollen.

The sciatic nerve runs down the lower back and down each of the legs, providing sensation to the lower extremities. The nerve can become inflamed or impinged due to degeneration of the spine, disease, or trauma. It does not cause an abnormal curvature of the spine.

Secret Key #1 - Time is Your Greatest Enemy

Pace Yourself

Wear a watch. At the beginning of the test, check the time (or start a chronometer on your watch to count the minutes), and check the time after every few questions to make sure you are "on schedule."

If you are forced to speed up, do it efficiently. Usually one or more answer choices can be eliminated without too much difficulty. Above all, don't panic. Don't speed up and just begin guessing at random choices. By pacing yourself, and continually monitoring your progress against your watch, you will always know exactly how far ahead or behind you are with your available time. If you find that you are one minute behind on the test, don't skip one question without spending any time on it, just to catch back up. Take 15 fewer seconds on the next four questions, and after four questions you'll have caught back up. Once you catch back up, you can continue working each problem at your normal pace.

Furthermore, don't dwell on the problems that you were rushed on. If a problem was taking up too much time and you made a hurried guess, it must be difficult. The difficult questions are the ones you are most likely to miss anyway, so it isn't a big loss. It is better to end with more time than you need than to run out of time.

Lastly, sometimes it is beneficial to slow down if you are constantly getting ahead of time. You are always more likely to catch a careless mistake by working more slowly than quickly, and among very high-scoring test takers (those who are likely to have lots of time left over), careless errors affect the score more than mastery of material.

Secret Key #2 - Guessing is not Guesswork

You probably know that guessing is a good idea. Unlike other standardized tests, there is no penalty for getting a wrong answer. Even if you have no idea about a question, you still have a 20-25% chance of getting it right.

Most test takers do not understand the impact that proper guessing can have on their score. Unless you score extremely high, guessing will significantly contribute to your final score.

Monkeys Take the Test

What most test takers don't realize is that to insure that 20-25% chance, you have to guess randomly. If you put 20 monkeys in a room to take this test, assuming they answered once per question and behaved themselves, on average they would get 20-25% of the questions correct. Put 20 test takers in the room, and the average will be much lower among guessed questions. Why?
1. The test writers intentionally write deceptive answer choices that "look" right. A test taker has no idea about a question, so he picks the "best looking" answer, which is often wrong. The monkey has no idea what looks good and what doesn't, so it will consistently be right about 20-25% of the time.
2. Test takers will eliminate answer choices from the guessing pool based on a hunch or intuition. Simple but correct answers often get excluded, leaving a 0% chance of being correct. The monkey has no clue, and often gets lucky with the best choice.

This is why the process of elimination endorsed by most test courses is flawed and detrimental to your performance. Test takers don't guess; they make an ignorant stab in the dark that is usually worse than random.

$5 Challenge

Let me introduce one of the most valuable ideas of this course—the $5 challenge:

You only mark your "best guess" if you are willing to bet $5 on it.
You only eliminate choices from guessing if you are willing to bet $5 on it.

Why $5? Five dollars is an amount of money that is small yet not insignificant, and can really add up fast (20 questions could cost you $100). Likewise, each answer choice on one question of the test will have a small impact on your overall score, but it can really add up to a lot of points in the end.

The process of elimination IS valuable. The following shows your chance of guessing it right:

If you eliminate wrong answer choices until only this many remain:	Chance of getting it correct:
1	100%
2	50%
3	33%

However, if you accidentally eliminate the right answer or go on a hunch for an incorrect answer, your chances drop dramatically—to 0%. By guessing among all the answer choices, you are GUARANTEED to have a shot at the right answer.

That's why the $5 test is so valuable. If you give up the advantage and safety of a pure guess, it had better be worth the risk.

What we still haven't covered is how to be sure that whatever guess you make is truly random. Here's the easiest way:

Always pick the first answer choice among those remaining.

Such a technique means that you have decided, **before you see a single test question**, exactly how you are going to guess, and since the order of choices tells you nothing about which one is correct, this guessing technique is perfectly random.

This section is not meant to scare you away from making educated guesses or eliminating choices; you just need to define when a choice is worth eliminating. The $5 test, along with a pre-defined random guessing strategy, is the best way to make sure you reap all of the benefits of guessing.

Secret Key #3 - Practice Smarter, Not Harder

Many test takers delay the test preparation process because they dread the awful amounts of practice time they think necessary to succeed on the test. We have refined an effective method that will take you only a fraction of the time.

There are a number of "obstacles" in the path to success. Among these are answering questions, finishing in time, and mastering test-taking strategies. All must be executed on the day of the test at peak performance, or your score will suffer. The test is a mental marathon that has a large impact on your future.

Just like a marathon runner, it is important to work your way up to the full challenge. So first you just worry about questions, and then time, and finally strategy:

Success Strategy

1. Find a good source for practice tests.
2. If you are willing to make a larger time investment, consider using more than one study guide. Often the different approaches of multiple authors will help you "get" difficult concepts.
3. Take a practice test with no time constraints, with all study helps, "open book." Take your time with questions and focus on applying strategies.
4. Take a practice test with time constraints, with all guides, "open book."
5. Take a final practice test without open material and with time limits.

If you have time to take more practice tests, just repeat step 5. By gradually exposing yourself to the full rigors of the test environment, you will condition your mind to the stress of test day and maximize your success.

Secret Key #4 - Prepare, Don't Procrastinate

Let me state an obvious fact: if you take the test three times, you will probably get three different scores. This is due to the way you feel on test day, the level of preparedness you have, and the version of the test you see. Despite the test writers' claims to the contrary, some versions of the test WILL be easier for you than others.

Since your future depends so much on your score, you should maximize your chances of success. In order to maximize the likelihood of success, you've got to prepare in advance. This means taking practice tests and spending time learning the information and test taking strategies you will need to succeed.

Never go take the actual test as a "practice" test, expecting that you can just take it again if you need to. Take all the practice tests you can on your own, but when you go to take the official test, be prepared, be focused, and do your best the first time!

Secret Key #5 - Test Yourself

Everyone knows that time is money. There is no need to spend too much of your time or too little of your time preparing for the test. You should only spend as much of your precious time preparing as is necessary for you to get the score you need.

Once you have taken a practice test under real conditions of time constraints, then you will know if you are ready for the test or not.

If you have scored extremely high the first time that you take the practice test, then there is not much point in spending countless hours studying. You are already there.

Benchmark your abilities by retaking practice tests and seeing how much you have improved. Once you consistently score high enough to guarantee success, then you are ready.

If you have scored well below where you need, then knuckle down and begin studying in earnest. Check your improvement regularly through the use of practice tests under real conditions. Above all, don't worry, panic, or give up. The key is perseverance!

Then, when you go to take the test, remain confident and remember how well you did on the practice tests. If you can score high enough on a practice test, then you can do the same on the real thing.

General Strategies

The most important thing you can do is to ignore your fears and jump into the test immediately. Do not be overwhelmed by any strange-sounding terms. You have to jump into the test like jumping into a pool—all at once is the easiest way.

Make Predictions

As you read and understand the question, try to guess what the answer will be. Remember that several of the answer choices are wrong, and once you begin reading them, your mind will immediately become cluttered with answer choices designed to throw you off. Your mind is typically the most focused immediately after you have read the question and digested its contents. If you can, try to predict what the correct answer will be. You may be surprised at what you can predict.

Quickly scan the choices and see if your prediction is in the listed answer choices. If it is, then you can be quite confident that you have the right answer. It still won't hurt to check the other answer choices, but most of the time, you've got it!

Answer the Question

It may seem obvious to only pick answer choices that answer the question, but the test writers can create some excellent answer choices that are wrong. Don't pick an answer just because it sounds right, or you believe it to be true. It MUST answer the question. Once you've made your selection, always go back and check it against the question and make sure that you didn't misread the question and that the answer choice does answer the question posed.

Benchmark

After you read the first answer choice, decide if you think it sounds correct or not. If it doesn't, move on to the next answer choice. If it does, mentally mark that answer choice. This doesn't mean that you've definitely selected it as your answer choice, it just means that it's the best you've seen thus far. Go ahead and read the next choice. If the next choice is worse than the one you've already selected, keep going to the next answer choice. If the next choice is better than the choice you've already selected, mentally mark the new answer choice as your best guess.

The first answer choice that you select becomes your standard. Every other answer choice must be benchmarked against that standard. That choice is correct until proven otherwise by another answer choice beating it out. Once you've decided that no other answer choice seems as good, do one final check to ensure that your answer choice answers the question posed.

Valid Information

Don't discount any of the information provided in the question. Every piece of information may be necessary to determine the correct answer. None of the information in the question is there to throw you off (while the answer choices will certainly have information to throw you off). If two seemingly unrelated topics are discussed, don't ignore either. You can be confident there is a relationship, or it wouldn't be included in the question, and you are probably going to have to determine what is that relationship to find the answer.

Avoid "Fact Traps"

Don't get distracted by a choice that is factually true. Your search is for the answer that answers the question. Stay focused and don't fall for an answer that is true but irrelevant. Always go back to the question and make sure you're choosing an answer that actually answers the question and is not just a true statement. An answer can be factually correct, but it MUST answer the question asked. Additionally, two answers can both be seemingly correct, so be sure to read all of the answer choices, and make sure that you get the one that BEST answers the question.

Milk the Question

Some of the questions may throw you completely off. They might deal with a subject you have not been exposed to, or one that you haven't reviewed in years. While your lack of knowledge about the subject will be a hindrance, the question itself can give you many clues that will help you find the correct answer. Read the question carefully and look for clues. Watch particularly for adjectives and nouns describing difficult terms or words that you don't recognize. Regardless of whether you completely understand a word or not, replacing it with a synonym, either provided or one you more familiar with, may help you to understand what the questions are asking. Rather than wracking your mind about specific detailed information concerning a difficult term or word, try to use mental substitutes that are easier to understand.

The Trap of Familiarity

Don't just choose a word because you recognize it. On difficult questions, you may not recognize a number of words in the answer choices. The test writers don't put "make-believe" words on the test, so don't think that just because you only recognize all the words in one answer choice that that answer choice must be correct. If you only recognize words in one answer choice, then focus on that one. Is it correct? Try your best to determine if it is correct. If it is, that's great. If not, eliminate it. Each word and answer choice you eliminate increases your chances of getting the question correct, even if you then have to guess among the unfamiliar choices.

Eliminate Answers

Eliminate choices as soon as you realize they are wrong. But be careful! Make sure you consider all of the possible answer choices. Just because one appears right, doesn't mean that the next one won't be even better! The test writers will usually put more than one good answer choice for every question, so read all of them. Don't worry if you are stuck between two that seem right. By getting down to just two remaining possible choices, your odds are now 50/50. Rather than wasting too much time, play the odds. You are guessing, but guessing wisely because you've been able to knock out some of the answer choices that you know are wrong. If you are eliminating choices and realize that the last answer choice you are left with is also obviously wrong, don't panic. Start over and consider each choice again. There may easily be something that you missed the first time and will realize on the second pass.

Tough Questions

If you are stumped on a problem or it appears too hard or too difficult, don't waste time. Move on! Remember though, if you can quickly check for obviously incorrect answer choices, your chances of guessing correctly are greatly improved. Before you completely give up, at least try to knock out a couple of possible answers. Eliminate what you can and then guess at the remaining answer choices before moving on.

Brainstorm

If you get stuck on a difficult question, spend a few seconds quickly brainstorming. Run through the complete list of possible answer choices. Look at each choice and ask yourself, "Could this answer the question satisfactorily?" Go through each answer choice and consider it independently of the others. By systematically going through all possibilities, you may find something that you would otherwise overlook. Remember though that when you get stuck, it's important to try to keep moving.

Read Carefully

Understand the problem. Read the question and answer choices carefully. Don't miss the question because you misread the terms. You have plenty of time to read each question thoroughly and make sure you understand what is being asked. Yet a happy medium must be attained, so don't waste too much time. You must read carefully, but efficiently.

Face Value

When in doubt, use common sense. Always accept the situation in the problem at face value. Don't read too much into it. These problems will not require you to make huge leaps of logic. The test writers aren't trying to throw you off with a cheap trick. If you have to go beyond creativity and make a leap of logic in order to have an answer choice answer the question, then you should look at the other answer choices. Don't overcomplicate the problem by creating theoretical relationships or explanations that will warp time or space. These are normal problems rooted in reality. It's just that the applicable relationship or explanation may not be readily apparent and you have to figure things out. Use your common sense to interpret anything that isn't clear.

Prefixes

If you're having trouble with a word in the question or answer choices, try dissecting it. Take advantage of every clue that the word might include. Prefixes and suffixes can be a huge help. Usually they allow you to determine a basic meaning. Pre- means before, post- means after, pro - is positive, de- is negative. From these prefixes and suffixes, you can get an idea of the general meaning of the word and try to put it into context. Beware though of any traps. Just because con- is the opposite of pro-, doesn't necessarily mean congress is the opposite of progress!

Hedge Phrases

Watch out for critical hedge phrases, led off with words such as "likely," "may," "can," "sometimes," "often," "almost," "mostly," "usually," "generally," "rarely," and "sometimes." Question writers insert these hedge phrases to cover every possibility. Often an answer choice will be wrong simply because it leaves no room for exception. Unless the situation calls for them, avoid answer choices that have definitive words like "exactly," and "always."

Switchback Words

Stay alert for "switchbacks." These are the words and phrases frequently used to alert you to shifts in thought. The most common switchback word is "but." Others include "although," "however," "nevertheless," "on the other hand," "even though," "while," "in spite of," "despite," and "regardless of."

New Information

Correct answer choices will rarely have completely new information included. Answer choices typically are straightforward reflections of the material asked about and will directly relate to the question. If a new piece of information is included in an answer choice that doesn't even seem to relate to the topic being asked about, then that answer choice is likely incorrect. All of the information needed to answer the question is usually provided for you in the question. You should not have to make guesses that are unsupported or choose answer choices that require unknown information that cannot be reasoned from what is given.

Time Management

On technical questions, don't get lost on the technical terms. Don't spend too much time on any one question. If you don't know what a term means, then odds are you aren't going to get much further since you don't have a dictionary. You should be able to immediately recognize whether or not you know a term. If you don't, work with the other clues that you have—the other answer choices and terms provided—but don't waste too much time trying to figure out a difficult term that you don't know.

Contextual Clues

Look for contextual clues. An answer can be right but not the correct answer. The contextual clues will help you find the answer that is most right and is correct. Understand the context in which a phrase or statement is made. This will help you make important distinctions.

Don't Panic

Panicking will not answer any questions for you; therefore, it isn't helpful. When you first see the question, if your mind goes blank, take a deep breath. Force yourself to mechanically go through the steps of solving the problem using the strategies you've learned.

Pace Yourself

Don't get clock fever. It's easy to be overwhelmed when you're looking at a page full of questions, your mind is full of random thoughts and feeling confused, and the clock is ticking down faster than you would like. Calm down and maintain the pace that you have set for yourself. As long as you are on track by monitoring your pace, you are guaranteed to have enough time for yourself. When you get to the last few minutes of the test, it may seem like you won't have enough time left, but if you only have as many questions as you should have left at that point, then you're right on track!

Answer Selection

The best way to pick an answer choice is to eliminate all of those that are wrong, until only one is left and confirm that is the correct answer. Sometimes though, an answer choice may immediately look right. Be careful! Take a second to make sure that the other choices are not equally obvious. Don't make a hasty mistake. There are only two times that you should stop before checking other answers. First is when you are positive that the answer choice you have selected is correct. Second is when time is almost out and you have to make a quick guess!

Check Your Work

Since you will probably not know every term listed and the answer to every question, it is important that you get credit for the ones that you do know. Don't miss any questions through careless mistakes. If at all possible, try to take a second to look back over your answer selection and make sure you've selected the correct answer choice and haven't made a costly careless mistake (such as marking an answer choice that you didn't mean to mark). The time it takes for this quick double check should more than pay for itself in caught mistakes.

Beware of Directly Quoted Answers

Sometimes an answer choice will repeat word for word a portion of the question or reference section. However, beware of such exact duplication. It may be a trap! More than likely, the correct choice will paraphrase or summarize a point, rather than being exactly the same wording.

Slang

Scientific sounding answers are better than slang ones. An answer choice that begins "To compare the outcomes..." is much more likely to be correct than one that begins "Because some people insisted..."

Extreme Statements

Avoid wild answers that throw out highly controversial ideas that are proclaimed as established fact. An answer choice that states the "process should used in certain situations, if..." is much more likely to be correct than one that states the "process should be discontinued completely." The first is a calm rational statement and doesn't even make a definitive, uncompromising stance, using a hedge word "if" to provide wiggle room, whereas the second choice is a radical idea and far more extreme.

Answer Choice Families

When you have two or more answer choices that are direct opposites or parallels, one of them is usually the correct answer. For instance, if one answer choice states "x increases" and another answer choice states "x decreases" or "y increases," then those two or three answer choices are very similar in construction and fall into the same family of answer choices. A family of answer choices consists of two or three answer choices, very similar in construction, but often with directly opposite meanings. Usually the correct answer choice will be in that family of answer choices. The "odd man out" or answer choice that doesn't seem to fit the parallel construction of the other answer choices is more likely to be incorrect.

Additional Bonus Material

Due to our efforts to try to keep this book to a manageable length, we've created a link that will give you access to all of your additional bonus material.

Please visit http://www.mometrix.com/bonus948/pance to access the information.

CPSIA information can be obtained
at www.ICGtesting.com
Printed in the USA
LVHW100747290719
625693LV00009B/120/P